What others are saying:

D1284479

"For more than thirty year̶s̶ ...man early warning system of commo̶...... dangers to workers. In *Designer Poisons*, she proves she is something even more rare: an understandable populist and common sense expert who can help all of us save our lives and health."

Gloria Steinem
Author, Feminist-Activist

"As a comprehensive guide book and analysis of the dangerous substances we welcome so casually into our lives, *Designer Poisons* is bound to be a critical source volume — indeed, no home (or place of work) should be without one."

Peter Matthiessen
Author-Naturalist

"Finally, the real facts we need to make our homes safer. Thank you!"

Frances Moore Lappé
Center for Living Democracy

"Cancer now strikes 1 in 3 Americans. In *Designer Poisons,* Marion Moses shows us how to reduce our risk of cancer and other diseases by reducing exposure to toxic pesticides at home. A skillful blend of wit, grit, and wisdom, this clear, practical guide can serve as a blueprint for change in our homes, our communities, and our country. Brava!"

Nancy Evans
Breast Cancer Action

"Protecting yourself and your family from toxic pesticides is not easy in today's toxic world. *Designer Poisons* is a great help in sorting through questions about toxic hazards and alternatives for which people want answers. Don't be misled by chemical product sales techniques and deficient legal standards. Use this book to make the right choices."

Jay Feldman
National Coalition Against
the Misuse of Pesticides

"You can't trust the manufacturers. You can't trust the government to protect us by banning dangerous pesticides. Fortunately, here comes Dr. Marion Moses' *Designer Poisons*, a source we can trust for information on how to protect ourselves."

Lois Marie Gibbs
Citizens Clearinghouse
for Hazardous Waste

Designer Poisons

How to Protect your Health and Home from Toxic Pesticides

by Marion Moses, M.D.

Author: Marion Moses

Title: Designer Poisons, How to Protect Your Health and
Home from Toxic Pesticides

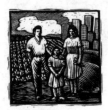

Publisher:

Pesticide Education Center
P.O. 420870
San Francisco, CA 94142-0870 U.S.A.
415/391-8511 Fax: 415/391-9159
e-mail pec@igc.apc.org

Cover Design: Linda Herman, Walking Stick Press
Cover Illustration: John Horn
Illustrations: Vincent Perez, page 22. Sharon Hour, page 23.
Typesetting: Joan Clayburgh, Victor Jimenez

ISBN 1-881510-15-8
First Printing June, 1995
412 pages, index, references, tables.
Copyright © 1995 by The Pesticide Education Center

To the memory of Cesar Chavez and Robert van den Bosch, visionaries and pathbreakers on the road to environmental health and sanity.

Table of Contents

About the Author

Marion Moses is a physician with many years experience investigating pesticide-related health problems in farmworkers and their families. Her concern about the increasing use of toxic chemicals for pest control in and around homes, and on lawns, and yards in urban and suburban areas led her to write this book. She was further motivated by the misleading advertising, marketing, and labeling of over-the-counter pesticides, that denies the consumer an effective informed choice. She is especially worried about health risks to children.

Dr. Moses received her medical degree from Temple University Medical School, completed her residency at the Mount Sinai Medical Center in New York City, and is board certified in occupational medicine. She has served on many government committees relating to the health effects of pesticides, and is consulting editor for several environmental journals. She founded the Pesticide Education center in 1988.

This book grew out of a collaborative urban pesticide use and reduction project between the Pesticide Education Center and the Pesticide Watch Education Fund, nonprofit organizations based in San Francisco.

About the Pesticide Education Center. The Pesticide Education Center (PEC) was founded in 1988 to educate the public about the hazards and health effects of pesticides. Much of the PEC's early work focused on developing videos and training manuals to educate farm workers about protecting themselves from toxic pesticides. The PEC makes presentations, develops curricular materials, and provides other services targeted to the needs of average citizens and workers throughout the country concerned about health risks of pesticide exposure. In some cases the PEC works directly with affected communities on specific problems. *Harvest of Sorrow,* a video produced by the PEC, received a Gold Apple Award from the National Educational Film and Video Festival in 1993.

About Pesticide Watch Education Fund. Pesticide Watch Education Fund works with California residents to safeguard our health against dangerous pesticides and promote safer alternatives. We are non-profit and non-partisan. Pesticide Watch helps individuals and groups combat the use of pesticides in our communities providing: education on state and federal pesticide regulations, organizing strategies to reduce the use of pesticides, referrals to legal, technical, and public health experts, and a network of others fighting similar battles to share ideas and band together on local, statewide and national issues.

Acknowledgements

This book grew out of a collaborative project between the Pesticide Education Center and the Pesticide Watch Education Fund. The author owes a great debt to Joan Clayburgh, director of Pesticide Watch. Her invaluable contributions include assisting with the San Francisco surveys, typesetting the WordPerfect 6.0 document in Pagemaker; and providing insightful and cogent suggestions throughout the gestation of the manuscript. Special thanks good friend, and still cheerful, collaborator.

We are grateful to the foundations whose grants made this book possible: the Richard and Rhoda Goldman Foundation, the Maximillian and Marion O. Hoffman Foundation, and the Elizabeth Ordway Dunn Foundation grant that enabled us to include Florida.

We thank The Apple Computer EarthGrants program for the donation of a MacIntosh IISi Computer and Laserwriter IIF, and the Environmental Support Center for the donation of a MacIntosh LCIII Computer used in preparing the book for publication.

We owe a great deal to the volunteers who gave up valuable time on weekends and after school and work to help us with the project. Their help includes collecting the survey data, entering them into the computer, and the tedious task of checking and correcting data entries. Our heartfelt thanks to: Martha Moses, Sara Martinez de Osaba, Danielle Hyatt, Peggy Scarborough, Mark Garzon, Chris Dunaway, Bob Bejnarowicz, Mara Beverwyck, Wendy Christiansen, Jim Delso, Kenwyn Derby, Alex Fitz, Hannah Gilberg, Molly Hodges, Abby Lewis, and Aloysha Ricards in the San Francisco Bay Area. Ann Mason, Judy Mekstraitis, and Carolyn Clark helped with the surveys in Sarasota, Florida. Monica Moore and Ann Lipow assisted with editorial comments and sound advice.

A special note of thanks to my assistant, Victor Jimenez, for his always good natured and skillful efficiency in data management, computer trouble shooting, and other invaluable assistance. My brother, Maron, and my sister, Martha, helped in many valued and indescribable ways that come only from family ties.

1

What this Book is About and How to Use It

Nature cannot be ordered about, except by obeying her.
Francis Bacon (1561-1626)

The purpose of this book is to help you choose pest control methods that are safer for you, your family, your pets, your neighbors, and the environment. It informs you of potential health hazards of widely available pesticide products and services. It recommends nontoxic or less toxic alternatives, which many consumers would use if they knew about them. We answer the following questions, and many others, about pesticides.

◆ What products that make the air in your home toxic for several months contain cancer causing pesticides? *(see pages 35, 50, 75, 113, 308).*

◆ Do home use pesticides cause cancer in humans? *(see pages 72-79).*

◆ What "fragrance free" product is 100% toxic? *(see page 249).*

◆ When is it safe for children and pets to play on a lawn sprayed with pesticides? *(see pages 29-30).*

◆ Can my children and pets be harmed by pesticides used on lawns? *(see pages 309-310).*

◆ What pesticide available over-the-counter has been linked to brain cancer and leukemia? *(see pages 75-76, 83-84)*.

◆ What pesticides can you buy that act like or interfere with estrogens (female hormones)? *(see page 84)*.

◆ What prescription lice shampoo contains a pesticide linked to brain cancer in children? *(see pages 75-76)*.

◆ What home use product labeled as "made from flowers" contains mostly other chemical pesticides? *(see page 33)*.

◆ What home use pesticide is contaminated with DDT? *(see page 80)*.

◆ What pesticide used to kill termites depletes the ozone layer? *(see page 280)*.

◆ Are pesticides containing "pine scent", "country fresh scent", or "lavender scent" safer? *(see page 28)*.

◆ Are "natural" products safer than synthetic chemical pesticides? *(see pages 106, 220)*.

◆ Aren't pesticides safe if you strictly follow the label directions? *(see pages 92, 94)*.

This book discusses basic information about pesticides in chapters two through five. Specific information about brand name over-the-counter products for indoor, outdoor, pet, and human use, is in chapters six through nine. Chapter ten discusses commercial use pesticides applied by professional pest control operators (exterminators). The last chapter briefly discusses and recommends some changes in pesticide law and policy.

Recommendations. We recommend that you read chapters two and three *before* you read chapters six through ten. We realize there is a lot of information in chapters four and five on acute and chronic health effects. Our purpose was not to overwhelm, but to give you concise information about health effects of pesticides that is difficult to find in one place. You may prefer to refer back and forth to different sections.

We encourage you to read all of the chapters, since useful information is dispersed throughout the book. If you do not have a lawn or a pet you can skip those chapters. Unless of course you have friends with lawns or pets, or in the future may have a lawn or a pet.

Chapter two describes what pesticides are, how they get into your body, and why children absorb more pesticides than adults. It discusses packaging, why foggers and aerosols are especially hazardous, and the problem of inert ingredients.

Chapter three discusses how to read a pesticide label, including what the warning words on the label mean. It also tells you what is not on the label that you need to know.

Chapter four discusses acute health effects of pesticides, from skin rashes to poisoning. It describes nerve-gas type pesticides, other classes of chemicals in over-the-counter products, and the health problems they can cause. It tells you what to do if you suspect a pesticide-related health problem, how to talk to your doctor, and discusses asthma and allergies related to pesticide exposure.

Chapter five is the longest chapter in the book. It discusses long-term health effects, including cancer, reproductive effects, and effects on the brain and nervous system. There is special emphasis on cancer in children related to their parents' use of pesticides in and around the home, and a discussion of breast cancer and pesticides.

Chapter six discusses indoor pests, cockroaches, ants, and fleas in particular. It tells you what nontoxic and least toxic alternatives are available and how to use them. A table listing indoor products by their brand names, specific ingredients, and chronic toxicity, concludes the chapter.

Chapter seven discusses outdoor pest problems, with an emphasis on lawn care. It tells you what nontoxic and least toxic alternatives are available for pests such as fire ants, cinch bugs, dandelions, and other pests. A table listing outdoor products by their brand names, specific ingredients, and chronic toxicity, concludes the chapter.

Chapter eight discusses pest problems on pets, focusing on fleas on cats and dogs. It tells you what nontoxic and least toxic alternatives are available and how to use them. A table listing pet products by their brand names, specific ingredients, and chronic toxicity, concludes the chapter.

Chapter nine discusses human pest problems, including use of insect repellents on children and adults, and treatment of lice. It recommends what products to avoid, safer alternatives, and how to use them.

Chapter ten describes products used by pest control professionals (exterminators, pest control operators) for indoor and outdoor use, including termite control. It discusses questions you should ask, and factors you should consider, before signing a contract for treatment of your home. A table listing the ingredients in commercial use pesticides with acute and chronic toxicity information concludes the chapter.

Chapter eleven gives a brief overview of pesticide law and policy regarding home use pesticides. It recommends changes that would better protect public health, especially children.

Exclusions and Qualifications

This book focuses on pesticides sold over-the-counter, and commercial use products applied by professional pest control operators (exterminators) in and around the home. It does not include cleaning products for use in bathrooms, kitchens, and general purpose cleaning, or swimming pool chemicals.

The brand name pesticides listed in the tables in chapters six through nine represent typical products available for direct sale to the public in the surveyed cities. They are not lists of all brand name home use pesticides available over-the-counter throughout the country.

It is beyond the scope of this book to include all of the potential pests found indoors, outdoors, on pets, and on humans. We discuss only the more common ones. There are several books and publications with more comprehensive information about pest problems. We refer to these sources in the appropriate sections in the text, and list them in an appendix of sources of further information.

Over-the-counter pesticides. The information on brand name pesticides was collected by volunteers from hardware stores, nurseries, supermarkets, variety stores, pet stores, and other retail outlets in San Francisco in 1994. Additional surveys were done in 1995 in Sarasota, Florida, Metarie, Louisiana (near New Orleans), and Colma, California (near San Francisco).

Commercial use pesticides. The information on pesticide use by professional pest control operators and exterminators, was gathered by volunteers at the San Francisco county agricultural commissioner's office. They copied a full year (1992-1993) of pesticide use reports filed by 157 commercial pest control companies licensed in the city and county. These Pesticide Use Reports, required by California law, are available to the public.

Such commercial pesticide use data is not available in Florida. We were unable to find any systematic source of pesticide use by companies that do pest control for hire. We did include information obtained from interviewing pest control companies, and talking to homeowners and condominium residents about pesticide use, especially for lawn care.

Pronunciation guide. Many of our readers will not be familiar with some terms used in this book. Pronouncing them properly makes it easier for you to talk to pest control operators, your doctor, and others. There is a pronunciation guide in Appendix A on page 319. This is the author's personal system, revised after trying it out on several people unfamiliar with medical and pesticide terminology. If you come up with a better "sound bite" for a particular entry, let us know and we will consider it for inclusion in later editions. We are considering making an audio cassette for a small additional charge, in which all of the terms in the pronunciation guide are read aloud. Let us know if you think this would be useful to you.

Please contact us. We like to hear from readers who have comments about the book, or suggestions for controlling pests in nontoxic or less toxic ways. While we cannot promise to answer each inquiry individually, we do read all our mail, and share what we learn with others. We will incorporate the most helpful suggestions in future editions.

2

Exposure to Pesticides

Its like playing Russian roulette. You pull the trigger and the gun doesn't go off, so it must be safe to pull the trigger again.

Richard P. Feynman (1918-1988)

Anxiety, fear, revulsion, total loss of composure, and other strong emotions, underlie attempts of many householders to control insects, weeds, and other pests they feel are threatening their personal patch of the planet. Intelligent, inquiring, and otherwise resourceful people, often give no thought to what is in those containers of designer poison they buy for use in their homes. Before going into detail about the acute and chronic health effects of pesticides in chapters three and four, we provide some background information on exposure to these toxic susbstances.

Economic poisons. Pesticides are toxic substances deliberately added to our environment to kill or harm living things. They can also kill or harm human beings. The 1947 federal pesticide law defined pesticides as "economic poisons." Pesticides are named according to the kind of pest they are used against. Table 2.1 shows some examples.

Pesticides come from two basic sources, synthetic chemicals and naturally occurring substances. Most pesticides are synthetic chemicals made from petroleum (petrochemicals), and are not found in nature. Natural sources of pesticides are flowers, plants, roots, fossils, elements, and biological agents.

Table 2.1

Type	Pests Used Against
Insecticides	Cockroaches, fleas, ants, flies, aphids, bees, beetles, bugs, caterpillars, centipedes, mosquitoes, moths, nematodes, spiders, termites, ticks, and other bugs, insects, and arachnids.
Herbicides	Weeds, grasses, woody plants, algae, and other vegetation.
Fungicides	Mildew, mold, rot, and other plant diseases
Rodenticides	Mice, rats, gophers, squirrels, and other vertebrates(animals with backbones).
Molluscicides	Snails, slugs, mussels, and other mollusks.

Most consumers know little or nothing about the chemicals in the pesticides they buy for home use. Most who pay for pest control services do not know what pesticides exterminators apply in their homes or on their property.

You might assume that using a pesticide according to the label directions will not harm you, your children, your pets, your neighbors, or the environment. This assumption may not be true. The law does not require full disclosure of potential health hazards of hundreds of chemicals in thousands of pesticides sold over-the-counter for home use.

You might also assume that a product approved by the EPA (Environmental Protection Agency) is safe. But in reality, the EPA does not allow chemical companies to market pesticide products as "safe." The EPA approves pesticides based on *efficacy*, not safety. Efficacy means the pesticide will do what the label says — kill insects, or weeds, or rats, or other pests.

Home Use Estimates. There are 94 million households in the U.S. The EPA estimates that 60 million of them (73%), use pesticides every year. In 1993, consumers spent $1.2 billion dollars to buy 71 million pounds of home pesticides. Figures 2.1 and 2.2 show these figures by category of use.

Figure 2.1

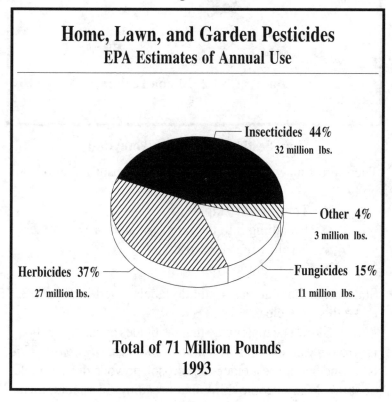

Home, Lawn, and Garden Pesticides
EPA Estimates of Annual Use

Insecticides 44%
32 million lbs.

Other 4%
3 million lbs.

Fungicides 15%
11 million lbs.

Herbicides 37%
27 million lbs.

Total of 71 Million Pounds
1993

Figure 2.2

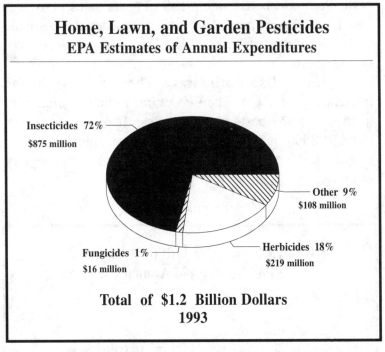

Home, Lawn, and Garden Pesticides
EPA Estimates of Annual Expenditures

Insecticides 72%
$875 million

Other 9%
$108 million

Fungicides 1%
$16 million

Herbicides 18%
$219 million

Total of $1.2 Billion Dollars
1993

How Pesticides Get into Your Body

There are four ways that pesticides are absorbed into your body:

♦ Through the skin
♦ Breathing into the lungs (inhalation)
♦ Swallowing (ingestion)
♦ Through the eyes

Statements from actual pesticide labels listed in Figure 2.3 make this very clear.

Skin. The major way that pesticides get into your body is *through your skin*. This *cannot be emphasized enough*. This is so whether the pesticide is an aerosol, powder, dust, granule, or spray. Many people think that breathing in vapors, mists, and sprays is the major way that pesticides get into their body.

You do inhale pesticides, but in lesser amounts than what goes through your skin.

Figure 2.3

Some Precautionary statements
from Pesticide labels

Avoid inhalation or contact with eyes or skin. Harmful if swallowed. May cause eye irritation.

Avoid eye contact. Wash thoroughly after handling.

Corrosive to eyes. Causes eye damage. Do not get in eyes. Harmful if swallowed.   Avoid contact with skin or clothing.

Do not apply to excessively sunburned or damaged skin. May cause skin reaction in rare cases.

Do not get in eyes, on skin, or clothing. Harmful if swallowed, inhaled, or absorbed through skin

Harmful if swallowed. May cause eye injury. Avoid contact with eyes and lips.

Harmful if swallowed. Avoid contact with eyes, skin, and clothing.

Harmful if absorbed through the skin. Avoid contact with skin, eyes, or clothing. Wash thoroughly with soap and water after handling.

May irritate eyes nose throat and skin. Avoid breathing dust or spray mist. Avoid contact with eyes, skin, and clothing.

Not intended for use by humans. Do not allow children to play with this collar.

Skin contact with this pesticide may be hazardous.

Figure 2.4

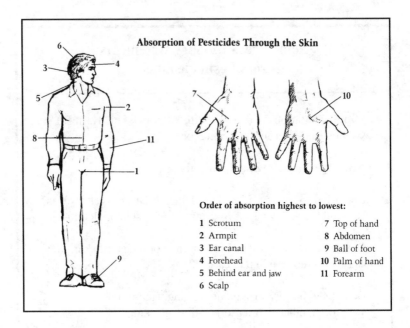

Absorption of Pesticides Through the Skin

Order of absorption highest to lowest:

1	Scrotum	7	Top of hand
2	Armpit	8	Abdomen
3	Ear canal	9	Ball of foot
4	Forehead	10	Palm of hand
5	Behind ear and jaw	11	Forearm
6	Scalp		

Pesticides differ in how fast they go through your skin, and in what amount. If your skin is wet, or you are sweating, or have a rash, a sore, or a cut, pesticides go through your skin faster and in greater amounts than if it were dry and undamaged. Some parts of the body absorb pesticides more readily than others – the genital area (scrotum), armpit (axilla), face, and neck in particular, as Figure 2.4 shows.

The skin is the largest organ in the body. Your skin is the major barrier and protective layer between you and the outside world. If you spill a pesticide directly on your skin, wash it off immediately. If your clothing gets damp or wet with a pesticide, remove it immediately, and thoroughly wash your skin. Otherwise you will continue to absorb the pesticide, as long as there is contact with your skin. The more concentrated the pesticide the more serious the potential for harm.

Children's skin exposure. Children have much more skin surface for their size than adults. Under similar conditions of exposure, children will absorb more than an adult, placing them at higher risk. Children can absorb pesticides residues from skin contact with contaminated carpet, furnishings, bed clothes, and other objects in the home. Infants and toddlers who wear less clothing have more exposed skin surface, are at even higher risk. The 'job' of children is to explore. Their

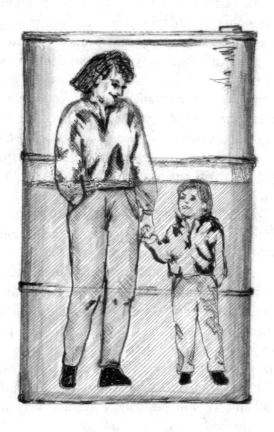

crawling, toddling, and other activities result in direct skin contact with contaminated floors, carpets, and other surfaces. Children also absorb pesticides from contact with pet collars, or residues on pets treated with pesticides.

Inhalation. How much you breathe into your lungs depends mostly on the size of the pesticide particles. The smaller the particles, the less likely they are to get trapped by your nose and upper air passages before they can get into your lungs. Because particles and mists from foggers, bombs, and aerosols are smaller than those from sprays, more can be breathed in. Dusts, granules, and most powders are large enough to get trapped before they get into your lungs.

How fast you are breathing (your respiratory rate), and the amount of ventilation also affect how much gets into your lungs. The faster you are breathing and the less circulating fresh air, the more you will breathe into your lungs.

Toxic vapors. Breathing in the particles and vapors is the major way that pesticides get into your body only for pesticides in the form of a gas – called fumigants. Home use pesticides that emit toxic vapors are solids, such as mothballs, moth bars and moth flakes, and no-pest strips. Some rodenticides give off a toxic gas when they react with moisture in the air.

The major use of fumigant type pesticides in the home is for termites. This is covered in chapter ten on commercial pest control companies, since the toxic gases can only be bought and applied by professional exterminators.

Children's inhalation exposure. Children are more at risk from breathing in pesticides than adults. Children have a higher respiratory rate, they take more breaths per unit of time. Under similar conditions of exposure, more particles will deposit into the lungs of children than adults. Studies show that using home foggers according to label directions can result in levels of pesticide exposure to children that exceed workplace standards for adults.

Swallowing. Swallowing is not a major way that home use pesticides get inside the body. An important exception is accidental ingestion, which can be life-threatening. Children are at much greater risk of swallowing pesticides accidentally. Most home use pesticides are not in child-proof containers, and are often stored where children can reach them.

Children can swallow small amounts of pesticides when playing with a treated pet or pet collars, while playing on a treated lawn or carpet, or other contaminated areas inside and outside the home. They get into everything and put everything into their mouths.

An EPA study in Florida of nine households with children six months to five years of age, found pesticides throughout the home environment. There were pesticide residues in indoor air, carpet dust, outdoor soil, and on the children's hands. The highest concentrations were in carpet dust.

Through the eyes. Pesticides can enter the body through the eyes. Because blood vessels are close to the surface, pesticides can then get into the blood stream and cause poisoning. However, the eyes are not a major way that home use pesticides enter your body. The most important problem is the potential for corrosive effects from direct splashes into the eyes, which can lead to scarring and potential blindness.

Types of Pesticide Packaging (Formulations)

Potential health hazards of home use pesticide depends on both the chemicals inside the pesticide container and the packaging, or type of formulation. There are four basic types of formulations:

◆ Foggers, bombs, and aerosols.
◆ Liquids and sprays.
◆ Dusts, granules, powders.
◆ Baits and traps.

Foggers, bombs and aerosols. We do not recommend any use of foggers, bombs, and aerosols. These broadcast sprays are designed to maximally penetrate the area being treated as thoroughly as possible. Residues settle out of the air and contaminate everything they contact. Contaminated floors, carpet, upholstery, drapes, furniture, and any objects in the treated area can become a source of continuing exposure. Foggers, bombs, and aerosols emit vapors, mists, and particles that are small enough to breathe directly into the lungs. They are also more likely to contain potentially harmful inert ingredients, including petroleum solvents. (See below for discussion of inert ingredients).

Liquids and sprays. Products with a finger or hand pump are potentially less hazardous than foggers, bombs, and aerosols because the spray is more directed and less likely to settle out on everything in the treated area. However, a lot depends on how toxic the pesticide is, how it is used, and whether you apply it directly from the container or mix it yourself. Pesticide concentrates you mix yourself are the most hazardous, because the percentage of pesticide active ingredient is high. Concentrated products that you dilute yourself may seem cheaper. However you should consider the hazards of mixing and applying them, and storing and disposing of what you do not use.

Dusts, granules powders. In general these products are less hazardous than foggers, bombs, aerosols and sprays. However, a lot depends on how toxic the pesticide is, how it is used, and whether it is applied directly from the container or requires mixing. Remember, pesticides you mix yourself are more concentrated, and the greater the concentration the greater the hazard. In general, powders are more hazardous than dusts and granules. This is because the particles are smaller and it is easier for them to settle out on the skin and enter the body.

Baits and traps. These products designed to attract and contain pests are the least hazardous. Traps are essentially nontoxic. Most baits do not give off harmful vapors, mists, sprays, or residues that contaminate the entire treated area. The pesticide stays in the container it comes in, relying on the pest coming to the bait or trap. We recommend the use of baits and traps whenever possible.

Inert ingredients. Home use products contain more than pesticides. So called "inert" ingredients, are added to dissolve the pesticide, to make it work better, to keep it from settling out, to make it stick better to surfaces it is applied to, or to make it last longer. These ingredients are called inert because they are not active as pesticides.

The term inert is a misnomer, since many inert ingredients are biologically active chemicals. Some inert ingredients are more toxic than the pesticide(s) they are mixed with. Some inerts make it easier for the pesticide it is mixed with to enter your body. The EPA does not require listing the names of inert ingredients on the pesticide label. By law, this information is proprietary – a trade secret. Chapter four discusses inert ingredients in more detail.

If the percentage of the active ingredient pesticide in a product is 0.25%, this seems like a very comforting small number. Remember, this means that there is 99.75% of something else inside that container – the inert ingredients. If the label does not disclose the names of the inert ingredients, how can the consumer make an informed choice of the least toxic product?

Number of ingredients. Many products contain two or more different pesticides. Pesticides mixed together can be more toxic than either one alone. The reason the manufacturer mixes pesticides and other chemicals is to make the product more harmful to the pest and get a better kill. This can also make it more harmful to the human beings who contact it.

More is not better when buying pesticides. Even when selecting a least toxic product, you should purchase the smallest amount that you need, in the lowest concentration. The more concentrated a pesticide is, the more harm it can cause. If a particular pesticide is 1% of one product and 20% of another, this means that there is twenty times more of the pesticide in the second product. An undiluted pesticide that requires you to mix it is a more toxic product that is one that already diluted.

If a pesticide is accidentally spilled or swallowed, the weaker the concentration, and the fewer the ingredients, the less likely it is to do serious harm. It is also easier for Poison Control Center personnel to advise you, and the emergency room doctor to treat any poisoning that might occur.

Remember that some nontoxic products may contain other ingredients that are toxic, so do not be misled. Selecting the least toxic or nontoxic products, formulations and methods are important steps in protecting your family.

Odor. Many pesticide products have a strong odor. This can be due to the pesticide, the inert ingredients, or a combination. Odor is *not* an indicator of how hazardous or potentially dangerous a pesticide is. Highly toxic products can be almost odorless, and less toxic products can have a strong odor. Just because you cannot smell a pesticide does not mean that it is not present in amounts that can enter your body or harm you.

Pesticide manufacturers often add pleasant smelling scents or perfumes to pesticides to mask the strong odor. This does *not* make the product less toxic. It is not a safety decision but a marketing gimmick to make the product more acceptable to the consumer. Products are often marketed as "fragrance free." This does *not* mean the product is less toxic. See the discussion of the skin repellent deet (Off!®) in chapter nine.

Drift. The movement of broadcast spray pesticides away from the site of application is called drift. The EPA ignores this serious problem when approving pesticides for home use. The agency approves labeling and marketing of home use pesticides without requiring any data on drift, environmental fate, or human exposure. The question is not *whether* pesticides drift – they do. The question is how far, how much, and for how long.

We know very little about drift in urban and suburban areas. Studies in agricultural areas show that 85 to 90% of broadcast sprays drift off target. They can drift in high concentrations for a mile or more, and in lower concentrations for up to 50 miles. This means that only 10 to 15% of the sprays actually reach the target pest. Much less than 1% of the pesticide used is actually needed to kill the pests. Current methods therefore can use 99% more poison than is needed, and apply them using primitive technology.

Home use exposures. Several studies show that human exposures from home use pesticides are higher than levels assumed safe, especially in children. The EPA has no information on how long lawn care pesticides persist in the soil. Nor do they require data on the exposures and risks to toddlers and children walking and playing on the lawn.

Yet label instructions for home use pesticides tell people to go back into the treated area, or children to play on a treated lawn when sprays have dried. This advice is based on no scientific data whatsoever. The following examples are from actual pesticides labels.

Figure 2.5

Precautionary statements from Pesticide labels

Do not allow children or pets to contact treated surfaces until spray has dried.

Do not allow children in treated areas until surfaces are dry.

There are no scientific studies to indicate that such label warnings are truly protective. Most such precautionary statements on pesticides labels therefore cannot be adequate as health and safety warnings. They are what is known as "boiler plate" generic language that applies to a wide range of products and activities. This is not science; it is marketing.

Environmental persistence. EPA studies show that urban soils have higher levels of pesticides than soil in agricultural areas. Pesticides residues in soil are tracked indoors and accumulate inside the home. House dust thus becomes a source of continuing contamination. Liquid pesticides can run off into the ground and be carried far from the site of application. Rain also carries pesticide residues away from the site of application. The EPA studies also show that residues can stay around much longer inside your house than outdoors. Persistence of pesticides in humans is discussed in detail in the chapters on acute and chronic health effects.

Storage and disposal. Home use pesticides in a garage, basement, or other household storage area, are serious potential health hazards – especially to children. Some pesticides become more toxic under storage conditions, particularly in hot weather. Stored toxic products increase the risk to your family, your neighbors and your community in case of storms, fires, floods, and earthquakes. Proper disposal is also a problem. Never pour pesticides into a sewer or septic system, or into the toilet, or down the drain. Never reuse an empty pesticide container for any purpose. Follow label instruction for disposal of the unused product and the empty container.

The following statements from pesticide labels are further indicators of the seriousness of drift, run off, and impact on humans, pets, and the environment beyond the treated area.

Figure 2.6

Some Precautionary statements from Pesticide labels

Do not use in hospitals or clinical rooms, such as patient rooms, wards, nurseries, operating or emergency areas. Do not use in any rooms where infants, or the sick or aged are, or will be present for any extended period of confinement.

Remove pets. Cover fish aquariums and plants before spraying.

This pesticide is highly toxic to birds, fish, and other wildlife.

Birds, especially waterfowl, feeding or drinking on treated areas can be killed.

This product is toxic to fish. Keep out of lakes, streams, or ponds.

This product is extremely toxic to fish and toxic to aquatic invertebrates. Drift or runoff may be hazardous to aquatic organisms in neighboring areas.

It keeps on killing with residual action even after you spray, for up to four weeks. Residual kill keeps on killing the roaches that return to the area that you have sprayed.

Do not graze treated area or feed clippings to livestock.

Do not apply when weather conditions favor drift from areas treated.

Do not contaminate water food or feed by storage or disposal.

Exercise caution when handling pesticides to prevent contamination of ground water supplies.

3

How to Read a Pesticide label

An expert is a man who tells you a simple thing in a confused way in such a fashion as to make you think the confusion is your own fault.

William B. Castle (b. 1897)

Pesticides have a common name and a chemical name, and there the simplicity ends. The common name, simpler and easier to remember, is often not on the pesticide label. The chemical name, longer and impossible to remember, is often the only name on the label.

Chemical name. For example, the insecticide with the common name "propoxur" is listed on one product only by its chemical name: *1-(1-methylethoxy)phenyl methyl-carbamate* (33 letters, 12 syllables). The insecticide with the common name "resmethrin" is listed on one product only by its chemical name: *([5-(phenylmethyl)-3-furanyl] methyl 2,2-dimethyl-3-(2 methyl -1- propenecyclopropane carboxylate* (69 letters, 24 syllables). This makes comparison shopping rather challenging.

Common name. We spare you (and ourselves) the chaos of pesticide naming by always using the common name. Since this common name might not be on the label, we prepared a cross reference of common names and chemical names (see Appendix F.1 and F.2 on page 373). However, the same pesticide ingredient can have more than one version of its chemical name. We list all the versions we came across. The cross references should help identify chemicals in products sold in your area not listed in our tables. A good rule of thumb – if you cannot figure out what is in it, don't buy it.

Active ingredients. The law requires the chemical name and percentage of each active ingredient pesticide to be on the label. They are listed in decreasing order of their percentage in the product.

Inert ingredients. The names of the inert ingredients are not on the label. They are listed only as the total percent in the product. Some products have a statement on the label that it contains petroleum distillates, or xylene grade aromatic solvents, or similar language. The brand name products in our survey that had these label statements are listed in Appendix D on page 366.

Misleading labels. Pesticide labels can be very misleading, even though they meet EPA standards (which is not difficult). For example there is a Raid™ product that has a very prominent statement on the label that reads *"This product contains pyrethrins, pyrethrins are made from flowers"*. When you look carefully at the small print you will see that the first ingredient is the nerve-gas insecticide, chlorpyrifos. There is three times more of it in the product than the pyrethrins from flowers.

The same pesticide active ingredient can be in many different brand name products, and many products contain more than one. Our survey found that a little more than half of the products contained one active ingredient, and one-fourth had three or more as Figure 4.1 shows.

Trade name products with similar names can have different ingredients. People often say the pesticide they used or were exposed to was "Raid" or "Black Flag". As Table 4.1 and 4.2 show, this is not very definitive information.

Our survey found twenty-five different Raid™ brand name products, which are listed in Table 4.1. These products contain two or more of twelve different pesticide ingredients: allethrin, chlorpyrifos, cyfluthrin, dichlorvos, MGK 264, permethrin, piperonyl butoxide, propoxur, pyrethrins, resmethrin, sulfluramid, and tetramethrin.

Figure 4.1

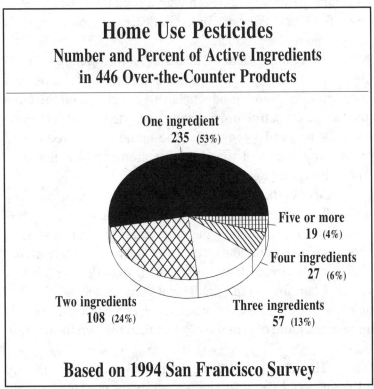

Home Use Pesticides
Number and Percent of Active Ingredients in 446 Over-the-Counter Products

One ingredient
235 (53%)

Five or more
19 (4%)

Four ingredients
27 (6%)

Two ingredients
108 (24%)

Three ingredients
57 (13%)

Based on 1994 San Francisco Survey

Our survey found twelve different Black Flag™ products, which are listed in Table 4.2. These products contain two or more of fifteen different pesticide ingredients: allethrin, chlorpyrifos, hydroprene, lethane, methoprene, methoxychlor, MGK 264, permethrin, phenothrin, piperonyl butoxide, propoxur, pyrethrins, unspecified pyrethroid, resmethrin, and tetramethrin.See the tables in chapters six through nine for the specific ingredients in these products.

Table 4.1

Raid™ Brand Name Products
From 1994 and 1995 Over-the-Counter Surveys

Raid Ant & Roach Home Insect Killer Formula II
Raid Ant & Roach Killer 6
Raid Ant Baits
Raid Flea Killer
Raid Flea Killer Plus Egg Stop Formula
Raid Flying Insect Killer Formula 5
Raid Fumigator Fumigating Fogger
Raid House & Garden Formula 11
Raid House and Garden Bug Killer
Raid House and Garden Bug Killer (from flowers)
Raid Indoor Fogger II
Raid Liquid Roach & Ant Killer Formula I
Raid Max Ant Bait
Raid Max Fogger
Raid Max Fogger II Penetrating Micro Mist
Raid Max Plus Egg Stoppers
Raid Max Plus Roach Bait IV
Raid Max Roach Bait
Raid Max Roach and Ant Killer
Raid Multibug Killer Formula D-39
Raid Roach Baits
Raid Wasp & Hornet Killer IV
Raid Wasp & Hornet Killer X
Raid Wasp and Hornet Killer III
Raid Yard Guard Outdoor Fogger Formula V

Precautionary statements. Precautionary statements on pesticide labels are discussed in chapter two on exposure, and chapter four on acute health effects.

Chronic toxicity. There is nothing on the label that indicates chronic toxicity as there is for acute toxicity. This is why we include a summary for each pesticide active ingredient in the tables in chapters six through ten.

Table 4.2

Black Flag™ Brand Name Products
From 1994 and 1995 Over-the-Counter Surveys

Black Flag Ant And Roach Killer
Black Flag Ant Control System
Black Flag Ant Roach Killer Formula B
Black Flag Flea Ender Fogger
Black Flag Flea Ender Fogger I
Black Flag Flea Ender Spray
Black Flag Flying Insect Killer I
Black Flag House & Garden Insect Killer
Black Flag Insect Spray
Black Flag Liquid Roach & Ant Killer
Black Flag Roach Ender Spray
Black Flag Wasp-Bee-Hornet Killer

Signal words. All pesticides have a signal word on the label that indicates how toxic it is. Table 4.3 shows the meaning of these signal words – Danger, Warning, and Caution. The Spanish version also appears on some labels.

Table 4.3

Signal Word	Meaning
Danger / Peligro	Highly toxic
Warning / Aviso	Moderately toxic
Caution / Precaución	Minimally toxic

These signal words refer to the *acute* hazard of the product – its potential to poison you immediately. They tell you nothing about chronic toxicity or potential long-term effects. If there is no signal word on the label, it means the product is not registered with the EPA as a pesticide. The signal word can be anywhere on the label and is sometimes very hard to find; it is usually on the front. A skull and crossbones on the label means a small amount of the pesticide can be fatal.

Proposition 65. California has a consumer disclosure law that requires a warning statement on retail products that contain chemicals known to cause cancer or birth defects. The law was passed by the voters as a ballot initiative – Proposition 65 – in 1986. Almost all home use pesticides are exempt from this requirement.

In our survey of hundreds of brand name products in San Francisco, only one pesticide had a Proposition 65 warning statement on the label. This pesticide, paradichlorobenzene, is a moth control product. The warning is also on the label for air freshener products containing paradichlorobenzene. Since air fresheners are not marketed as pesticides they have no EPA registration number, and are not regulated under the pesticide law. Figure 4.2 shows the actual wording.

Figure 4.2

Proposition 65 Warning Statement

Notice. California has determined that a chemical contained in this product causes cancer based on tests performed on laboratory animals. *(From the labels for Enoz Cedar-ize moth bar- which contains 99.35% paradichlorobenzene, and Excell Cedar-Pine Scented Closet Freshener- that contains 99.5%).*

EPA Registration Number

All pesticides must be registered by the Environmental Protection Agency (EPA) before they can be sold. Each brand name product has its own unique EPA registration number which must be on the label. This registration number identifies the manufacturer, formulator and distributor of the product. It tells you nothing about how toxic the pesticide is. The number can be anywhere on the label, and sometimes is very hard to find. It is most often in the lower left hand corner on the back of the label, and is always listed as EPA Reg. No.

Registered products. There are approximately 21,000 brand name pesticide products registered with the EPA. They contain one or more of 825 different active ingredient pesticide chemicals and 2,000 different inert ingredients. This includes all uses – agriculture, industrial, commercial, and home.

Pesticide companies. Major pesticide manufacturers in the U.S. include Dupont, DowElanco, Monsanto, American Cyanamid, and FMC. European manufactures whose products are widely sold in the U.S. include Rhône-Poulenc (France), ICI Americas (England), and Ciba Geigy (Switzerland). Both U.S. and foreign companies sell pesticides to hundreds of smaller companies who mix and package them under their own labels and brand names. According to the EPA, there are 120 major producers, 9,500 formulator/producers and 17,200 distributors (wholesalers) of pesticides in the U.S.

No EPA number. If there is no EPA registration number, it means that the product is not registered as a pesticide by the EPA. Such products include Roach Motels™, rat and mouse traps, sticky fly paper, herbs or plant oils, and other products.

Some products contain ingredients identical to pesticides, but are not marketed as pesticides. If the active ingredient is not used as a pesticide, the product will not have an EPA registration number. An example from our survey is products containing paradichlorobenzene, the active ingredient in mothballs. Enoz- Cedar-ize Moth Bar with 99.35% paradichlorobenzene has an EPA registration number. Excell Cedar-Pine Scented Closet Freshner, which contains 99.5%, does not. As discussed above, both have a Proposition 65 warning statement on the label.

4

Acute Health Effects of Pesticides

To say, for example, that a man is made up of certain chemical elements is a satisfactory description only for those who intend to use him as a fertilizer.

Herbert J. Muller (b. 1905)

There are two major ways that pesticides affect human health. They can cause short-term acute effects, or long-term chronic effects. Exposure to pesticides can also worsen existing health problems and medical conditions.

Acute Toxicity of Pesticides

Acute toxicity refers to short-term adverse health effects that occur close in time of exposure to the toxic substance. Usually this is within a few minutes to a few hours – at the most a few days. The types of acute effects that pesticides can cause include the following:

◆ *Irritant effects*: stinging, burning, itching of the eyes, nose, throat, skin.

◆ *Skin effects*: contact dermatitis – rashes, blisters, skin burns.

◆ *Eye effects*: chemical conjunctivitis; abrasion or ulceration of the cornea; corrosive damage with scarring and blindness.

◆ *Systemic effects*: mild, moderate, and severe poisoning.

Irritant effects. Irritant effects are the most frequent acute effects of pesticide exposure. The most common effects are stinging, burning, and itching of the eyes, nose, throat, or skin. The cause can be the pesticide, the inert ingredient, or a combination. You should assume that any pesticide product can potentially cause irritant effects in some individuals. Sometimes the pesticide label tells you that the product contains an eye or skin irritant.

Irritant effects can occur in everyone exposed if the dose is high enough. Some people are affected sooner than others who tolerate a higher dose. Irritant effects are signs of a local reaction, the pesticide is affecting the part of the body it comes in direct contact with.

Skin effects. Dermatitis is the medical term for inflammation of the skin. It is called contact dermatitis if the cause is a substance outside the body coming in contact with the skin. There are two kinds of contact dermatitis – the irritant type, which is very common, and the allergic type, which is much less common.

Irritant contact dermatitis is very common from pesticide exposure. Depending on the nature and intensity of the exposure, pesticides can cause rashes, blisters, and skin burns. Irritant effects are not the same as allergic reactions. Allergic reactions to pesticides are discussed in more detail below.

Eye effects. The most common effect is conjunctivitis (similar to pink eye). Pink eye is caused by a bacteria or virus. When the cause is a chemical it is called chemical conjunctivitis.

If pesticides splash directly into the eyes they can cause severe damage to the cornea – the clear part of the eye that covers the iris and pupil. It is a very delicate and fragile tissue. Pesticides and inert ingredients can cause a corneal abrasion or ulcer – mild or moderate damage to the layers of the cornea. With complete removal of the pesticide from the eye and proper treatment, the cornea should heal completely. However if the pesticide or inert ingredient substance is corrosive and is not thoroughly removed it can cause permanent scarring that can lead to blindness.

This is why all of the label statements instruct you to rinse the eyes for 15 minutes if pesticides get into your eyes. If all of the pesticides and inert ingredients are not removed, they can stick to the corneal tissues and cause serious damage.

Systemic effects. Systemic effects are toxic effects that occur after the pesticide gets inside the body and into the blood stream. Such poisoning can occur with or without irritant or skin effects. Different classes of pesticides present different signs and symptoms of poisoning, and can require specific management as summarized below.

Major Classes of Insecticides

Most of the highly toxic home use pesticides are insecticides. This is because humans share some similarities with insects. For example, we have an enzyme in our nervous system affected by certain pesticides – and so do cockroaches, ants, flies and other insects. The enzyme is called cholinesterase (coal-in-ESTER-ace) and is discussed in detail below.

Most insecticides belong to one of four classes of chemicals. Home use insecticides are listed below according to these four classes, and the rest by use groups.

◆ *Chlorinated hydrocarbons*: DDT, the best known member of this class, was first marketed in the U.S. in 1945. At the time of its ban in 1972 it was one of the most widely used pesticides in the country. DDT and related pesticides were the main target of Rachel Carson's 1962 book, *Silent Spring*.

◆ *Organophosphates*: The first of these nerve-gas type pesticides was marketed in the1940s. They were developed by the Germans researching chemical warfare agents during World War II.

♦ *Carbamates*. These pesticides are also nerve-gas type pesticides and were first marketed in the U.S. in 1956.

♦ *Pyrethrum, pyrethrins, and synthetic pyrethroids*. Pyrethrum and pyrethrins are made from flowers (a type of chrysanthemum). Synthetic pyrethroids are chemical imitations of these natural products. Synergists are chemicals added to this class of insecticides to increase their killing power.

♦ *Fumigants*. Fumigants are pesticides in the form of a gas or vapor. Home use products include solids, flakes, and strips that emit vapors slowly over time as well as products that release a toxic gas on contact with moisture in the air or soil.

♦ *Natural substances*. This category includes basic elements, inorganic compounds, plant alkaloids and other botanicals.

♦ *Insect growth regulators*. These products are a form of birth control for insects and interfere with their ability to grow and develop normally.

♦ *Biological control agents*. These products are made from living organisms, including antibiotics, bacteria, nematodes, beneficial insects, fungi, and viruses.

♦ *Inert ingredients*. These are ingredients in pesticide products that are not active as pesticides.

Acute health effects of Insecticides

A summary of acute health effects related to exposure to different classes of insecticides follows. The examples are the pesticides from our surveys, both over-the-counter and commercial use. Pesticides used only by professional pest control operators, not available over-the-counter, are listed separately as commercial use. All of the pesticides are listed alphabetically by common name. The names inside the parentheses are trade names if they have the symbol ®, and another common name if they do not.

Because a particular health effect or condition is not discussed in this section does not mean that pesticide exposure cannot cause it. It is beyond the scope of this book to list all known and possible human health effects of pesticides.

Chlorinated hydrocarbons

Examples (over-the-counter). Dicofol (Kelthane®), dienochlor (Pentac®), endosulfan (thiodan); lindane (gamma-HCH, Kwell®), methoxychlor.

Examples (commercial use). There were no chlorinated hydrocarbon pesticides used exclusively in commercial pest control.

Mode of action. These pesticides attack the brain and nervous system.

Local effects. Can cause irritant reactions and rashes, including allergic reactions.

Systemic effects. The hallmark of poisoning from this class of pesticides is convulsions (seizures). Other signs and symptoms of poisoning include: headache, dizziness, nausea, vomiting, incoordination, tremor, mental confusion, and jerky muscle movements (myoclonus). Convulsions can occur without the other symptoms. Lindane is the most toxic of the chlorinated hydrocarbons used in home use products in the U.S.. There are deaths from toxic encephalopathy (severe damage to the brain) reported in infants and children from skin application of lindane.

Antidote. There is no specific antidote to poisoning. Treatment includes decontamination (removing contaminated clothing, washing the pesticide from the skin and hair, pumping it out of the stomach, if swallowed), seizure control, treatment of signs and symptoms, and support of respiration, blood pressure, and other body systems.

Absorption and excretion. Most are readily absorbed through the skin and excreted in the urine. Dicofol, dienochlor, endosulfan (thiodan), and methoxychlor do not accumulate and are not stored for any length of time. Dicofol is contaminated with DDT that does accumulate, and stays in the body for many years. Lindane and its break down products (metabolites) α-HCH, and β-HCH accumulate and persist in body tissue, primarily fat.

Blood tests. Can be detected in the blood (serum), and tests are done in most toxicology laboratories. Except for lindane, it is unlikely that residues will be found if the exposure occurred a week or more prior to the test, unless there were unusual exposure conditions.

Other comments. Lindane, DDT, and related compounds are also found in breast milk and fat at much higher levels than in the blood. Chlorinated hydrocarbons pass from mother to fetus across the placenta, and are also found in semen.

Organophosphates and Carbamates
(Nerve-gas type)

Examples (over-the-counter). *Organophosphates:* acephate (Orthene®), chlorpyrifos (Dursban®), diazinon, dichlorvos (DDVP), dimethoate, malathion, tetrachlorvinphos. *Carbamates:* bendiocarb (Ficam®), carbaryl (Sevin®), methomyl, propoxur (Baygon®).

Examples (commercial use). *Organophosphates*: dicrotophos, fenamiphos (Nemacur®), propetamphos (Safrotin®), sulfotep (Bladfume). *Carbamates*: methiocarb (Measurol®), oxamyl (Vydate®).

Mode of action. These pesticides attack the brain and nervous system, and are similar to nerve-gas. They affect a vital chemical in the nervous system, an enzyme called cholinesterase. The brain and nerves cannot function without this enzyme. Nerve-gas type pesticides inhibit the activity of cholinesterase (decrease the level in the nervous system) which causes the poisoning.

Many organophosphates do not affect cholinesterase directly. The pesticides pass through the liver which changes them into simpler chemicals called metabolites. One of these metabolites, called an oxon, is more toxic than the original pesticide. It is this oxon form of the organophosphate that affects the cholinesterase level. Examples are chlorpyrifos-oxon (from chlorpyrifos) and malaoxon (from malathion).

The enzyme in the liver that is needed to make the toxic oxon metabolite is called an oxonase. Our genes determine how much of this enzyme we have in our bodies. Some people have lower levels than others. Differing levels of this enzyme could explain why some people have worse reactions from organophosphate exposure than others. However, we know very little about this because appropriate studies have not been done.

Local effects. Can cause irritant reactions and rashes.

Systemic effects. The nerve-gas pesticides include the most toxic pesticides known. They are the leading cause of human poisoning and deaths from pesticides in the U.S. and throughout the world. Table 4.1 lists the signs and symptoms of systemic poisoning from nerve-gas type pesticides.

Antidote. The antidote to poisoning by organophosphate and carbamate pesticides is the drug atropine. There is another drug called 2-PAM (Protopam®), which is an antidote to organophosphate but not carbamate poisoning. 2-PAM must be given within 24 to 48 hours after poisoning to be effective. The emergency room doctor will know about these drugs.

If the health warning on the label includes the statement *Atropine is an antidote, this product contains a cholinesterase inhibiting pesticide*, or similar language, then the product contains a nerve-gas type organophosphate or carbamate pesticide. However some products that contain nerve-gas type pesticides may not have a statement about atropine or cholinesterase inhibition on the label. Make sure you take the pesticide container with you to the doctor or the emergency room. If the exposure is from a commercial application you should get the name of the pesticide from the exterminator.

Table 4.1

Signs & Symptoms of Nerve-gas Type Pesticide Poisoning
(Organophosphates and Carbamates)

Mild Poisoning

Headache	Blurry vision
Dizziness	Excess sweating
Fatigue	Excess salivation (drooling)
Nausea	Muscle pain, cramping
Vomiting	Abdominal pain
Chest pain	Diarrhea

Moderate Poisoning

Generalized weakness	Confusion
Difficulty walking	Difficulty concentrating
Difficulty talking	Small pupils (miosis)
Muscle twitching	

Severe Poisoning

Loss of consciousness	Cyanosis (turns blue)
Convulsions	Tiny pupils (marked miosis)
Difficulty breathing	Coma
Involuntary urination	Death
Involuntary defecation	

Absorption and excretion. Most are readily absorbed into the body, and excreted in the urine within twenty-four to thirty-six hours. They do not accumulate in the body and are unlikely to be found in fatty tissue or breast milk, except under unusual exposure conditions.

Blood tests. There is a blood test for poisoning by nerve-gas type pesticides called a cholinesterase test. The test does *not* measure pesticides in the blood but the cholinesterase activity level. Sometimes the doctor resists doing a cholinesterase test if there are no signs of severe poisoning. You should strongly urge the doctor to do the test if the following conditions are met:

1. An exposure to a pesticide known to affect cholinesterase activity has occurred.

2. The exposure occurred within the last two weeks or less.

3. There are indications of a health problem potentially related to the exposure.

It is important that the doctor administer and interpret the cholinesterase test properly. Appendix B on page 324 discusses cholinesterase testing in more detail.

Urine tests. If the exposure was recent, a test called urinary alkylphosphates can detect whether or not organophosphate pesticide residues remain in the body. The urine must be collected as soon as possible after the exposure – within 24 to 48 hours. It is not a test for a *specific* pesticide, but for the residues and metabolites (break down products) of certain organophosphates. The ones used in home products are detected by this test. The test is not done in hospital laboratories, and the urine must be sent to a special laboratory. It may be difficult to get your doctor to agree to do this test, and some insurance companies may not pay for it.

Pyrethrins, Pyrethrum, and Synthetic Pyrethroids

Examples (over-the-counter). *Pyrethrins and pyrethrum:* the label will have the name as is, pyrethrins or pyrethrum. *Synthetic pyrethroids:* allethrin, cyfluthrin, fenvalerate, flucythrinate, permethrin, phenothrin, resmethrin, tetramethrin, trihalothrin.

Examples (commercial use). cypermethrin, fluvalinate, lambda-cyhalothrin

Mode of action. Pesticides in this group attack the brain and nervous system. They do not affect cholinesterase the way nerve-gas pesticides do, and are usually less toxic.

Local effects. Irritation of the eyes, nose and throat, and also skin itching, burning, and rashes. Direct contact with the skin can cause stinging, burning, itching, tingling, numbness, and other unpleasant sensations. Can cause severe allergic reactions. Some doctors who are misinformed may tell you that only the plant-based products cause allergies and not the synthetic pyrethroids. While it is true that the flower-based natural products contain allergens that cross-react with ragweed and other pollens, both the natural and synthetic forms can cause allergies.

Systemic effects. Most are not highly acutely toxic and are unlikely to cause serious poisoning unless swallowed. Signs and symptoms of systemic poisoning include tremor, salivation (drooling), vomiting, diarrhea, and irritability to sound and touch. People with asthma can have severe reactions to this class of pesticides.

Antidote. There is no specific antidote to poisoning. Treatment includes decontamination (removing contaminated clothing, washing the pesticide from the skin and hair, pumping it out of the stomach, if swallowed), treatment of signs and symptoms, and support of respiration, blood pressure, and other body systems.

Absorption and excretion. They are poorly absorbed into the body and rapidly excreted, mostly in the urine. They do not accumulate.

Blood and urine tests. There are no readily available blood or urine tests.

Fumigants

Examples (over-the-counter). Metam-sodium (Vapam®) releases methyl isothiocyanate gas (MITC) on contact with moisture in the soil. Zinc phosphide releases phosphine gas on contact with water vapor in the air.

Examples (commercial use). Methyl bromide, chloropicrin, sulfuryl fluoride (Vikane®).

Mode of Action. Fumigants are powerful tissue poisons that can severely injure any tissue they come into contact with.

Local effects. Irritant effects such as burning and itching of the eyes, skin and respiratory tract (breathing passages), including cough, and nose bleeds. Can cause vesiculation (small blisters), and severe second or third degree chemical burns of the skin, the severity of the injury depends on the duration of contact with the skin. Chloropicrin is a tear gas (lacrimator) added as a warning agent to methyl bromide, which is odorless.

Systemic effects. Fumigants are pulmonary irritants and can cause severe injury to the lungs. Signs and symptoms of poisoning include headache, dizziness, nausea vomiting, tremor, difficulty breathing, cough, restlessness, muscle twitching, and seizures (convulsions). Sulfuryl fluoride can cause severe kidney damage. People who recover from poisoning from methyl bromide can have permanent damage to the brain and nervous system, including changes in personality and temperament. If death occurs, it is usually from pulmonary edema (fluid leaking into the lungs) resulting in asphyxiation (suffocation).

Antidote. There are no specific antidotes and if the poisoning is severe, emergency life support may be needed to save the victim's life.

Blood and urine tests. Victims of methyl bromide poisoning have a greater amount of inorganic bromide in their blood (serum) than the usual background level. Fluoride is high in the blood (serum) of victims of sulfuryl fluoride poisoning. There are no readily available blood or urine tests for exposure to the other fumigants, although there are breakdown products excreted in the urine.

Absorption and excretion. Fumigants are rapidly absorbed through the lungs, stomach (gut) and skin. They are excreted from the body through the lungs (by exhaling the vapors) and in the urine.

Other Comments. Naphthalene (flakes) and paradichlorobenzene (mothballs, moth bars) emit vapors continuously until used up. Pest strips contain a resin strip impregnated with dichlorvos (DDVP) which vaporizes into the air for several months. These pesticides have fumigant action but do not cause severe lung injury and systemic poisoning when used according to label directions.

Natural substances

Examples (over-the-counter). arsenic, boric acid, diatomaceous earth (amorphous silica), neem (azadirachtin), nicotine (Black Leaf 40®), silica gel (silicon dioxide).

Examples (commercial use). Liquid nitrogen.

Mode of action. *Diatomaceous earth* (made from fossils – diatoms), and silica gel kill insects by drying them out; they absorb the waxy coating on the insects' protective outer cover, called the cuticle. *Neem* is a tree oil that kills insects by unknown mechanisms. *Boric acid* is a tissue and stomach poison if swallowed. *Nicotine* is the most acutely toxic of this group of pesticides. It attacks the brain, nervous system, and nerve-muscle connections, but does not affect cholinesterase the way nerve-gas pesticides do. *Arsenic* acts as a tissue poison by combining with sulfur and phosphate in proteins and enzymes, interfering with their normal function. *Nitrogen* is a gas (78% of the air we breathe) which freezes when compressed into a liquid. It is used to freeze termites to death.

Local effects. *Arsenic* can cause skin problems but is unlikely to so do from home use pesticides where problems arise from a child swallowing a bait. *Boric acid* powders are not absorbed through the skin but can be mildly irritating (including borax). Any pesticide product can potentially cause skin irritation or rash in some individuals.

Systemic effects. *Arsenic:* acute poisoning results from ingestion (swallowing) the pesticide. The breath and stool (bowel movements, feces) can smell like garlic; there is abdominal pain, and watery diarrhea that might have blood in it. The nervous system, heart, liver, kidneys, and bone marrow can also be affected. *Boric acid:* acute poisoning results from ingestion (swallowing) the pesticide. If only a small amount is swallowed there may be no symptoms. Vomiting, abdominal pain, and diarrhea are common symptoms when they do occur. *Nicotine:* the signs and symptoms of mild to moderate nicotine poisoning are very similar to those from nerve-gas type pesticides (organophosphates and carbamates) – excess salivation (drooling), nausea, vomiting, and miosis (small pupils). Severe poisoning results in muscle paralysis, shock (collapse of the heart and vascular system with drastic lowering of blood pressure), and respiratory paralysis. *Liquid nitrogen:* An exterminator applying liquid nitrogen died from suffocation (lack of oxygen) while working in an enclosed wall space without any ventilation. There is no danger to the home owner after the gas dissipates since it is a normal part of the air we breathe. *Diatomaceous earth, silica gel,* and *neem* have no apparent significant toxicity for humans.

Antidote. BAL (dimercaprol) is an antidote to arsenic poisoning; D-penicillamine is another antidote that can be used if the victim is not allergic to penicillin. There is no specific antidote to nicotine poisoning, but atropine can control the excess secretions. Treatment includes decontamination (removing contaminated clothing, washing the pesticide from the skin and hair, syrup of ipecac or pumping the stomach if swallowed), treatment of signs and symptoms, and support of respiration, blood pressure, and other body systems.

Absorption and excretion. *Boric acid* is poorly absorbed through the skin and is excreted in the urine in about 24 hours. *Nicotine* is readily absorbed and is transformed by the liver into several simpler chemicals (metabolites) which are excreted into the urine within a few hours. They do not accumulate. *Arsenic* is also excreted in the urine.

Blood and urine tests. Borates (from *boric acid*) can be measured in the blood (serum) and the urine. *Arsenic* is also found in the urine. Cotinine is the major metabolite of *nicotine* found in the urine.

Other comments. The diatomaceous earth registered for use as a pesticide is *not* the same product as that used as a filtering agent in swimming pools. These products are *not* interchangeable. The swimming pool product is higher in free silica, the crystalline form that can cause scarring of the lungs (silicosis).

Biological control agents

Examples (over-the-counter). Avermectin (abamectin, Avid®), B.T. (Bactospeine®, Dipel®).

Mode of action and acute health effects. *Abamectin* is an antibiotic with a narrow spectrum of activity. *B.T.* is Bacillus thuringiensis, bacteria with exotoxins toxic to insects. These agents have a narrow spectrum of activity, that is, their toxicity is specific to the particular target pest they are being used against. They are the least likely to pose a human health hazard. However any product can potentially be an irritant or cause local skin reactions, allergies, or other acute reactions.

Insect growth regulators

Examples (over-the-counter). methoprene (Altosid®, Precor®), kinoprene (Enstar®), hydroprene (Gencor®).

Mode of action and acute health effects. In general these chemicals do not pose a high acute toxicity risk to human beings. Their toxic action is very specific to disruption of reproduction of the insect by affecting growth and development. However any product can potentially be an irritant or cause local skin reactions, or other acute reactions.

Table 4.2 is a selected list of insecticides discussed in the acute health effects section above.

Table 4.2

Some Examples of Home Use Pesticides by Common name
(with brand and other names)

Chlorinated hydrocarbons
Dicofol (Kelthane®)
Dienochlor (Pentac®)
Endosulfan (Thiodan)
Lindane (gamma-HCH)
Methoxychlor

Synthetic Pyrethroids
Allethrin
Cyfluthrin
Fenvalerate
Flucythrinate
Permethrin
Phenothrin
Resmethrin
Tetramethrin

Natural substances
Arsenic
Boric acid
B.T. (Dipel®)
Diatomaceous earth
Neem (azadirachtin)
Nicotine
Silica gel

Organophosphates
Acephate (Orthene®)
Chlorpyrifos (Dusrban®)
Diazinon
Dichlorvos (DDVP)
Dimethoate
Disulfuton
Malathion
Tetrachlorvinphos

Carbamates
Bendiocarb (Ficam®)
Carbaryl (Sevin®)
Carbofuran (Furadan®)
Propoxur (Baygon®)

Fumigants / Fumigant Action
Metam-sodium (Vapam®)
Methyl-bromide
Naphthalene
Paradichlorobenzene
Sulfuryl fluoride (Vikane®)
Zinc phosphide

Acute health effects of Other Pesticides

The following discussion includes the acute health effects of skin repellents, herbicides, fungicides, rodenticides, and inert ingredients.

Skin Repellents

Examples. Deet (Off!®, dimethyl-toluamide)

Mode of action. It is applied directly to the skin to repel mosquitoes, ticks, fleas, gnats, biting flies, and chiggers.

Local effects. Can cause a severe skin reaction in some individuals.

Systemic effects: Deet is very toxic to the brain and nervous system. Signs and symptoms of mild poisoning include headache, restlessness, irritability, crying spells in children, and other changes in behavior. In more severe poisoning there can be slurring of speech, tremor (shakiness), convulsions, and coma. Deet has caused death in children from absorption through the skin applied repeatedly and/or in a high concentration. There is a report of a five year old child at a day camp who had a major seizure (convulsion) without any other symptoms shortly after deet was applied to his skin.

There are rare reports of deet causing a severe allergic reaction called anaphylaxis, or anaphylactic shock. This is the same kind of allergic reaction some people get from bee stings; it can lead to death if not treated promptly.

Antidote. There is no specific antidote to poisoning. Treatment includes decontamination (removing contaminated clothing, washing the pesticide from the skin and hair, pumping it out of the stomach, if swallowed), seizure control, treatment of signs and symptoms, and support of respiration, blood pressure, and other body systems.

Absorption and excretion. Deet can be rapidly absorbed if the skin is sunburned, damaged, or irritated. It is excreted mostly in the urine. It does not accumulate.

Blood and urine tests. There are no readily available blood or urine tests.

Other comments. Our survey found a product that was 100% deet (Back Woods Off!). This makes it a 100% toxic product. See chapters nine and eleven for recommendations about deet, and alternatives.

Herbicides

Examples (over-the-counter). Aciflurofen (Goal®), atrazine, benefin, 2,4-D® (Weed-b-Gon®), 2,4-DP, DCPA (Dacthal®), Dalapon, dicamba, diquat, EPTC, fluazifop-butyl (Fusilade®), glyphosate (Roundup®), MCPA, MCPP, MSMA, napropamide (Devrinol®), oryzalin (Surflan®), sodium chlorate, atrazine, prometon, trichlopyr, trifluralin (Treflan®).

Examples (commercial use). Bromacil (Hyvar), bromethalin, cacodylic acid, chlormequat, chlorsulfuron (Telar®, Glean®), dichlobenil (Casaron®, Dyclomec®), diuron, metolachlor, oxadiazon (Ronstar®), pronamide (Kerb®), simazine, sulfometuron-methyl (Oust®), trifluralin (Treflan®). *Plant growth regulators*: Daminozide (B-nine®, Alar®), ethephon (Ethrel®), maleic hydrazide, mefluidide (Embark), naphthaleneacetic acid (NAA).

Mode of action. Herbicides kill plants by affecting chemical reactions and metabolic pathways that do not exist in human beings. Plant growth regulators act like plant hormones and slow down or speed up growth.

Local and systemic effects. Most can cause irritant effects in the eyes, skin, nose and throat. Some can also cause allergic reactions in sensitive individuals. In general, they are not highly toxic and are unlikely to cause serious poisoning under usual conditions of exposure. Systemic poisoning could occur if a concentrated form gets in the eyes or on the skin, or they are swallowed.

Antidote. There is no specific antidote to poisoning. Treatment includes decontamination (removing contaminated clothing, washing the pesticide from the skin and hair, pumping it out of the stomach, if swallowed), treatment of signs and symptoms, and support of respiration, blood pressure, and other body systems.

Absorption and excretion. Most are excreted into the urine within one to four days after exposure. They do not accumulate in the body.

Blood and urine tests. There are no readily available blood or urine tests.

Other comments. A problem with most herbicide products is the false sense of security in buying and using them. Because they are not acutely toxic and do not cause immediate apparent illness they are considered "safe". The greater concern with this group of chemicals is their chronic toxicity discussed further in chapter five.

Fungicides

Examples (over-the-counter). anilazine (Dyrene®), benomyl (Benlate®), captan, chlorothalonil (Daconil®), copper compounds, PCNB, sulfur, thiram, triadimefon (Bayleton®), triforine (Funginex®).

Examples (commercial use). Aliette (Fosetyl-al), dazomet (Basamid®), dicloran (DCNA, Botran®), fenarimol (Rubigan®), fenbutatin oxide (hexakis,Vendex®), iprodione, lime sulfur, mancozeb, metalaxyl (Ridomil®), oxycarboxin (Plantvax®), piperalin (Pipron®), thiophanate-methyl, vinclozolin (Ronilan®).

Mode of action. Fungi do not share any attributes with human beings; therefore, fungicides tend to have low acute toxicity for humans.

Local effects. Most are eye and skin irritants, and can cause skin rashes. As a group they are the most likely to cause allergic skin reactions, and can sensitize the skin at low levels.

Systemic effects. Because of their low acute toxicity, fungicides are unlikely to cause serious poisoning. Of the examples listed, thiram can cause an unusual reaction. It is chemically similar to antabuse, a pill taken by alcoholics who are trying to quit. If they drink while taking the pill they get nausea, vomiting, pounding headache, dizziness, difficulty breathing, abdominal pain, and profuse sweating, among other symptoms. The same problem is possible with home use of thiram while drinking alcohol, but has only been reported in workers.

Antidote. There is no specific antidote to poisoning. Treatment includes decontamination (removing contaminated clothing, washing the pesticide from the skin and hair, pumping it out of the stomach, if swallowed), treatment of signs and symptoms, and support of respiration, blood pressure, and other body systems.

Absorption and excretion. Most are poorly absorbed into the body and excreted primarily in the urine. They do not accumulate.

Blood and urine tests. There are no readily available blood and urine tests.

Other comments. A problem with many fungicides is the false sense of security in buying and using them. Because they are not acutely toxic and do not cause immediate apparent illness they are considered to be safe. The greater concern with this group of chemicals is their chronic toxicity which is discussed in chapter five.

Rodenticides

Examples (over-the-counter). *Anticoagulants.* brodifacoum, bromadiolone, chlorophacinone, diphacinone, warfarin. *Fumigant.* zinc phosphide. *Botanical:* strychnine.
Examples (commercial). Aluminum phosphide, dikegulac sodium (Atrinal®), magnesium phosphide, pindone (Pival®, Pivalyn®).

Mode of Action. The *anticoagulants* are blood thinners and cause internal bleeding. On contact with moisture in the air, zinc phosphide releases the toxic gas phosphine that damages biological tissues. Strychnine (a natural toxin also known as nux vomica) violently attacks the nervous system.

Systemic effects. The anticoagulants and strychnine are in the form of baits. The risk of poisoning is from ingestion (swallowing.) The anticoagulants can cause nosebleeds, bruises, and blood in the urine and stool, depending on the amount ingested. If large amounts are swallowed it can be fatal. *Strychnine* causes violent seizures (convulsions) which can cause asphyxiation and death. *Phosphine gas* released from zinc and magnesium phosphide causes severe irritation of the lungs. If the dose is high enough it can cause pulmonary edema (fluid in the lungs) which can be fatal.

Antidote. Vitamin K_1 is the antidote to poisoning with the anticoagulants. There is no antidote to strychnine. Treatment includes seizure control, support of respiration, and kidney dialysis if needed. There is no antidote to phosphine. Management includes treatment of signs and symptoms, and support of respiration, blood pressure, and other body systems.

Absorption and excretion. Most are poorly absorbed into the body and excreted primarily in the urine. They do not accumulate.

Blood tests. The anticoagulants affect a clotting factor in the blood called prothrombin. The prothrombin time test determines when the clotting ability of the blood is back to normal. There are no readily available blood or urine tests for strychnine or phosphine.

Inert ingredients

Examples. Petroleum distillates, toluene, xylene, alcohols, glycols, ethers.

Mode of action. Inert ingredients are added to pesticides to dissolve, emulsify, or stabilize them, or to facilitate spreading, sticking, and penetration of the pesticide.

Local health effects. Irritation of the eyes and skin.

Systemic health effects: The most serious problems occur when the pesticide/inert ingredient is swallowed. There is danger of chemical pneumonia (also called hydrocarbon pneumonitis) from aspiration of even tiny amounts into the lungs if the victim vomits, if vomiting is induced, or the stomach is pumped. Signs and symptoms of chemical pneumonia are fever, rapid heart beat, rapid breathing, and cyanosis (turns blue). This type of pneumonia can be fatal, and recovery can take several weeks. Many inerts are chlorinated hydrocarbons that can cause damage to the liver, heart, and kidneys.

Antidote. There is no specific antidote to poisoning.

Absorption and excretion: Are not persistent and do not accumulate.

Blood and urine tests. The standard tests should be done to determine if there is damage to the liver, heart, or kidneys.

Allergic reactions to Pesticides

We now move from the discussion of potential health effects related to specific classes and types of pesticides, to a more general discussion of allergies, asthma, and other medical conditions.

An allergy is a reaction of the immune system to a material that is foreign to the body. The foreign material is called an allergen or an antigen. Hay fever, for example, is an allergy to antigens such as ragweed, grasses, and pollen.

Allergic dermatitis occurs when the skin becomes sensitized to an allergen. Poison oak and poison ivy are plants that can cause this type of allergy. Pesticides can also sensitize the skin and cause allergic dermatitis.

Sometimes there will be a statement on the label that the pesticide causes allergic reactions. But most label language is not this direct and clear. If you see one of the statements in

Figure 4.1, or similar statements on a pesticide label, it means that the pesticide can cause allergic reactions.

Figure 4.1

> ## Label Warning Examples Indicating a Pesticide Can Cause Allergic dermatitis
>
> This product is a skin sensitizer. *(from a label for the fungicide Daconil® (chlorothalonil))*.
>
> May cause skin reaction in rare cases. *(from a label for the skin repellent deet (Off!®)*
>
> May cause contact sensitization following repeated contact with skin of susceptible individuals. If sensitization reactions result,contact a physician. *(from a label for the insecticide diazinon)*.
>
> Frequent or repeated exposure to this product may cause allergic reactions in some people. Skin contact with this pesticide may be hazardous.*(From a label for the insecticide / miticide dicofol [Kelthane®])*.

Sensitization does not occur with the first exposure to the pesticide allergen or sensitizer. It takes time for the immune system to develop the memory cells that will react to a future exposure. If the pesticide is only a weak allergen it may take several more exposures before the immune system overreacts. It can take many years of exposure to a sensitizer before a person becomes sensitized and exhibits an allergic reaction.

Once a person has become sensitized to a chemical, it takes a much smaller amount to cause a future allergic reaction. Sometimes people who are sensitized to an allergen cannot tolerate even the tiniest amount of exposure.

If exposure continues, the attacks can come on sooner, last longer, and become increasingly severe. The only treatment is to avoid any exposure to the pesticide allergen. A person suffering from allergic sensitization can often avoid exposures in their own home, but often have no control over exposures from use by their neighbors, at their workplace, or environmental exposures.

Any pesticide can theoretically cause an allergic reaction. However, some are more likely to do so than others. Products that contain pyrethrins and pyrethrum that come from flowers, and synthetic pyrethroids can cause allergic reactions. Those who already have hay fever are more likely to be affected. Table 4.3 lists home and commercial use pesticides found in our survey that are reported to be sensitizers, or cause allergic dermatitis.

Table 4.3

Pesticides Reported to Cause Allergic dermatitis	
Anilazine (Dyrene®)	DDVP (dichlorvos)
Benomyl (Benlate®)	Malathion
Captan	Maneb
Chlorothalonil (Daconil®)	Naled (Dibrom®)
Dazomet	PCNB(pentachloronitrobenzene)

Patch Tests. There is a test that can determine if you are allergic to a specific pesticide, called a patch test. However, this test is almost never done. The pure form of the pesticide needed for the test are not made available to allergists by the manufacturers.

If a person knew they were allergic to a specific pesticide they could try to avoid exposure to it. Much could be learned about pesticide allergens if the patch test were widely available. However, in some individuals, even if the test were available it shouldn't be done. In some people even the tiny amount used in the test could cause a very serious reaction.

A severe allergic reaction, called anaphylaxis or anaphylactic shock, can rarely be caused by pesticides. This is the same kind of allergic reaction some people have to bee stings and can lead to death if not treated promptly.

Pesticides and Asthma

People with asthma can have very severe reactions to pesticides. They can have problems at low levels of exposure that have no apparent effect on people without these conditions. This is especially true in children.

The pesticides most likely to precipitate an asthma attack are the pyrethrins and pyrethroid class of pesticides, and the organophosphate and carbamate nerve-gas type pesticides. However, *any* pesticide or inert ingredient can be a potential problem.

If pesticides are causing or aggravating asthma attacks, the only way to prevent them is to avoid *any* exposure to the pesticide causing the problem. While the asthmatic can often do this in their own home, they often have no control over exposures from their neighbor's use, use in schools, at work or other environmental exposures.

Effects on Medical Conditions

Pesticide exposure can aggravate existing health problems. Anyone who is already ill, has a chronic disease, or is taking daily medications can be more at risk from exposure to toxic chemicals, including pesticides.

We do not know as much as we should about the contribution of pesticides to existing health problems and conditions. There are several reasons for this. Patients may forget to tell the doctor about recent pesticide exposures, even though they meant to. Patients may not even think about pesticide exposure as being useful information to tell the doctor. All too often, the patient does tell the doctor, but the doctor ignores or dismisses their concerns. Nor do doctors always think to ask their patients about pesticide exposure.

Medications. Some people taking medication for ulcers, epilepsy, heart disease, or other conditions can be affected by pesticides at a much lower exposure level than if they were not taking the medication. You should make sure your doctor knows about any recent toxic exposures, including pesticides, if you are taking medication regularly, and are having unexplained health problems.

Alcohol can also interact with pesticides, since the combination of alcohol and pesticides puts an additional burden on the liver and kidneys.

Those with liver or kidney problems may be at greater risk from pesticide exposure. The liver is very important in detoxifying pesticides in the body. It breaks them down into simpler chemicals (usually, but not always less toxic), so the body can get rid of them, mostly through the kidneys into the urine.

Nonspecific Signs and Symptoms

Most of the signs and symptoms of mild or moderate pesticide poisoning are nonspecific. This means that other illnesses and conditions can cause similar signs and symptoms. This can make it difficult to determine if a recent pesticide exposure is contributing to a health problem.

An example of a nonspecific symptom is a headache. The headache could be from high blood pressure, meningitis, migraine, stress, sinusitis, or a brain tumor. A doctor determines what is causing your headache by finding out how often you get it, how long you have had it, what other symptoms you have, and doing a physical examination and medical history. Since headache is a very common problem, the doctor will usually make a decision about whether to proceed with x-rays, blood, urine, and other tests depending on how sick you are and whether he or she suspects a serious health problem.

The nonspecific symptoms of mild or moderate pesticide poisoning include headache, nausea, vomiting, dizziness, and stomach cramping, among others. It is rare for there to be just one symptom – there are usually two or three or more. It may be hard to differentiate mild or moderate pesticide poisoning from the flu, an upset stomach, gastroenteritis, or other common health problems.

Many doctors know very little about pesticides and their potential health effects. Medical students and residents in training are taught very little about environmental and occupational toxic exposures except for asbestos and lead. The only experience they may have is learning how to treat life-threatening poisoning when someone accidentally or suicidally swallows a pesticide. So it is not surprising that a doctor might not consider pesticide exposure a problem unless it is life-threatening.

Seeing the doctor. It is important to see a doctor promptly if you suspect a pesticide-related health problem in you or your child. You should tell the doctor your suspicions, the name of the pesticide, and the circumstances of the exposure. This is especially important with asthma and allergies, since avoidance of future exposures is so important. If a pesticide precipitates an attack it should be documented in the medical record. That way the information is available to other doctors for continuing care and follow-up.

Documentation. Make sure your problem and concerns are either written down or clearly organized in your head so you can tell the doctor. Remember, doctors are not famous for being patient listeners, especially when dealing with something they may know very little about, or think is not a serious problem.

This documentation in your medical record or your child's is very important. Even if you are not certain, or do not know the exact name of the pesticide(s), you should tell the doctor as much as you know or suspect so it becomes part of the medical record. This can be very helpful if the problem does not resolve, or if you have to do a lot of doctor shopping to get someone to pay attention to your problem. Make sure you include the following:

1. What happened – exact date and circumstances of the exposure (be brief and concise).
2. What pesticide(s) was involved – if you have the container take it with you (inside a plastic bag).
3. The time relationship between signs and symptoms of illness and exposure to the pesticide.

Be prompt. Often people wait weeks, or sometimes months, after an exposure to seek medical attention. By this time the trail is usually cold. The more time that elapses, the less likely that the doctor can determine if a current acute health problem is pesticide-related. It is unlikely that new symptoms that first develop weeks or months later are due to a past exposure. In general, with removal from exposure and proper treatment, acute effects resolve with apparent complete recovery.

The emergency room. Since there are so many different chemicals used as pesticides, *it is very important to take the container with you* to the emergency room for a pesticide-related problem. Doctors in emergency rooms and poison control centers usually know more about pesticides than other doctors. But even they cannot optimally treat you if they do not know what pesticide(s) you were exposed to.

California reporting law. California has a law that requires physicians to report pesticide-related illness, both confirmed and suspected. Either the health department or agricultural commissioner must be notified. Your doctor may fail to do this, or sometime even refuse when you request it. You should remind the doctor that this is the law.

First Aid

You should not improvise or use home remedies to treat suspected pesticide poisoning. The most important source of information for first aid and emergency treatment is the pesticide label.

We hope that before you bought the pesticide, you read the precautionary statements and health warnings on the label. If not, we hope that you read them before you used the product in or around your home, or on yourself, your children, or your pet. If not, we hope you will do so in the future.

Preventing exposure. The most important first step is to immediately stop any further exposure to and absorption of the pesticide. If exposure and absorption continue, the problem can only get worse. Statements on the label tell you how to do this.

Figure 4.2

Immediate Steps to Prevent Further Exposure
(Statements from Pesticide labels)

If on skin, wash promptly with soap and water. Rinse thoroughly.

In case of contact, immediately remove contaminated clothing or shoes. Flush skin with plenty of water.

For eyes flush with water for at least 15 minutes and get medical attention.

Remove victim to fresh air. Apply artificial respiration if indicated.

It is important to use cool water for the initial decontamination of the skin. You do not want to use warm or hot water since it will speed up absorption of the pesticide through the skin.

Inducing vomiting. If the pesticide was swallowed, it is very important to follow the label directions about whether or not to make the person vomit. If you cause someone to vomit, some of the material they are throwing up (called vomitus) can get into the lungs. This can result in severe damage to the lungs causing aspiration pneumonia. Some examples of label statements about what do if a pesticide is swallowed are listed in Figure 4.3.

Figure 4.3

What to Do if a Pesticide is Swallowed
(Examples of Label Statements)

Call a physician immediately. Drink one or two glasses of water and induce vomiting by touching the back of the throat with finger. Repeat until vomit fluid is clear.

Drink one or two glasses of water and induce vomiting by touching back of throat with finger.

Do not induce vomiting or give anything by mouth if person is unconscious or convulsing.

Note to Physicians: Solvent presents aspiration hazard. Gastric lavage is indicated if material was taken internally. *(Gastric lavage means to pump the stomach.)*

Do not induce vomiting. Call a physician or Poison Control Center immediately.

Do not induce vomiting or give anything by mouth to an unconscious person.

Note to Physician: Inducing vomiting as first aid may result in an increased risk of chemical pneumonia or pulmonary endema [sic] caused by aspiration of the hydrocarbon solvent. Vomiting should be induced only under professional supervision.

The administration of milk or other fat-based demulcents which might enhance absorption is to be avoided.

Many pesticides contain petroleum solvents or other chemicals that can cause serious damage if they are aspirated into the lungs. The resulting chemical pneumonia (also known as hydrocarbon pneumonitis) is a medical emergency and can be very difficult to treat.

Appendix D on page 366 lists the brand name pesticides that state on the label that they contain petroleum byproduct inert ingredients .

Depending on the seriousness of the problem you should call your family doctor, contact the local poison control center, take the victim to an emergency room, or call 911.

5

Chronic Health Effects of Pesticides

Heredity is nothing but stored environment.
Luther Burbank (1849-1926)

Chronic toxicity refers to long-term health effects that occur months or years after the toxic exposure. Chronic effects can be delayed consequences of past exposures, or a result of continuing low-level exposures over time.

Many pesticides in home use products are known to cause chronic toxicity in laboratory animals – including cancer, birth defects, genetic damage, brain damage, and effects on the liver, lungs, kidneys, bone marrow, and other body systems. Pesticides are therefore a potential cause of chronic health effects in human beings.

This chapter has two parts, one on chronic health effects in humans, and the other on chronic toxicity in laboratory animals.

Part I. Chronic Health Effects of Pesticides

Human health studies show associations between pesticide exposure and chronic health effects in humans including the following:

- ◆ Cancer and other tumors.
- ◆ Brain and nervous system damage.
- ◆ Reproductive effects – birth defects, stillbirth, spontaneous abortion, infertility.

◆ Adverse effects on other body systems, such as the liver, kidneys, lungs, and other body organs.

Chronic health effects from pesticides are potentially more serious than acute effects. By the time a chronic disease manifests itself, it is too late to do anything about past exposures. Chronic diseases may not be curable, can lead to disability, and can severely affect quality of life.

Clinical latency. The major characteristic of chronic toxicity is a period of time when the disease is silent. This disease-free interval, when there is no evidence of a health problem, is known as clinical latency. The period of clinical latency can be months for birth defects, or years for cancer.

The risk of pesticide-related chronic effects depends on the intensity, nature, and duration of past exposures. This chapter summarizes the most important studies of pesticide exposure and chronic health effects in humans. It is beyond the scope of this book to discuss all potential chronic health effects.

Pesticide Epidemiology

This section briefly discusses epidemiology and pesticide exposure studies. You can skip to the next section on children without missing any important health information if this topic doesn't interest you.

Definition. Epidemiology is the study of diseases and their causes. Epidemiology studies groups of people, or populations, not individuals. There are different kinds of epidemiological studies, but they all do the same thing – make comparisons.

Types of studies. Some studies compare the health of groups with a specific *exposure* (the cases), to groups without the exposure (the controls) to find out if there are any differences. For example, studies of smokers (the cases) compared to nonsmokers (the controls) find that smokers are much more like to have lung cancer than nonsmokers. Another way of saying this is that smokers are at greater risk, or have a much higher risk of lung cancer.

Another way to do a comparison study is to study a group with a specific *disease* (the cases) and compare them to a group without the disease (the controls) to find out if there are any differences in exposure. For example, studies of people with lung cancer (the cases) compared to people without lung cancer (the controls) find that people with lung cancer are much more likely to be smokers than people without lung cancer.

Pesticide exposure. In pesticide exposure studies, it is not as easy to define the cases (groups exposed to pesticides), and the controls (groups not exposed to pesticides). There are no groups in the population without some exposure to pesticides. This is because of the large amounts used (about 1.2 billion pounds a year in the U.S.), and the ways they are applied. Pesticides contaminate everything and everyone they contact. Residues are found in air, water, soil, rain, fog, snow, food, livestock, wildlife, and human beings, even newborn babies. This makes it very difficult to find control groups without any exposure to pesticides for comparison purposes. The only way to do a study in this situation, is to compare groups with different amounts of exposure.

Populations with heavy pesticide exposure include exterminators, landscape maintenance workers, highway sprayers, farmers, farm workers, and chemical workers. Groups with minimal exposure are those who do not work directly with pesticides and whose exposures are similar to background levels for the rest of the population.

Human versus animal studies. Studies in humans are not the same as studies in experimental animals. In chronic toxicity studies, rats or other animals are divided into two groups; one group is administered the pesticide, and the other is not. After completion of the study (if done properly) the data are used to find out if the pesticide causes specific diseases or chronic effects, and if so at what dose.

Unlike laboratory animals, humans have exposure to a variety of pesticides from different sources. These exposures can change significantly over time since humans do not live under rigid conditions of laboratory experimentation.

In reporting results of studies in humans, investigators include their confidence in the findings by applying statistical tests to the data. They also indicate whether their findings confirm or challenge findings of other related studies.

Epidemiological studies provide critical information about the risks to human health from pesticides. There are many studies that implicate pesticides in chronic health effects in humans. Some of them are discussed below.

Cancer and pesticides. Pesticide exposure is implicated in several types of cancer in humans. We know this from epidemiological studies of the following populations:

◆ Workers with occupational exposure to pesticides.
◆ Children whose parents have occupational exposure to pesticides.
◆ Populations living in agricultural areas of heavy pesticide use.
◆ Children whose parents use pesticides inside and outside the home.

The focus of this book is not the exposure of workers occupationally exposed to pesticides. We discuss these exposures in a brief summary of the types of cancers reported. Our discussion of cancer and pesticides is in three parts:

◆ Childhood cancer and parents' home use of pesticides.
◆ Cancer in children and parents' exposure to pesticides on the job.
◆ Cancer in adults who are not occupationally exposed to pesticides.

Cancer in Children

Age at the time of first exposure is the most important risk factor in chronic health effects. Low levels of exposure that seem to have no apparent effect in adults, can affect the fetus, infant, and prepubertal child. Although we have already discussed the reasons children are at high risk, we summarize them here to refresh your memory.

◆ Their body cells are rapidly differentiating, growing and maturing.

◆ They have less mature liver and other enzyme systems to detoxify chemicals.

◆ They have a less mature immune system to protect them.

◆ They have much more skin surface for their size and at comparable exposure levels will absorb more through their skin than adults.

◆ They are more likely to have direct skin contact with contaminated floors, carpets, and other surfaces in the treated area because of crawling, toddling, and exploring type of activities.

◆ They take more breaths per unit of time (have a higher respiratory rate); at comparable exposure levels, more particles will deposit into their lungs than in adults.

◆ They can swallow significant amounts from ingesting contaminated house dust, and mouthing and chewing on contaminated objects in treated areas.

Leukemia

Los Angeles. In a study done in Los Angeles, California, children were four times more likely to have leukemia (cancer of the white blood cells), if their parents used pesticides in the home once a week or more, compared to children whose parents did not. The children were six times more likely to have leukemia if their parents used garden pesticides (includes herbicides) once a month or more. If it was the mother who used garden pesticides, the risk for leukemia was nine times greater. The children in the study were diagnosed with acute lymphocytic leukemia between 1980 and 1984. The specific pesticides used by the families were not identified.

Denver. In a study done in Denver, Colorado, children were three times more likely to have leukemia if their parents used pest-strips in the home. There was a slight increase in risk if the parents used pesticides in the yard but it was not statistically significant.

Travis Air Force Base. There is a report from Travis Air Force Base Medical Center in California of four children with leukemia (three with acute lymphocytic and one with juvenile chronic myelogenous type). The common exposure was their parents' use of household aerosol insecticide sprays. The most prolonged exposure was in a child with juvenile chronic myelogenous leukemia, whose parents sprayed his mattress twice a week for most of his life.

Aplastic anemia

There are reports of pesticide exposure as a cause of aplastic anemia (failure of the bone marrow to produce any blood cells including red cells, white cells, and platelets, which can be fatal). The reports are fewer since the banning of chlorinated hydrocarbon pesticides such as DDT, dieldrin, and chlordane. Aplastic anemia can be a precursor of leukemia or other blood disorders.

Lindane. While any pesticide could theoretically cause aplastic anemia, most of the reported cases are linked to lindane. This is the only one of the persistent chlorinated hydrocarbons in the DDT family that is still in use. Two recent reports include aplastic anemia in a child whose parents used lindane to treat his head lice; and a 21 year old man who applied it daily for three weeks to treat scabies.

Travis AFB. The report from Travis Air Force Base mentioned above under leukemia, included eleven children with aplastic anemia. The most common exposure was to household aerosol sprays containing DDVP® and Baygon. Both DDVP, the pesticide ingredient in pest-strips, and propoxur (the common name for Baygon®) found in over-the-counter aerosols, cause cancer in animals; both are considered probable human carcinogens by the EPA.

Kwell ® . You may be familiar with lindane as a 1% shampoo or liquid sold under the brand name Kwell® for the treatment of lice and scabies. It is no longer marketed under this name, but is available generically by prescription. However, you can buy a *20%* insecticide formulation over-the-counter (Ortho Lindane Borer and Leaf Miner Spray®). Lindane, which causes cancer in animals, is discussed in more detail in chapter seven on outdoor use pesticides, and in chapter nine on human use. Its use as a lice treatment is also mentioned below in the discussion of childhood brain cancer.

Brain Cancer

Baltimore. In a study done in Baltimore, Maryland, children were twice as likely to have primary brain cancer if their parents used insecticides in the home, than children whose parents did not. When the children with brain cancer were compared to children with other types of cancer no differences were found. This suggests that pesticide exposure is related to other kinds of cancer in children besides the brain cancer that was being studied. The children in the study were diagnosed with cancer between 1965 and 1975.

Denver. Children were almost twice as likely to have brain cancer if their parents used pest-strips in the home. There was also a very slight increase in risk if the parents used yard pesticides, or if the home had been exterminated, but it was not statistically significant.

Columbia, Missouri. In a study done in Columbia, Missouri, children were six times more likely to have brain cancer if their parents used pesticides inside or outside the home, than healthy children whose parents did not. The highest risk found in the study was for children whose parents used a bomb or fogger indoors; these children were six times more likely to have brain cancer when compared to healthy children. If the parents used no-pest strips, their children were five times more likely to have brain cancer. The parents' use of flea collars on pets increased the likelihood of brain cancer in their children by five and a half times; and any termite treatment by three times. Use of insecticides in a yard, garden, or orchard increased the likelihood of brain cancer in the children two to three times.

Lindane for head lice. Children treated with lindane for head lice were almost five times more likely to have brain cancer compared to children without cancer, but the difference was not significant The children in the study were diagnosed with brain cancer between 1985 and 1989 (twenty with astrocytoma, eleven with medulloblastoma, fourteen with a mix of other types).

Missouri family use. A telephone survey was done of pesticide use in the 238 Missouri families with children up to ten years of age included in the brain cancer study described above. Of the families studied, 45 had children with brain cancer, 108 children with other kinds of cancer, and 85 healthy children who were friends of the children with brain cancer.

Almost all the cancer families (98%) used pesticides at least once a year up to the time their children were diagnosed with cancer; two thirds used them more than five times a year. Eighty percent of the families used pesticides during the pregnancy with the affected child, 70% during the first six months of life of their child. The cancer families generally avoided more extensive pesticide treatments in the home with spray liquids and bombs during pregnancy, but continued to use pest-strips and pet flea collars.

Soft Tissue Sarcoma and Lymphoma

In a study done in Denver, Colorado, children whose parents used pesticides in their yards, were four times more likely to have a rare type of cancer, soft tissue sarcoma. There was a slight increase in lymphoma in children whose parents used pest-strips, but it was not statistically significant.

St. Jude's Hospital

At St. Jude's hospital in Memphis, Tennessee, the mothers of 1,270 children with cancer were asked questions about factors that might contribute to their child's cancer. Living in a home with a garden where pesticides were used increased the risk of cancer in the children. The children's cancers were diagnosed between 1979 and 1986; there were 620 with leukemia, 230 with lymphoma, and 404 with other cancers.

Neuroblastoma

There is a report of five cases of neuroblastoma diagnosed at the same pediatric hospital in Ohio in 1975. (Neuroblastoma, a cancerous tumor of immature nerve cells usually found in the chest or abdomen, is one of the most common cancers in children two years of age and younger). All of the children had prenatal or extensive environmental exposure to chlordane.

Chlordane is a persistent chlorinated hydrocarbon that was the major pesticide used for termite control until it's ban in 1988. Estimates are that more than 30 million homes in the U.S. were treated at least once with this pesticide. Chlordane is still manufactured in the U.S. for export.

Cancer in Children and Parents Occupation

Studies of parents exposed to pesticides at work show that their children are more likely to have cancer than children whose parents do not have occupational exposure to pesticides. The types of cancer reported in the children include leukemia, bone cancer, and brain cancer. The younger the child the greater the risk.

Leukemia

United States. The U.S. Children's Cancer Study Group found that children younger than five were eleven times more likely to have acute nonlymphocytic leukemia if their parents were exposed to pesticides on the job, compared to children whose parents were not exposed. If the children were older than five, they were twice as likely to have leukemia.

If the father was exposed to pesticides on the job for 1,000 days or more, his child was almost three times more likely to have leukemia, compared to children whose fathers were not exposed. There was also increased likelihood of leukemia if the child had direct exposure to pesticides, and if the mother had exposure to home use pesticides during her pregnancy with the child.

Japan. A study done in Japan found that children were more likely to have acute lymphoblastic leukemia if their fathers or their mothers worked in agriculture. The risk was even higher if exposure to pesticides occurred during the pregnancy with the affected child.

Bone Cancer

A study done in five San Francisco Bay Area counties of Ewing bone sarcoma, found that children were six times more likely to have bone cancer if their father was exposed to pesticides, compared to children whose fathers were not exposed.

The children were almost nine times more likely to have bone cancer if their father was working in agriculture during the six-month period before the child was conceived, and up to the time the child was diagnosed with cancer.

Brain Cancer

A study done in Columbus, Ohio, found that children whose parents worked in agriculture were almost three times more likely to have primary brain cancer, when compared to children whose parents worked in other industries. The risk was higher if the parents worked in agriculture in the six-month period before the child was conceived, and during the pregnancy with the affected child.

Wilm's Tumor

In a study done in Brazil, children were three times more likely to have Wilm's tumor if their parents were farm workers and used pesticides frequently, compared to children whose parents were not farm workers with pesticide exposure.

Cancer in Adults

It is a great irony that Rachel Carson died of breast cancer in 1964, two years after the publication of Silent Spring. Her book was a powerful indictment of DDT and similar chlorinated hydrocarbon pesticides. She specifically targeted the ability of this class of pesticides to accumulate and persist in the human body, especially in fatty tissue. She discussed the similarity of these pesticides to estrogens – female hormones.

Carson predicted future cancers if use and exposure continued. She warned against assuming that low-level human and environmental contamination was safe and the risks acceptable, calling pesticides "elixirs of death."

Breast cancer. The biggest risk factor for breast cancer is being female. Forty-six thousand women die of breast cancer every year in the U.S., and about three hundred men. One-hundred eighty-thousand women are newly diagnosed with breast cancer every year, and about one thousand men. The biggest known risk factors for the disease are estrogens, female hormones. There are four major sources of estrogens.

♦ Natural estrogens: the female hormones found in the human body.

♦ Phytoestrogens (FIE-toe-ess-troh-gens): plant estrogens found in nature, especially soybeans and other legumes. "Phyto" is Greek for plant. These estrogens are probably protective, that is, eating them decreases the risk of breast cancer.

♦ Synthetic estrogens - such as DES (diethylstilbestrol), a nonsteroidal chemical with estrogenic activity. In the past, DES was used as a medication to prevent miscarriage, resulting in risk of vaginal cancer and other abnormalities in the progeny. It is currently used in animal husbandry (fattening cattle before slaughter).

♦ Xenoestrogens (ZEE-no-ess-troh-gens): substances that are not normally found in the human body, or in nature, that act like or mimic estrogens. "Xeno" is Greek for foreign or strange. Exposure to these estrogens may increase the risk of breast cancer.

Xenoestrogenic pesticides. Pesticides in current use that are xenoestrogens include: endosulfan (thiodan), lindane, methoxychlor, and dienochlor. All these pesticides were found in over-the-counter products in our surveys. See Appendix C on page 328 for the brand name products containing them.

Banned pesticides that are xenoestrogens include DDT, dieldrin, chlordane (transnonachlor, oxychlordane), heptachlor, and hexachlorobenzene. Pesticides in current use contaminated with them include dicofol (Kelthane®) – contaminated with DDT, and chlorothalonil (Daconil®), Dacthal, and PCNB – contaminated with hexachlorobenzene. All these pesticides were found in over-the-counter products in our surveys. See Appendix C on page328 for the brand name products containing them.

DDT and DDE. Although DDT was banned in the U.S. in 1972, its residues are still in our bodies. DDE is the breakdown product of DDT found in blood, fat, breast milk, and other body tissues in human beings throughout the world. It takes a very long time, several decades, to eliminate DDE from our bodies. Almost all of us living on planet earth today will take residues of DDE, and other chlorinated hydrocarbon pesticides in the DDT family, with us to our graves.

DDE and breast cancer. There are several recent studies suggesting that DDE may be a risk factor for breast cancer. Three of these studies were done in the U.S., one in Finland, and one in Israel.

Connecticut. A study done in Connecticut in 1987, measured the amounts of DDT, DDE, hexachlorobenzene, oxychlordane, transnonachlor and PCBs, in women having a biopsy for a lump in their breast. The purpose of the study was to find out if the twenty women who turned out to have breast cancer, had higher levels of the chemicals in their breast tissue, than the twenty women whose tumors were benign.

Total DDT, DDE, and PCBs were significantly higher in the women with breast cancer. Hexachlorobenzene, oxychlordane, and transnonachlor were also higher in the women with cancer but the difference was not statistically significant. The number of cases is too small to draw any conclusions, and these findings must be confirmed by additional studies on larger populations.

New York. A study done in New York City in 1991, measured the amount of DDE and PCBs in stored blood samples from women with breast cancer. The investigators compared 58 women diagnosed with cancer (after the samples were taken) to 171 women without cancer.

DDE was significantly higher in the breast cancer patients than in the women without cancer. PCBs were also higher in the women with breast cancer, but the difference was not statistically significant. The numbers of cases is small, but the findings are consistent with the Connecticut study for DDE.

San Francisco. A study was done in San Francisco in 1990, of the amount of DDE and PCBs in stored blood samples (collected in the 1960s), from fifty white, fifty black, and fifty Asian women who later developed breast cancer. The women, members of the Kaiser Health Plan, were compared to women who did not develop cancer.

The results were similar to the New York study, for white and black women, but not for Asian women. DDE levels were higher in white and black women with breast cancer, consistent with the Connecticut study and New York study.

The author interpreted the study as showing no evidence of DDE as a risk factor for breast cancer. This is not a correct interpretation of the study. The data show breast cancer risk increases with increasing levels of DDE – in black and white women, consistent with the other studies. Asian women are known to have a lower risk of breast cancer. The author reported on the group analysis only, without a separate analysis of white and black women together.

Finland. A study was done in Helsinki in 1985 and 1986 of environmental chemicals in the breast fat of 48 women with breast cancer, collected at the time of surgery. The chemicals measured were: several polyaromatic hydrocarbons (PAHs), several chlorinated hydrocarbon pesticides, and polychlorinated biphenyls (PCBs).

A significantly higher level of β-HCH, a metabolite of the pesticide hexachlorocyclohexane (lindane), was found in the women with breast cancer. Higher levels of DDE, hexachlorobenzene, and PCBs were also found in the breast cancer cases, but they were not statistically significant from those in the women without breast cancer.

Unfortunately the investigators chose autopsy fat from 38 women who died in accidents as the comparison group, which limits the conclusions that can be drawn.

Israel. Israel is the only country that has ever reported a *decrease* in the number of deaths from breast cancer. Compared to the previous ten years, 8% fewer women died overall between 1976 and 1986. The decreases were only in younger women: 34% fewer deaths in women 25 to 35 years old, 10% fewer in those 45 to 54, and 24% fewer in those 55 to 64. There was an increase in older women: 3% more deaths in women 65 to 74 years old, and 25% more in those 75 and older.

The authors suggest the decrease may be related to the banning of two chlorinated hydrocarbon pesticides, lindane and DDT in 1978. The pesticides were heavily used in dairy farming; very high levels were in milk sold to the Israeli public. DDE levels averaged 177 parts per million (ppm), the lindane metabolites α–HCH and β-HCH averaged 1,019 ppm, and 341 ppm respectively. The average levels in U.S. cow's milk during the same period were: 30 ppm for DDE, 10 ppm for α–HCH, and 20 ppm for β-HCH. By 1980, there was a 98% decrease in the levels of α–HCH, and a 43% decrease in DDE in cow's milk. See Appendix I for an explanation of ppm.

This mortality study, performed ten years after the change in exposure, is what is known as an ecological study. There were no measurements of the actual levels of pesticides in blood or breast tissue of Israeli women with and without breast cancer. There was no investigation of whether the women with and without breast cancer actually drank the milk. No tissue was kept from the women who died; there was no data about other risk factors for breast cancer, or about occupational and other environmental exposures potentially related to breast cancer.

It is an intriguing report, adding useful information about the potential role of pesticides as risk factors for breast-cancer. The lack of exposure data limits the conclusions that can be drawn from this study. However, it is consistent with the previous ones in suggesting a relationship between breast cancer and pesticides.

Endocrine disrupters. Toxic substances that can disrupt hormone action in the body, even though they do not act like estrogens, are called endocrine disrupters. Pesticides that cause breast (mammary) tumors in laboratory animals, but are not xenoestrogens fit into this category. The pesticides found in our survey that cause mammary tumors in animals include the insecticides DDVP, naled and flucythrinate, and the herbicides atrazine, cyanazine, and ethafluralin.

Figure 5.1 lists pesticides found in our surveys that are xenoestrogens and endocrine disrupters. The list includes pesticides contaminated with DDT and hexachlorobenzene which are no longer used as pesticides.in the U.S. See Appendix C on page 328 for the brand name products containing these active ingredient pesticides.

Figure 5.1

Pesticides in Current Use
Xenoestrogens and Endocrine Disrupters
(Based on 1993 to 1995 Surveys)

Insecticides	Herbicides	Fungicides
DDVP (dichlorvos)	Atrazine	Chlorothalonil [2]
Dicofol [1]	Cyanazine	Dacthal [2]
Dienochlor	Ethafluralin	PCNB [2]
Endosulfan	Simazine	
Flucythrinate	Trifluralin	
Lindane		
Methoxychlor		

1=Contaminated with DDT 2=Contaminated with Hexachlorobenzene

---

Ovarian Cancer

In a study done in Italy, women were almost three times more likely to have cancer of the ovary (malignant epithelial type) if they lived in an area of potential exposure to the herbicides atrazine and simazine (in the same chemical family). These herbicides, heavily used on corn, are widespread contaminants of ground water in the area.

About atrazine. Atrazine is an endocrine disrupter which causes breast tumors in laboratory animals. More pounds of this herbicide are used in the U.S. than any other according to EPA estimates (its major use is on corn). Atrazine can persist in soil for several years, and is a groundwater contaminant throughout the Midwestern states.

Atrazine is not sold over-the-counter in California. However, we found it widely available over-the-counter in Florida and Louisiana for use on lawns. Chapters seven and ten discuss atrazine as a home use pesticide.

Occupational Cancer

There are many studies that show an association between pesticide exposure and certain types of cancer in workers occupationally exposed to pesticides. These studies were done in farmers and other agricultural workers, exterminators, landscape maintenance workers, roadside sprayers, and workers in factories where pesticides are manufactured or formulated. These groups have much higher exposures than the average person, which is why they were studied in the first place.

The types of cancer associated with pesticides in these studies include non-hodgkin lymphoma, leukemia, brain cancer, pancreatic cancer, multiple myeloma, stomach cancer, testicular cancer, prostate cancer, lung cancer, and liver cancer.

Effects on the Reproductive System

Many factors affect fertility and the ability to conceive and carry a healthy child to term. Major ones include age, health, genetic, and nutritional status of the parents, their occupation, and their use of alcohol, tobacco, medications, and drugs. We know that viruses, drugs, ionizing radiation, and genetic abnormalities account for about one third of all birth defects; for sixty-five percent of the cases the cause is unknown.

Placental Transfer. Most pesticides readily cross the placenta after they are absorbed into the body. Potential adverse effects of pesticide exposure include birth defects, spontaneous abortion (miscarriage), stillbirth (baby is born dead), sterility and infertility.

Sterility/infertility. DBCP (dibromochloropropane) is the only pesticide *proven* to cause reproductive damage in humans. Men working at a chemical plant in northern California where the soil fumigant was manufactured and formulated were found to be sterile (no sperm at all), or infertile (very low sperm counts), because of their exposure to the pesticide. The levels of exposure did not cause poisoning or any symptoms of health problems, and the men were otherwise healthy.

Drinking Water. A study was done of birth defects in Fresno County, California, where thousands of drinking water wells are contaminated with DBCP. No relationship was found between birth defects and levels of DBCP in the water. The study did not determine the actual DBCP exposure of the women who delivered children with birth defects, compared to women who delivered normal babies. DBCP was banned in the U.S. in 1979, except for pineapple in Hawaii where it was banned in 1985.

A settlement was recently announced that several chemical companies will pay Fresno County $21 million dollars for cleaning up of the city water supply which is still contaminated with DBCP. One-hundred million more is committed in the future. In addition to its effects on sperm, DBCP is also an animal carcinogen.

Occupational exposure. Most human health studies of reproductive effects of pesticides have been done in men and women (mostly men) exposed to pesticides in their work including: cropduster pilots, roadside sprayers, pest control operators, exterminators, agricultural workers, and chemical workers.

The most frequent adverse effects in which the mother was studied include limb reduction defects (missing fingers, toes, hand, feet, arms, legs), and stillbirth (the baby is born dead). It is possible that more birth defects are not found because the pesticide is toxic to the embryo or fetus, which dies early in the pregnancy and is spontaneously aborted. The results of most studies have not found strong effects for most pesticides and the findings have not been consistent.

Accidents and spills. The transportation of pesticides can result in toxic spills such as the railroad tank car derailment near Dunsmir, California in 1991. This spill released about 13,000 gallons of the highly toxic pesticide, metam-sodium, which causes birth defects in animals. Fish and all other life along a fifty mile stretch of river were killed. Metam-sodium is available over-the-counter as Vapam®. Chapter four discusses MITC, the toxic gas emitted by metam-sodium.

EPA requirements. The EPA requires studies in rats and rabbits to find out if pesticides cause birth defects, spontaneous abortion, still birth, infertility, or genetic damage. These tests are supposed to be done *before* a pesticide is marketed. The tables in chapters five through eight show that many pesticides in home use products cause reproductive or genetic damage in laboratory animals. The tables also show that many home use pesticides are on the market without the tests the law requires.

Home use pesticides. There are no studies in humans of reproductive effects of home use pesticides. It can be difficult or impossible to prove that a specific pesticide exposure caused a particular adverse reproductive effect in humans. Many people may not even think about home use pesticides being a health risk at all.

Avoiding exposure. It is very important that you and your partner avoid pesticides and other toxic exposures not only during a pregnancy but prior to conception. There is evidence that toxic exposure of the father and the mother *prior* to conception can affect pregnancy outcome. Because a pesticide causes reproductive or genetic effects in animals, does not mean it will cause similar effects in humans.

Seeing the doctor. If you suspect that pesticide exposure may be affecting your pregnancy, it is very important that you tell your doctor. Make sure to tell him or her the name of the pesticide and the circumstances of the exposure. Insist that your doctor record your concerns on your medical record, even if the doctor is skeptical or feels that your exposure has nothing to do with any problems you might have. If patients report potential problems, and doctors become more aware of them, in time we will obtain better information on the role of pesticide exposure in reproductive problems in humans.

The first trimester. The first three months of pregnancy are when the organ systems are developing in your baby. This is the time of greatest risk for structural defects, for example missing arms and legs or a hole in the heart. Since the nervous system continues to develop throughout pregnancy, pesticides can continue to affect the developing brain and nervous system for all nine months.

Another area of public health concern related to pesticides are the effects on the brain and nervous system in both adults and children.

Effects on the Brain and Nervous system

We know much less about chronic effects of pesticides on the brain and nervous system than about acute effects. Delayed effects can occur from long term low-level exposures that do not cause acute poisoning. Chronic effects can also be signs and symptoms that persist (called sequelae) after an episode of poisoning, often for years.

There are anecdotal reports of behavioral effects such as anxiety, difficulty in concentrating, memory deficits, personality changes and other more subtle effects in the pesticide literature. There are also some early reports of mental illness or severe psychological disturbances in workers who applied pesticides. Follow-up studies done several years later of pesticide poisoning victims, show that neurological sequelae do occur.

Follow-up studies of poisoning victims. One-hundred persons who had been seriously poisoned by pesticides (mostly organophosphates) were investigated an average of nine years later. The poisoning cases were compared to one-hundred nonpoisoned controls similar in age, race, and sex, to find out if there were any differences in the function of their brain and nervous system. The parts of the nervous system tested were muscles (motor), sensations (sensory), balance (cerebellum), mood, memory, personality (neurobehavioral) and cognitive ability (intelligence, reasoning).

Those poisoned in the past (the cases) were significantly different from the nonpoisoned group (the controls). They did worse on tests of memory, mood, and the ability to abstract (reason). They were twice as likely to show scores consistent with brain damage or dysfunction. Their scores on personality tests showed greater distress and complaints of disability.

Another study found that a group severely poisoned by organophosphate pesticides in the past, had persistent nervous system defects in function. These defects were not found in the nonpoisoned comparison group. The poisoned subjects did much worse on tests of the parts of the brain that deal with hearing (auditory attention), vision (visual memory, visual-motor speed), intelligence (problem solving), and tests of brain-muscle coordination (motor steadiness, reaction time, and dexterity).

The percentage of people poisoned by pesticides who develop clinically significant neurological sequelae is not known.

Brain wave studies. The brain has electrical impulses that can be measured by an electroencephalograph (EEG). Such brain wave studies could be an excellent additional source of information on the impact of pesticide exposure on the brain. Unfortunately there are very few epidemiological studies of people occupationally exposed to or poisoned by neurotoxic pesticides that include an EEG. This is not only because of the expense, but also the complexity of interpreting brain wave studies. One study showed that there were some disturbances in rhythm, especially an increase in beta wave activity.

Chronic neurological diseases. There are several studies that implicate pesticide exposure as a risk factor for Parkinson disease (a movement disorder of older people characterized by rigid muscles, tremor, and difficulty walking). This chronic disease, which is expected to increase as the population ages, appears to be increasing in younger age groups.

Parkinson disease. There are studies that implicate pesticides in Parkinson disease. Several reports from Quebec, Canada, found there were more cases in agricultural areas with heavy pesticide use. These studies found more cases of Parkinson disease in younger people in rural areas compared to urban areas.

There are also reports relating pesticide applicators' exposure to the development of Parkinson disease later in life. There is a report of two young agricultural workers with a Parkinson-like illness who had exposure to a magnesium-containing fungicide (maneb). A recent study found that pesticide exposure was more likely to be a risk factor when Parkinson disease is diagnosed at the age of fifty or younger.

Other chronic diseases. There are human studies that suggest environmental toxic exposures may have an impact on other neurological diseases. This includes choreoathetosis (abnormal twisting movements of the head, arms, legs, and other parts of the body), amyotrophic lateral sclerosis (a wasting disease of muscle also known as Lou Gehrig disease), and dementia of both the Alzheimer and non-Alzheimer type. Pesticides have not been well studied in this regard.

Impact of neurotoxic pesticides. The explosion in the use of chemical pesticides is a post World War II phenomenon. Most of the neurotoxic chlorinated hydrocarbon pesticides such as DDT, aldrin, dieldrin, chlordane and heptachlor, which persist in human tissues and the environment, are banned in the U.S. (see chapter 11 for a list of banned pesticides). Residues are still present in our bodies. They are found in blood, fat, breast milk, and other tissues, although the quantities are decreasing over time.

Other pesticides which can damage the nervous system, the nerve gas type organophosphates and carbamates, do not persist in human tissue, and are quickly eliminated by the body into the urine.

Fetal Exposures. Both kinds of pesticides, those that persist and those that do not, can affect the brain and nervous system. Especially vulnerable to toxic insult are the brain and nervous system of the fetus and developing child. Adults living today who were born before the middle 1940s got their first exposures to modern pesticides as adults. Those born between 1946 and 1974, the era of the heaviest and most widespread use of pesticides highly toxic to the brain and nervous system, were first exposed as infants, often while still inside the womb. Pesticide residues are found in umbilical cord blood in newborn infants from all over the world.

Neurodevelopmental effects. You might assume that using over-the-counter pesticides according to label directions will not result in potentially harmful exposures to the fetal and infant brain. This assumption may be unwarranted for three reasons.

♦ The EPA does not require pesticide companies to test home use products for potential neurotoxic effects in the fetus and developing child. As discussed in detail earlier in this book, the fetus and developing child are more susceptible than adults to toxic exposures.

♦ Pesticide label warnings only relate to acute poisoning, not to potential long-term effects.

♦ The label warnings that do exist are not based on scientific studies of what actually happens in the home environments with legal use according to the label. There are almost no data on actual level of pesticide residues, how long they persist, and the potential for absorption of infants and children, whose exposure patterns are very different from adults.

Acute vs. chronic effects. Because you use a pesticide according to label directions and do not notice any immediate illness or other acute effects, does not mean that potential long term effects are not occurring. The fact that most home pesticide use does not cause immediate observable illness may lead to a false sense of security about these toxic exposures.

Low levels of neurotoxic pesticide exposure to the developing brain can potentially affect it in complex and subtle ways, which are difficult to observe and measure. Such potential effects can be on the development of cognitive functions such as memory, judgement, and intelligence, as well as on personality, mood, and behavior.

Animal data. Although there are no pesticide-related neuro-developmental studies of the human fetus and infant, the animal data are very clear. Exposure of the fetus and very young animal to neurotoxic chemicals in amounts that do not cause poisoning can permanently damage the brain and nerve cells. Such exposures can affect brain function in ways that may not cause obvious clinical disease.

Allowing exposures to neurotoxic pesticides based on untested, invalid, and potentially harmful assumptions of safety, is tantamount to using the human fetus and infant as a guinea pig. We have more than enough data on other neurotoxic chemicals to know that we should prevent all avoidable exposures to neurotoxic pesticides in any amount to the most vulnerable among us.

Public Health Implications

Most human exposures to pesticides are from legal, accepted use. This makes the findings of chronic health effects in humans, especially children, of grave public health concern. Pesticides are applied in ways that maximize opportunities for pollution, contamination, drift, and run off.

Once we release these toxins into our environment we cannot take them back. Many will persist in the environment and in biological tissues for many future generations. There is eventual global dispersion of pesticides used anywhere in the world. The result is continuing low-level contamination of the earth and all its living creatures.

Part II. Chronic toxicity of Pesticides
in Laboratory Animals

The EPA essentially ignores chronic toxicity in the regulation of home use pesticides. There are no signal words on the label, as there are for acute effects, to alert the consumer to potential chronic effects of the pesticides they purchase.

If the information we provide you here on the chronic toxicity potential of pesticides in home use products is incomplete, it is because the required animal studies are incomplete, not done, or we were unable to find any information from our sources.

Legal requirements. The federal pesticide law requires that animal studies of chronic toxicity be done before a pesticide is registered by the EPA. These studies are performed by the companies that manufacture the pesticides, who then submit them to the EPA. The EPA then evaluates the studies to determine if the data are complete and meet all legal requirements. If the pesticide is approved by the EPA, it is registered with label and use requirements.

USDA. Most of the pesticides on the market today were first registered in the 1950s and 1960s when the U.S. Department of Agriculture (USDA) was in charge of administering the pesticide law. In her book *Silent Spring,* Rachel Carson aimed her most pointed attacks against the USDA administration of the pesticide law. She was particularly critical of the failure to test pesticides scientifically for potential long-term effects.

EPA. In 1972 responsibility for administration of the pesticide law was transferred from the USDA to the newly created EPA (thank you, Rachel). The EPA is an improvement over the USDA (which in this case is not difficult). However, the state of pesticide regulation continues to be a national joke, or would be if anyone in Washington had a sense of humor on this issue (which we assure you they do not). We leave this topic now, but discuss the deficiencies of chronic toxicity testing, and other regulatory matters at greater length in chapter eleven.

Sources of data. There is no single source available from EPA of the chronic toxicity of all the active ingredients the Agency registers as pesticides in the U.S.. Nor is there a readily available retrieval system to access the data in EPA files. The EPA pesticide registration process is often in a state bordering on anarchy.

California data. There is an excellent source of information on chronic toxicity of pesticides which we rely on heavily in this book. It includes many, but not all, of the pesticides used in home use products found in our survey. This source of information is the continuing evaluation by State of California toxicologists of chronic toxicity studies of pesticides registered for use in the state. California is the only state which has its own pesticide registration program, with additional requirements to those of federal EPA.

Chronic toxicity tables. Our sources of information for the chronic toxicity tables in this book are listed below. Even when using all of them together, we were still left with a large number of pesticides and categories of chronic toxicity for which there are no readily available data.

◆ State of California medical toxicology summaries issued by the California Environmental Protection Agency (Cal-EPA). See Chapter eleven for a discussion of the California law (SB-950, the Birth Defects Prevention Act of 1984) mandating these evaluations.

◆ EPA Fact Sheets: These fact sheets are available for some active ingredient pesticides. They are not always up-to-date but sometimes may be the only information available.

- EPA Position Documents available for some active ingredient pesticides.
- EPA Reregistration Evaluation Documents (REDs), available for some active ingredient pesticides.

From these sources, we let you know whether or not the EPA or the State of California knows or suspects that an active ingredient pesticide causes chronic toxicity in laboratory animals. Remember that these evaluations are based on studies done by the companies that manufacture the pesticides.

To give you the information on chronic toxicity in as orderly a fashion as possible, we list the active ingredient pesticides by their common name in a table for each of the classes and groups of pesticides. We then inform you of the findings for three categories of chronic toxicity as follows:

- **Cancer/tumors.** This category lists the potential for the pesticide to cause tumors in laboratory animals. Tumors can be benign or malignant; another name for a malignant tumor is cancer. An agent that causes tumors is called an oncogen (ONK-oh-gen), and is oncogenic (onk-oh-GEN-ick). An agent that causes cancer is called a carcinogen (car-SIN-oh-gen), and is carcinogenic (CAR-sin-oh-gen-ick). Our ratings include both oncogens and carcinogens.

- **Reproductive damage.** This category lists the potential for the pesticide to cause birth defects, stillbirth, or the equivalent of spontaneous abortion in humans (laboratory rats resorb their fetuses and do not abort them as humans do). An agent that causes structural birth defects is called a teratogen (teh- RAT-oh-gen), and is teratogenic (teh-rat-oh-GEN-ick).

◆ **Genetic damage.** This category lists the potential for the pesticide to cause changes in or damage to genes, chromosomes, and DNA (deoxy-ribonucleic acid, pronounced dee-OXY RYE-bow-new-clay-ick acid). An agent that causes changes in genetic material is called a mutagen (MUTE-ah-gen), and is (mute-ah-GEN-ick). Changes in genetic material are called mutations (mew-TAY-shuns).

There are three possible ratings for each active ingredient pesticide in each chronic toxicity category. These same ratings are used in the pesticide brand name tables in chapters six through ten. The explanation of these ratings is as follows:

◆ An 'x' means that the pesticide is known or is suspected to cause an adverse chronic toxic effect.

◆ A dash '-' means that there are not enough data to determine whether the active ingredient pesticide causes or is suspected to cause an adverse chronic toxic effect. This could be because the studies have not been done, or the studies available were not done properly. Such missing or inadequate data are known as a data gaps. This category also includes pesticides that we could not find any chronic toxicity information for in our sources.

◆ An open dot 'o' means that sufficient data on the active ingredient exists indicating it does not cause an adverse effect. The dot could mean the EPA has waived or does not require data in this category; or that the chemical is on the FDA's (Food and Drug Administration) GRAS list (Generally Regarded As Safe).

Summary of chronic toxicity data. There were 146 active ingredient pesticides found in over-the-counter products in our surveys. We list the chronic toxicity data for them in Appendix G on page 391. Figure 5.2 below summarizes the chronic toxicity findings for these over-the-counter ingredients. The commercial use summary is in chapter ten.

Figure 5.2

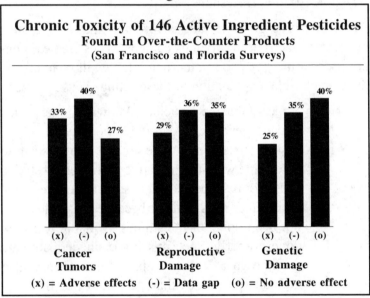

As you can see from Figure 5.1, one-third of the pesticides surveyed are known or suspect animal carcinogens; close to one-third are known or suspect reproductive toxins, and one-fourth are known or suspected to cause genetic damage.

Of great concern is the large percentage of pesticides for which required toxicity data are missing. There are no cancer data for 40% of the pesticides, no reproductive data for 36%, and no genetic data for 35%. These data gaps mean untested or inadequately tested products, and are especially worrisome because of the exposures of children and the fetus.

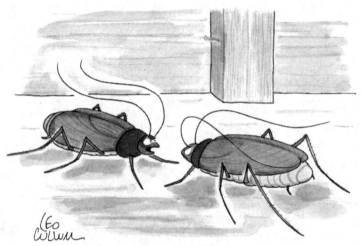

"I got over DDT, and I'll get over you!"

6

Indoor Use Pesticides

If the only tool you have is a hammer, all problems begin to look like nails.

Mark Twain (1835-1910)

If you go to the kitchen for a midnight snack and discover a scurrying cockroach when you turn on the light, or see a line of ants alongside the dish drainer, or just learned your carpet is flea infested; it is no comfort to you to know that 99% of all insects are beneficial or harmless.

The fact that cockroaches and ants inhabited the planet long before humans, and are likely to survive long after we are gone; and that zapping the creatures with the latest in designer poisons doesn't work in the long run, is the furthest thing from your mind.

Enough already, you want them dead, and you want them dead now. In the heat of the moment, you are not interested in long-term solutions to your pest problem. You are not thinking about the health and environmental implications of reaching for that can of designer poison.

What are these products that are so widely available? There is some good news but mostly bad news. This chapter discusses indoor use pesticides in three sections.

- A brief description of the use, formulations, ingredients, and chronic toxicity of active ingredients in indoor use pesticides found in our surveys.
- A general discussion of nontoxic alternatives to chemicals and least toxic chemical control methods for the most common indoor pests -- cockroaches, ants, and fleas.
- Tables listing brand name products with their use, label ingredients, and chronic toxicity summary for the active ingredient. Table 6.1 includes survey data from 1994, and Table 6.2 from 1995. Since the tables are long, we put them at the end of the chapter to make it easier for you to use them.

Termite control is discussed in chapter ten on commercial pest control services, pesticides for use on pets in chapter eight.

Part I: General Survey Findings

In our over-the-counter surveys the majority of indoor use products were insecticides, with a small percentage of insect growth regulators (IGRs). Rodenticides that kill mice and rats accounted for the remainder. Figure 6.1 shows the actual percentages.

Type of formulations. Unfortunately, a large percentage of the products were aerosols and foggers, followed by liquids and sprays. Figure 6.2 shows that almost two thirds of the products were these broadcast sprays, which are the most polluting. Baits, powders, dusts, and granules which are limited to the site of application, were a much smaller percentage. For a discussion of the different types of formulations see chapter two.

Figure 6.1

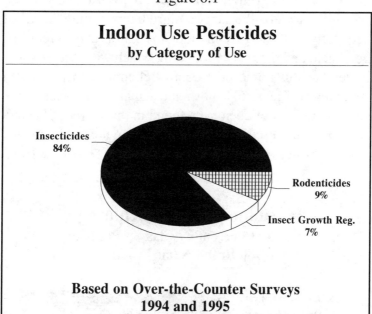

Indoor Use Pesticides
by Category of Use

Insecticides
84%

Rodenticides
9%

Insect Growth Reg.
7%

**Based on Over-the-Counter Surveys
1994 and 1995**

Figure 6.2

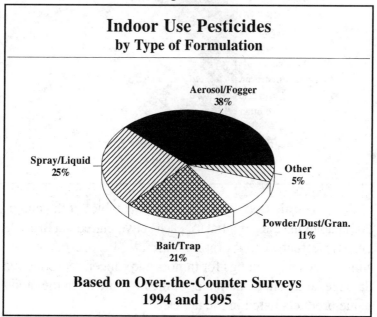

Indoor Use Pesticides
by Type of Formulation

Aerosol/Fogger
38%

Spray/Liquid
25%

Other
5%

Powder/Dust/Gran.
11%

Bait/Trap
21%

**Based on Over-the-Counter Surveys
1994 and 1995**

Active ingredients in pesticide products. Synthetic pyrethroids were the active ingredients found the most frequently, followed by organophosphates, and pyrethrins. Boric acid and diatomaceous earth, which we discuss below as very useful home pest control chemicals, were found infrequently. Figure 6.3 shows the actual percentages of the different classes of chemicals found in the survey. Chapters three and four discuss the health effects of these ingredients.

Figure 6.3

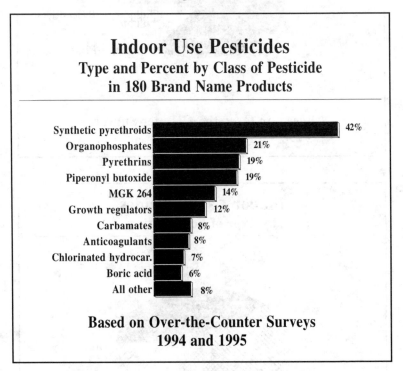

Chronic toxicity summary. The tables at the end of this chapter list the potential for each active ingredient to cause chronic effects in laboratory animals. Figure 6.4 below summarizes the findings for tumors and cancer, reproductive damage, and genetic damage for the ingredients in the brand name products listed in the tables.

Figure 6.4

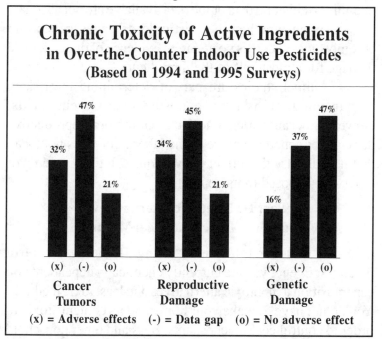

Chronic Toxicity of Active Ingredients
in Over-the-Counter Indoor Use Pesticides
(Based on 1994 and 1995 Surveys)

Cancer
Tumors

Reproductive
Damage

Genetic
Damage

(x) = Adverse effects   (-) = Data gap   (o) = No adverse effect

Figure 6.4 shows that one-third of the active ingredient pesticides are known or suspect to cause tumors or cancer in animals (x). There are data gaps for almost one-half of the pesticides – either no data or inadequate data to determine whether the pesticide causes cancer (-). There is no apparent evidence for tumor formation for only one-fifth of the ingredients (o).

The figure also shows that one-third of the active ingredients are known or suspect to cause reproductive damage (x). There are data gaps for close to half of the pesticides – either no data or the data available is inadequate to determine whether the pesticide causes reproductive damage. There is no apparent evidence of reproductive damage for only one-fifth of the ingredients.

Finally, Figure 6.4 shows that about one-sixth of the active ingredient pesticides are known or suspected to cause genetic damage. There are data gaps for a little more than one-third – either no data or the data available are not adequate to determine whether the pesticide damages genes and chromosomes. There is no apparent evidence of direct genetic damage for almost half of the ingredients.

Animal studies are part of determining the risk to human populations from exposure to toxic chemicals. However, because a chemical causes tumors, reproductive damage, or genetic damage in the laboratory, does not mean that it will cause that effect in everyone using the product or otherwise exposed to its contents.

Part II: Nontoxic alternatives and Least Toxic Chemical Methods

It is never too late to change toxic pest control practices. Even if you are currently chemically dependent you can transition to nontoxic alternatives and least toxic methods. You do not have to make your home and its contents toxic in order to control cockroaches, ants, fleas and other household pests. You can solve your indoor pest problems without using aerosols, bombs or foggers. You can do it without using nerve-gas type of pesticides or synthetic pyrethroids, or other toxic broadcast sprays.

Most indoor pest problems can be solved using the preventive strategies described below, and when necessary, selective use of powders, dusts, and baits that do not give off vapors or leave residues. These formulations can be used in ways that maximize contact with the pest, without posing a threat to humans and pets, and without contaminating your home and its contents.

Natural products. You should not assume that because a product is 'natural' or made from flowers, plants, or roots, that it is nontoxic. Compounds found in nature include toxics such as arsenic, strychnine, and nicotine. Also remember that nontoxic products are often mixed in with more toxic pesticides, synergists, and inert ingredients.

The Jimmy Durante principle. Making the changes needed to prevent household pests from reproducing in large numbers requires changes in human behavior. It is very important to apply the Jimmy Durante principle -- everybody has to get into the act! Everyone in the home needs to understand the importance of depriving the pest of food, water, and other conditions that allow them to continue to reproduce in large numbers. You do not have to be the world's best housekeeper, but you do have to be consistent about certain things. Think of it as brushing and flossing your teeth – a great pay off for a minimal amount of daily effort.

There are two cardinal rules to follow for nontoxic and least toxic pest control:

◆ Don't panic, remember you're bigger than they are.
◆ Be patient, it takes time to get things under control.

Cockroaches. In order to control cockroaches in your home you must think prevention as well as treatment. By using a few simple strategies you can effect long-term control without using toxic sprays. While boric acid is very effective in the control of roaches, it should be used selectively and along with two other important controls.

1. Prevent entry into your home by repairing, caulking, and otherwise sealing points of entry such as cracks and crevices and holes around pipes. Don't forget outside your house where telephone wires and TV cables enter. You should also screen vents and windows.

2. Remove sources of food and water. This means that you should clean up food wastes immediately and don't leave dirty dishes in the sink. Garbage should be taken out daily, and pet food should not be left out. If you feel you must leave your pet's food bowl out then put it in a larger bowl of soapy water to form a moat; this will prevent the roaches from getting

to the food. Remember, roaches can get water from leaky pipes and sink traps.

3. Boric acid powder, bait, gel and paste are excellent treatments when used along with the strategies of preventing entry and reducing access to food and water. Such an approach can result in a happy resolution to your cockroach problem. Boric acid is toxic and should not be used in ways that it can be ingested. Make sure it is applied only in cracks, crevices, and other areas inaccessible to children and pets.

You can use sticky traps placed around the rooms where the cockroaches are to get the numbers down until the boric acid starts to work. The traps also let you know where to concentrate your control efforts, and serve as a monitor of how effective they are. I can assure you that the combined strategy of sticky traps, control of food waste, and boric acid works. Almost every apartment I have ever lived in was cockroach infested and I was able to get rid of them within a month. I never saw another in my apartment, although they were elsewhere in the building. Preventive strategies and boric acid work, you just have to be patient and help it along by not allowing conditions conducive to roach reproduction.

If you feel you must use commercial pest control services please read chapter ten before you make your decision. Don't allow yourself to be talked into using toxic broadcast sprays because it is easier for the exterminator.

Ants. You probably do not want to hear this, but most indoor ants are your friends (except for carpenter ants which are not). Ants prey on other insects, including fleas and subterranean termites, and are great recyclers of decayed organic material and aerators of soil. So while you want to get them out of your kitchen you should limit total warfare against them in the yard. Fire ants and other stinging ants are an exception; they are discussed in the next chapter on outdoor pests.

The measures discussed under cockroaches will also control ants – preventing entry and removing sources of food. You should follow the trail and see where they are coming from and then seal or caulk the entry point (use petroleum jelly (Vaseline™) until you can do it permanently with silicone). Then wipe or spray the area with a soapy solution, or a fifty-fifty mix of vinegar and water. All of these will remove the scent trail and discourage them from returning.

There are ant bait stations for use indoors that contain boric acid or arsenic that you can put in the areas where ants are coming from. These same products are available as ant stakes for use outside. The ants will take the pesticide back to the colony and being the social creatures they are, share it. So be patient and give it time to work. Both of these ingredients are toxic when ingested so make sure you place the baits and stakes where they are not accessible to children and pets.

Fleas. A home with a pet is a home with fleas. The more pets the more fleas since they thrive where there are readily available sources for their blood meals. Flea eggs which drop off the pet after they are hatched can lie dormant for many months. They infest the carpet, tiny crevices in the floor, house dust, pet bedding, and pet sleeping areas. If your pet is allowed outdoors, fleas will be brought in from the outside, and you should treat indoors and outdoors and your pet at the same time. If your pet is confined indoors, it is much easier to control the problem.

Flea control is a matter of reducing their numbers to a tolerable level for your pet, yourself, and other household members. Total eradication is unlikely under most conditions under which pets and humans share the planet. Attempting total eradication may require methods which are toxic to your pet and that can create serious health and contamination problems in your home.

While there is probably a Nobel Prize out there for whoever finds a nontoxic, easy way to control fleas, don't be intimidated. You will be amazed at what you can achieve with soap and water, a flea comb, a vacuum cleaner, diatomaceous earth, and a washing machine. More importantly, you can do it without using toxic sprays. The discussion below concerns strategies for flea control in the home. See chapter eight for a discussion of the pesticides used directly on pets.

The mainstay of household flea control includes preventive strategies as well as direct controls. One of the most important strategies is to treat your home, pet area and bedding, and your pet all at the same time. If your pet is allowed outdoors, include the yard in your plan.

Fleas are very attracted to anything white. An excellent way to get an idea of the severity of the flea infestation is to apply the white sock test. Walk around while wearing knee high socks (not stockings) and if fleas are present they will jump on your socks almost immediately. Laying down a white cloth will have the same effect. This is a good way to find out what parts of your house or yard need more vigorous treatment than others, and also to monitor how you are doing. This is especially useful outdoors if you have a big yard.

The items you need to take on the fleas are all nontoxic: soap and water, a pet grooming comb, diatomaceous earth (*not* the pool filter type), a vacuum cleaner, a washing machine, and time to groom and shampoo your pet. A summary follows:

◆ Thorough and frequent vacuuming (daily if necessary) of both carpeted and non-carpeted areas throughout your house is essential. An initial steam cleaning should be done, which can significantly reduce flea populations.

◆ If you have a carpet you can treat it with diatomaceous earth. The treatment will last for about a year before you have to treat again. See below for how to use it.

♦ Pet bedding should be laundered in hot water regularly, weekly if possible, and more often if necessary. Don't use pet bedding that can't be washed.

♦ Use soapy solutions to clean your pet's sleeping areas, both inside and outside. It is a good idea to confine your pet to a specific area of the house as this will make cleaning and control efforts much easier and more effective.

♦ Shampoo your pet regularly using soap (not detergent).

♦ Spray insecticidal soaps, or soap solutions you prepare yourself (not detergent) in the areas outside in your yard where you find large flea populations.

♦ Groom your pet daily using a flea comb, and drown the fleas you comb out in soapy water. If daily is not possible, groom at least twice a week.

Diatomaceous earth. Do not use the diatomaceous earth sold for use in swimming pool filters. It has been heated in processing and contains free silica which causes lung disease. Buy the agricultural product, available in nurseries. Avoid diatomaceous earth that is formulated with pyrethrins or piperonyl butoxide, since it is effective without these toxic substances.

You should remove the furniture (treat half the room at a time if you can't take it all out) and pour the diatomaceous earth all around the corners of the room, or edge of the rug if it is not a wall to wall carpet. Wear a dust mask when you do this, as you would for any nuisance dust. Then make a big "X" from the middle of the carpet out to the corners. With a broom sweep the diatomaceous earth thoroughly into the carpet. Wait three days and then vacuum thoroughly.

Soaps. It is important to use real soap and not detergent. We are told that Dr. Bronner's Castile Soap is effective, either the bar or the liquid. Safer® insecticidal soaps are true soaps. Remember, though, not to buy a product that has pyrethrins or piperonyl butoxide, since they are toxic and not needed to achieve adequate control. Read the label carefully if you decide to use an insecticidal soap.

About insect growth regulators. Insect growth regulators (IGRs) are a form of birth control for insects. They mimic or interfere with juvenile hormones necessary for normal growth and development. Their major advantage is their selectivity; IGRs target specific insects and spare nontarget beneficial species. Pest control professionals like them very much because they can be used together with a direct killing insecticide to eradicate both adult and larval stages.

IGRs pose much less of a health threat because they attack insect hormones that are not present in human beings. Because of their selectivity and low toxicity, IGRs are known as third generation pesticides. First generation pesticides are the stomach poisons such as arsenic; second generation pesticides are neurotoxins such as the organophosphates and chlorinated hydrocarbons, and synthetic pyrethroids.

However much we approve of the excellent qualities of IGRs, we cannot recommend most of the products available over-the-counter. Methoprene, the IGR found most often in our survey, was in eighteen products. Unfortunately, all of them were broadcast sprays -- eleven foggers and aerosols, and seven sprays or liquid. All of these products contained more toxic active ingredients in addition to methoprene. A synthetic pyrethroid was in thirteen of the eighteen products and pyrethrins in four. As discussed in chapter two on acute health effects, synthetic pyrethroids are toxic to the nervous system, and both the pryrethroids and pyrethrins can cause health problems in people with asthma, allergies, or sensitivity to chemicals.

While methoprene itself has no apparent chronic toxic effects, it can be mixed in with other active and inert ingredients that do. The synergist piperonyl butoxide was in four products, and MKG 264 in three. All of the formulations contained inert ingredients, but because they were not listed on the label we can't tell you what they are.

As much as methoprene seems to be an ideal agent, we cannot recommend it because of the company it keeps, and the way it is formulated. If it were a non-broadcast spray without other toxic ingredients, it would be an excellent choice for least toxic pest control strategies. See Appendix C for the brand name products containing this active ingredient.

Toxic air in your home. We alert you to two types of products found in our survey that work by making the air in your home toxic. We cannot recommend these products under any circumstances. One of the products is the pest strips which contain DDVP (dichlorvos), a nerve-gas type organophosphate insecticide. The pest strip emits toxic vapors for about four months, and has been linked to cancer in children as discussed in chapter four. Paradichlorobenzene, the active ingredient in mothballs, is the second product we do not recommend. Also marketed as a closet air freshener, it continues to emit toxic vapors until the solid is used up. It is also a carcinogen. See Appendix C on page 328 for brand name products containing DDVP and paradichlorobenzene.

Other pests. It is beyond the scope of this book to discuss all of the potential indoor pests you may encounter in your home. Fortunately there is an excellent book that does just that. It is called *Common-Sense Pest Control*, is encyclopedic and highly recommended. Appendix J on page 403 tells you how to obtain it.

Part III: Brand Name Product Listing

As you consider your purchases of pest control products, remember that pesticide residues from broadcast sprays accumulate in house dust which can be a significant source of exposure for infants and toddlers.

About piperonyl butoxide (puh-PAIR-uh-nill bew-TOX-ide): As you will see in the tables, the synergist piperonyl butoxide is an active ingredient in many products containing pyrethrins and synthetic pyrethroids. Piperonyl butoxide is also known by the initials PBO.

The chronic toxicity data in Table 6.1 and Table 6.2 show data gaps for piperonyl butoxide for cancer and birth defects. Two recent reports in the open literature show that piperonyl butoxide causes liver cancer and birth defects in rats. The EPA (Environmental Protection Agency) has not included these findings in assessing piperonyl butoxide. We want you to know this since this ingredient is in so many products. See Appendix C on page 328 for the brand name products that contain it.

About MGK-264. Another widely used synergist is MGK-264, which may be listed on the label by its chemical name -- bicycloheptene dicarboximide. MGK-264, often used in place of, or along with piperonyl butoxide, causes chronic toxic effects as well. You will see in the tables, both synergists can be in the product at a higher percentage than the other active ingredients. All the surveyed brand name products containing MGK-264 are listed in Appendix C on page 328.

About chlorpyrifos (clor-PEER-ah-foss). The nerve-gas type insecticide chlorpyrifos (Dursban®) is one of the most widely used indoor pesticides. We are very concerned about the increasing and widespread use of this nerve-gas type pesticide. Not only is it toxic to the nervous system but it persists longer than other organophosphate pesticides. Unfortunately it is often applied directly to carpets and other home furnishings.

We think you should know that the EPA has fined the manufacturer of this pesticide, DowElanco, almost three quarters of a million dollars, a large fine by EPA standards. The company did not report health problems it knew about to the EPA as the law requires.

We state over and over in this book that it is *not* necessary to use nerve-gas type pesticides to control your home pest control problems. We say it once again. Read the labels and avoid these products. We list all the products in our survey that contain nerve-gas type pesticides (organo-phosphates and carbamates) in Appendix C on page 329.

Listing of brand name products. The products listed in Table 6.1 and Table 6.2 are typical of pesticides marketed for control of common household pests. The listing does not represent all of the indoor use pesticide products available throughout the country.

Table 6.1 includes products from a 1994 survey in the city and county of San Francisco. Table 6.2 includes *additional* products from 1995 surveys in Sarasota, Florida, in Metarie, Louisiana (near New Orleans), and in Colma, California (near San Francisco). An explanation of the abbreviations and other terms used in the tables immediately precedes them.

Key to Brand Name
Product Table

Use

Her = Herbicide   **Mul** = Multiple Uses
IGR = Insect Growth Regulator   **PGR** = Plant Growth Regulator
Fun = Fungicide   **Rep** = Repellent
Mol = Molluscicide   **Rod** = Rodenticide

Formulation

Aer = Aerosol   **Gel** = Gel
Bat = Bait   **Grn** = Granule
Bar = Barrier   **Liq** = Liquid
Bom = Bomb   **Lot** = Lotion
Col = Collar   **Pel** = Pellet
Dus = Dust   **Pow** = Powder
Fer = Fertilizer   **Sld** = Solid
Fog = Fogger   **Spr** = Spray
Fom = Foam   **Stp** = Strip
Fum = Fumigant   **Tap** = Tape
Gas = Gas   **Trp** = Trap
Rep = Repellent   **Tab** = Tablet

Label Word

D = Danger
W = Warning
C = Caution
N = Not required or not on label

Class

CB = Carbamate   **PY** = Pyrethrin
CH = Chlorinated hydrocarbon   **SP** = Synthetic pyrethroid
OP = Organophosphate   **SY** = Synergist

Tumors/Cancer

A tumor is an abnormal growth of tissue that can be benign or malignant. Another name for a malignant tumor is cancer. Substances that cause cancer are called *carcinogens*. Substances that cause tumors are called *oncogens*.

Repro. Damage

Reproductive damage refers to effects such as death of the embryo or fetus (equivalent to spontaneous abortion and stillbirth in humans), low birth weight, sterility/infertility. It also includes birth defects such as structural defects such as missing arms or legs, or hole in the heart, spina bifida etc. Substances that cause birth defects are called *teratogens*.

Genetic Damage

Genetic damage refers to effects on genetic material including genes, chromosomes, and DNA.

(X) = Possible adverse effect

(-) = Either no data available or information available is not sufficient to make a determination

(0) = Adequate data and no adverse effect noted.

* Sources for the above chronic toxicity data are from Cal-EPA SB-950 Toxicology Summaries, U.S.EPA Factsheets, U.S.EPA R.E.Ds (Registration Eligibility Documents), and scientific journals.

Table 6.1
Indoor Use Pesticides - 1994

Brand Name	Use	Formulation	Inert Ingredients
A			
Ace Hardware Dursban Insect Killer	Ins	Liq	93.38%
Ace Hardware Flying Insect Killer II	Ins	Aer	99.60%
Ace Hardware Home Fogger	Ins	Fog	99.45%
Antrol Ant Killer Formula II	Ins	Liq	98.00%
B			
Black Flag Ant And Roach Killer	Ins	Aer	99.50%
Black Flag Ant Control System	Ins	Bat	99.50%
Black Flag Ant Roach Killer Formula B Water Based	Ins	Aer	98.89%
Black Flag Flea Ender Fogger	IGR Ins	Fog	99.43%
Black Flag Flea Ender Fogger I	Ins	Aer	99.12%
Black Flag Flea Ender Spray	IGR Ins	Aer	99.78%
Black Flag Flying Insect Killer I	Ins	Aer	99.30%
Black Flag Insect Spray	Ins	Liq	98.05%
Black Flag Liquid Roach & Ant Killer	Ins	Spr	99.05%
Black Flag Roach Ender Spray	Ins IGR	Aer	99.36%

Label Word	Class	Active Ingredients	Tumors/Cancer	Repro. Damage	Genetic Damage
W	OP	Chlorpyrifos 6.62%	o	o	x
C	SP	Tetramethrin 0.25%	x	x	o
	SP	Phenothrin 0.15%	x	-	o
C	OP	Chlorpyrifos 0.5%	o	o	x
	SP	Allethrin 0.05%	o	o	o
C		Boric acid 2%	-	x	x
C	CB	Propoxur 0.5%	x	o	o
C	OP	Chlorpyrifos 0.5%	o	o	x
C	SP	Pyrethroid 0.28%	-	-	-
	SP	Permethrin 0.24%	x	x	o
	SY	Piperonyl butoxide* 0.59%	-	-	o
W		Methoprene 0.07%	o	o	o
	SP	Permethrin 0.5%	x	x	o
C		Pyrethrins 0.05%	x	x	x
	SY	MGK 264 0.4%	x	x	o
	SP	Permethrin 0.43%	x	x	o
C		Methoprene 0.02%	o	o	o
		Pyrethrins 0.2%	x	x	x
	SY	Piperonyl butoxide* 1%	-	-	o
	SY	MGK 264 1%	x	x	o
C	SP	Tetramethrin 0.4%	x	x	o
	SP	Phenothrin 0.3%	x	-	o
C	CH	Methoxychlor 0.75%	-	x	-
		Lethane 1%	-	-	-
		Oil unspecified 0.2%	-	-	-
C	SP	Allethrin 0.05%	o	o	o
	SY	MGK 264 0.4%	x	x	o
	OP	Chlorpyrifos 0.5%	o	o	x
W	SP	Permethrin 0.25%	x	x	o
		Hydroprene 0.39%	-	-	-

Table 6.1

Indoor Use Pesticides - 1994

Brand Name	Use	Formulation	Inert Ingredients
Black Leaf Ant Killer Powder	Ins	Pow	95.00%
Blue Lustre Flea Killer for Carpets	Ins	Pow	98.90%
C			
Carpet Magic Household Flea & Tick Killer	Ins	Spr	99.30%
Combat Ant & Roach Killer 2	Ins	Aer	99.48%
Combat Ant Control System	IGR	Trp	99.10%
Combat Ant Killing System	IGR	Bat	99.10%
Combat Roach Killing System	IGR	Trp	98.35%
Combat Room Fogger 1	Ins	Aer	99.40%
Combat Superbait Brand Insecticide Patented Action Ant Control	Ins	Bat	99.00%
Combat Superbait Insecticide Patented Action Roach Control	Ins	Trp	98.35%
Cooke Ant Barrier	Ins	Spr	99.19%
D			
d-Con Bait Pellets	Rod	Bat	99.99%
d-Con Mouse-Prufe II	Rod	Bat	99.99%
d-Con Pellets Kills Rats & Mice	Rod	Bat	99.97%
d-Con Ready Mixed Bait Bits	Rod	Bat	99.99%
d-Con d-stroy Roach Killing Station	Ins	Bat	99.50%
Defend Home & Carpet Spray	Ins	Spr	99.00%
Dr. X Roach Killer Dry Spray Formula	Ins	Spr	98.00%

Label Word	Class	Active Ingredients	Tumors/Cancer	Repro. Damage	Genetic Damage
C	OP	Diazinon 5%	o	x	x
C		Pyrethrins 0.1%	x	x	x
	SY	Piperonyl butoxide* 1%	-	-	o
C		Pyrethrins 0.11%	x	x	x
	SY	Piperonyl butoxide* 0.22%	-	-	o
	SY	MGK 264 0.37%	x	x	o
C		Pyrethrins 0.05%	x	x	x
	SY	MGK 264 0.25%	x	x	o
	SP	Permethrin 0.22%	x	x	o
C		Hydramethylnon 0.9%	o	x	o
C		Hydramethylnon 0.9%	o	x	o
C		Hydramethylnon 1.65%	o	x	o
W	SP	Tetramethrin 0.2%	x	x	o
	SP	Permethrin 0.4%	x	x	o
C		Hydramethylnon 1%	o	x	o
C		Hydramethylnon 1.65%	o	x	o
C		Pyrethrins 0.05%	x	x	x
	SY	Piperonyl butoxide* 0.26%	-	-	o
	OP	Chlorpyrifos 0.5%	o	o	x
C		Brodifacoum 0.01%	-	-	-
C		Brodifacoum 0.01%	-	-	-
C		Warfarin 0.03%,	o	x	o
C		Brodifacoum 0.01%	-	-	-
C	OP	Chlorpyrifos 0.5%	o	o	x
C	SP	Permethrin 1%	x	x	o
C	SP	Pyrethroid 2%	-	-	-

Table 6.1

Indoor Use Pesticides - 1994

Brand Name	Use	Formulation	Inert Ingredients
E			
Eatons A-C Formula 90	Rod	Bat	99.99%
Enforcer 7 Month Flea Spray For Homes	Ins	Spr	99.74%
Enforcer Ant Kill Granules	Ins	Grn	95.00%
Enforcer Flea Fogger	Ins	Aer	99.43%
Enforcer Flea Fogger II	Ins	Fog	99.33%
Enforcer Flea Killer For Carpets II	Ins	Pow	99.50%
Enforcer Four Hour Fogger X	Ins	Aer	99.11%
Enforcer Mouse Kill III	Rod	Bat	99.99%
Enforcer Rat & Mouse Bars	Rod	Bat	99.99%
Enforcer Rat & Mouse Bars II	Rod	Bat	99.99%
Enforcer Rat & Mouse Killer	Rod	Bat	99.99%
Enforcer Rat Bait V Kills Rats & Mice	Rod	Bat	99.99%
Enforcer Rat Kill	Rod	Bat	99.99%
Enoz Cedar-Ize Moth Bar	Ins	Sld	00.35%
Enoz Plastic Hang-up Moth Case With Para-Cake	Ins	Sld	00.65%
Excell Moth-Tek Paper Covered Moth Ball Hangers	Ins	Sld	00.50%
G			
Grants Ant Control	Ins	Bat	99.54%
Grants Kills Ants Insect Granules	Ins	Grn	99.50%
Green Thumb Home Insect Fogger	Ins	Aer	99.42%

Label Word	Class	Active Ingredients	Tumors/Cancer	Repro. Damage	Genetic Damage
C		Chlorophacinone 0.01%	-	-	-
C		Methoprene 0.01%	o	o	o
	SP	Permethrin 0.25%	x	x	o
C	OP	Diazinon 5%	o	x	x
C		Methoprene 0.07%	o	o	o
	SP	Permethrin 0.5%	x	x	o
C		Methoprene 0.09%	o	o	o
	SP	Permethrin 0.58%	x	x	o
C	SP	Permethrin 0.5%	x	x	o
C		Pyrethrins 0.05%	x	x	x
	SY	MGK 264 0.4%	x	x	o
	SP	Permethrin 0.44%	x	x	o
C		Bromadiolone 0.01%	-	-	-
C		Brodifacoum 0.01%	-	-	-
C		Brodifacoum 0.01%	-	-	-
C		Chlorophacinone 0.01%	-	-	-
C		Chlorophacinone 0.01%	-	-	-
C		Brodifacoum 0.01%	-	-	-
C	CH	Paradichlorobenzene 99.65%	x	x	o
C	CH	Paradichlorobenzene 99.35%	x	x	o
C	CH	Paradichlorobenzene 99.5%	x	x	o
C		Arsenic trioxide 0.46%	x	x	x
C	OP	Chlorpyrifos 0.5%	o	o	x
C	SP	Tetramethrin 0.2%	x	x	o
	SP	Permethrin 0.38%	x	x	o

Table 6.1

Indoor Use Pesticides - 1994

Brand Name	Use	Formulation	Inert Ingredients
H			
Holiday Bug Bomb I	Ins	Aer	99.11%
Holiday Indoor Fogger	Ins	Fog	97.95%
Holiday Roach Control System	Ins	Bat	99.50%
Holiday Tick And Flea Killer	Ins	Aer	99.30%
Hot Shot Flea & Tick Killer	Ins	Aer	98.49%
Hot Shot Flying Insect Killer Formula 411	Ins	Aer	99.60%
Hot Shot Fogger 3	Ins	Fog	99.40%
Hot Shot Mouse & Rat Killer	Rod	Bat	99.97%
Hot Shot Roach & Ant Killer 4	Ins	Aer	99.70%
Hot Shot Roach & Ant Killer 5	Ins	Aer	99.45%
I			
Insectigone Ant Killer	Ins	Pow	15.00%
Insectigone Crawling Insect Killer	Ins	Pow	15.00%
Insectigone Earwig Killer	Ins	Pow	15.00%
Insectigone Roach and Ant Killer	Ins	Pow	15.00%

Label Word	Class	Active Ingredients	Tumors/Cancer	Repro. Damage	Genetic Damage
C		Pyrethrins 0.05%	x	x	x
	SY	MGK 264 0.4%	x	x	o
	SP	Permethrin 0.44%	x	x	o
C	CB	Propoxur 1%	x	o	o
	OP	Dichlorvos 0.5%	x	o	x
		Pyrethrins 0.05%	x	x	x
	SY	Piperonyl butoxide* 0.25%	-	-	o
	SY	MGK 264 0.25%	x	x	o
C	OP	Chlorpyrifos 0.5%	o	o	x
C	SP	Tetramethrin 0.4%	x	x	o
	SP	Phenothrin 0.3%	x	-	o
C	SP	Allethrin 0.16%	o	o	o
	SP	Pyrethroid 0.1%	-	-	-
	SY	MGK 264 1.25%	x	x	o
C	SP	Tetramethrin 0.25%	x	x	o
	SP	Pyrethroid 0.15%	-	-	-
C	SP	Tetramethrin 0.2%	x	x	o
	SP	Permethrin 0.4%	x	x	o
C		Warfarin 0.03%	o	x	o
C	OP	Chlorpyrifos 0.25%	o	o	x
	SP	Allethrin 0.05%	o	o	o
C	OP	Chlorpyrifos 0.5%	o	o	x
	SP	Allethrin 0.05%	o	o	o
C		Diatomaceous earth 85%	o	o	o
C		Diatomaceous earth 85%	o	o	o
C		Diatomaceous earth 85%	o	o	o
C		Diatomaceous earth 85%	o	o	o

Table 6.1
Indoor Use Pesticides - 1994

Brand Name	Use	Formulation	Inert Ingredients
L			
Lilly Miller Ant Killer Plus	Ins	Pow	99.00%
M			
Maki Rat & Mouse Bait Packs (pellets)	Rod	Pel	99.99%
N			
Nu-MRK Nu-Method Ant & Roach Killer Made by Professionals	Ins	Aer	99.45%
O			
Ortho Ant Killer Bait	Ins	Bat	99.75%
Ortho Ant-Stop Ant Killer Spray	Ins	Aer	99.60%
Ortho Flea-B-Gon Flea Killer Formula II	Ins	Aer	99.85%
Ortho Flying & Crawling Insect Killer Formula	Ins	Aer	99.48%
Ortho Household Insect Killer Formula II	Ins	Aer	99.60%
Ortho Total Flea Control	Ins	Fog	99.42%
Ortho-Klor Ant Killer Dust	Ins	Dus	99.00%
P			
Pest Strip	Ins	Stp	80.00%
Pic Ant Trap	Ins	Trp	91.00%
Pic Boric Acid Roach Killer III	Ins	Pow	1.00%
Power House Ant & Roach Killer	Ins	Aer	99.50%
R			
Raid Ant & Roach Home Insect Killer Formula II	Ins	Liq	99.50%

Label Word	Class	Active Ingredients	Tumors/Cancer	Repro. Damage	Genetic Damage
C	CB	Bendiocarb 1%	-	x	x
C		Bromadialone 0.01%	-	-	-
C	OP	Chlorpyrifos 0.5%	o	o	x
	SP	Resmethrin 0.05%	x	x	o
C	CB	Propoxur 0.25%	x	o	o
C	SP	Tetramethrin 0.2%	x	x	o
	SP	Phenothrin 0.2%	x	-	o
W	SP	Tetramethrin 0.05%	x	x	o
	SP	Phenothrin 0.1%	x	-	o
C	SP	Allethrin 0.32%	o	o	o
	SP	Phenothrin 0.2%	x	o	o
C	SP	Tetramethrin 0.25%	x	x	o
	SP	Phenothrin 0.15%	x	-	o
C	SP	Methoprene 0.08%	o	o	o
	SP	Permethrin 0.5%	x	x	o
C	OP	Chlorpyrifos 1%	o	o	x
C	OP	Dichlorvos 20%	x	o	x
C		Boric acid 9%	-	x	x
C		Boric acid 99%	-	x	x
C	OP	Chlorpyrifos. 0.5%	o	o	x
C	OP	Chlorpyrifos 0.5%	o	o	x

Table 6.1

Indoor Use Pesticides - 1994

Brand Name	Use	Formulation	Inert Ingredients
Raid Ant & Roach Killer 6	Ins	Aer	99.10%
Raid Ant Baits	Ins	Bat	99.97%
Raid Flea Killer	Ins	Aer	97.82%
Raid Flea Killer Plus Egg Stop Formula	Ins IGR	Aer	97.78%
Raid Flying Insect Killer Formula 5	Ins	Aer	99.21%
Raid Fumigator Fumigating Fogger	Ins	Fog	87.40%
Raid Indoor Fogger II	Ins	Fog	96.33%
Raid Liquid Roach & Ant Killer Formula I	Ins	Spr	99.27%
Raid Max Ant Bait	Ins	Bat	99.50%
Raid Max Fogger	Ins	Fog	97.82%
Raid Max Roach & Ant Killer	Ins	Aer	97.85%

Label Word	Class	Active Ingredients	Tumors/Cancer	Repro. Damage	Genetic Damage
C	SP	Permethrin 0.2%	x	x	o
		Pyrethrins 0.2%	x	x	x
	SY	Piperonyl butoxide* 0.5%	-	-	o
C	OP	Chlorpyrifos 0.03%	o	o	x
C		Pyrethrins 0.14%	x	x	x
	SY	Piperonyl butoxide* 1%	-	-	o
	SP	Tetramethrin 0.06%	x	x	o
	SY	MGK 264 0.98%	x	x	o
C	SP	Pyrethrins 0.14%	x	x	x
	SP	Tetramethrin 0.06%	x	x	o
	SY	Piperonyl butoxide* 1%	-	-	o
	SY	MGK 264 1%	x	x	o
		Methoprene 0.01%	o	o	o
C	SP	Allethrin 0.15%	o	o	o
	SP	Pyrethroid 0.14%	-	-	-
	SY	Piperonyl butoxide* 0.5%	-	-	o
W	SP	Permethrin 12.6%	x	x	o
C	SP	Tetramethrin 0.54%	x	x	o
	SP	Permethrin 0.41%	x	x	o
		Pyrethrins 0.05%	x	x	x
	SY	Piperonyl butoxide* 1%	-	-	o
	SY	MGK 264 1.67%	x	x	o
C	OP	Chlorpyrifos 0.25%	o	o	x
		Pyrethrins 0.08%	x	x	x
	SY	Piperonyl butoxide* 0.4%	-	-	o
C		Sulfluramid 0.5%	-	-	-
C	SP	Cyfluthrin 0.1%	-	-	o
	SY	MGK 264 1%	x	x	o
	SY	Piperonyl butoxide* 1%	-	-	o
		Pyrethrins 0.08%	x	x	x
C	SP	Cyfluthrin 0.1%	-	-	o
	CB	Propoxur 1%	x	o	o
	SY	Piperonyl butoxide* 1%	-	-	o
		Pyrethrins 0.05%	x	x	x

Table 6.1

Indoor Use Pesticides - 1994

Brand Name	Use	Formulation	Inert Ingredients
Raid Max Roach Bait	Ins	Bat	99.00%
Raid Multibug Killer Formula D-39	Ins	Spr	99.60%
Raid Roach Baits	Ins	Bat	99.50%
Rid-A-Bug Flea & Tick Killer Brand TF5	Ins	Liq	99.50%
Ringer Crawling Insect Attack	Ins	Spr	99.56%
Ringer Flea & Tick Attack Contains Pyrethrum	Ins	Liq	99.34%
roach prufe	Ins	Pow	1.00%
S Safer Flea & Tick Attack Premise Spray Ready-To-Use	Ins	Spr	98.99%
Sergeants Indoor Fogger	Ins	Aer	99.28%
Sergeants Rug Patrol Carpet Insecticide and Freshener	Ins	Pow	97.89%
Spectracide Indoor Fogger 2	Ins	Aer	99.40%
Starbar 1% Indoor Concentrate	IGR	Liq	99.00%
T TAT Ant Trap	Ins	Trp	99.75%
TAT Roach Killer VI	Ins	Bat	98.00%
Term-Out	Ins	Spr	99.72%
Terro Ant Killer II	Ins	Bat	94.60%
Thrifty Ant & Roach Killer	Ins	Aer	99.65%
Thrifty Flying Insect Killer	Ins	Aer	99.60%

Label Word	Class	Active Ingredients	Tumors/Cancer	Repro. Damage	Genetic Damage
C		Sulfluramid 1%	-	-	-
C	SP	Allethrin 0.3%	o	o	o
	SP	Resmethrin 0.1%	x	x	o
C	OP	Chlorpyrifos 0.5%	o	o	x
C	OP	Chlorpyrifos 0.5%	o	o	x
C		Pyrethrins 0.04%	x	x	x
	SY	Piperonyl butoxide* 0.4%	-	-	o
C		Pyrethrins 0.06%	x	x	x
	SY	Piperonyl butoxide* 0.6%	-	-	o
C		Boric acid 99%	-	x	x
C		Pyrethrins 0.01%	x	x	x
		Potassium salts of fatty acids 1%	o	o	o
C	SP	Fenvalerate 0.4%	x	x	o
	SY	MGK 264 0.17%	x	x	o
	SY	Piperonyl butoxide* 0.1%	-	-	o
		Pyrethrins 0.05%	x	x	x
C	SP	Phenothrin 0.48%	x	-	o
	SY	Piperonyl butoxide* 1.63%	-	-	o
C	SP	Tetramethrin 0.2%	x	x	o
	SP	Permethrin 0.4%	x	-	o
C		Methoprene 1%	o	o	o
C	CB	Propoxur 0.25%	x	o	o
C	CB	Propoxur 2%	x	o	o
C	SP	Resmethrin 0.28%	x	x	o
C		Boric acid 5.4%	-	x	x
C	SP	Resmethrin 0.2%	x	x	o
	SP	Allethrin 0.15%	o	o	o
C	SP	Tetramethrin 0.2%	x	x	o

Table 6.1
Indoor Use Pesticides - 1994

Brand Name	Use	Formulation	Inert Ingredients
Timed Release 120 Day Flea Halt! House & Carpet Spray	Ins	Spr	99.50%
V			
Victor Liquid Ant Killing System	Ins	Liq	95.00%
Victory Carpet & Household Spray with Dursban	Ins	Aer	99.45%
Victory Carpet Powder Flea & Tick Killer	Ins	Pow	97.80%
Victory Household Flea and Tick Killer	Ins	Spr	99.50%
Victory Veterinary Formula Indoor Fogger with Dusrban	Ins	Fog	99.45%
W			
Walgreens Ant & Roach Killer Contains Dursban	Ins	Aer	99.18%
Walgreens Roach & Flea Fogger	Ins	Fog	99.11%
Walgreens Roach Control System	Ins	Trp	98.00%
Warf With Diphacinone	Rod	Bat	99.99%
X			
X-O-Trol Flea & Tick Fogger	IGR Ins	Fog	98.29%
X-O-Trol Flea & Tick Household Spray	IGR Ins	Spr	98.89%

Label Word	Class	Active Ingredients	Tumors/Cancer	Repro. Damage	Genetic Damage
C	OP	Chlorpyrifos 0.5%	o	o	x
C		Boric acid 5%	-	x	x
C	OP	Chlorpyrifos. 0.5%	o	o	x
	SP	Allethrin 0.05%	o	o	o
C		Pyrethrins. 0.2%	x	x	x
	SY	Piperonyl butoxide* 2%	-	-	o
C	OP	Chlorpyrifos 0.5%	o	o	x
C	OP	Chlorpyrifos 0.5%	o	o	x
	SP	Allethrin 0.05%	o	o	o
C	OP	Chlorpyrifos 0.5%	o	o	x
	SP	Allethrin 0.05%	o	o	o
	SY	Piperonyl butoxide* 0.1%	-	-	o
	SY	MGK 264 0.17%	x	x	o
C	SP	Permethrin 0.44%	x	x	o
		Pyrethrins 0.05%	x	x	x
	SY	MGK 264 0.4%	-	x	o
C	CB	Propoxur 2%	x	o	o
C		Diphacinone 0.01%	-	-	o
C		Fenoxycarb 0.66%	o	o	o
	SP	Permethrin 0.5%	x	x	o
		Pyrethrins 0.05%	x	x	x
	SY	Piperonyl butoxide* 0.5%	-	-	o
C		Fenoxycarb 0.06%	o	o	o
	SP	Permethrin 0.5%	x	x	o
		Pyrethrins 0.05%	x	x	x
	SY	Piperonyl butoxide* 0.5%	-	-	o

Table 6.1
Indoor Use Pesticides - 1994

Brand Name	Use	Formulation	Inert Ingredients
Z			
Zap-A-Roach	Ins	Pow	0.00%
Zodiac Fleatrol Carpet Spray	IGR Ins	Aer	97.78%
Zodiac Fleatrol Flea Spray	IGR Ins	Spr	98.61%
Zodiac Fleatrol Fogger	IGR Ins	Fog	99.42%
Zodiac Fleatrol Fogger (Kills Larvae)	IGR Ins	Fog	99.33%
Zodiac Fleatrol Indoor Spray	IGR Ins	Spr	99.74%
Zodiac Fleatrol Premise Spray	IGR Ins	Aer	99.42%
Zodiac House & Kennel Fogger	Ins	Fog	99.50%
Zodiac Super Tick & Fly Spray	Ins	Spr	96.10%

Label Word	Class	Active Ingredients	Tumors/Cancer	Repro. Damage	Genetic Damage
C		Boric acid 100%	-	x	x
C		Methoprene 0.02%	o	o	o
		Pyrethrins 0.2%	x	x	x
	SY	Piperonyl butoxide* 1%	-	-	o
	SY	MGK 264 1%	x	x	o
C		Methoprene 0.25%	o	o	o
		Pyrethrins 0.18%	x	x	x
	SY	Piperonyl butoxide* 0.36%	-	-	o
	SY	MGK 264 0.6%	x	x	o
C		Methoprene 0.08%	o	o	o
	SP	Permethrin 0.5%	x	x	o
C		Methoprene 0.09%	o	o	o
	SP	Permethrin 0.58%	x	x	o
C		Methoprene 0.01%	o	o	o
	SP	Permethrin 0.25%	x	x	o
C		Methoprene 0.08%	o	o	o
	SP	Permethrin 0.5%	x	x	o
W	SP	Permethrin 0.5%	x	x	o
W	SP	Permethrin 0.2%	x	x	o
		Pyrethrins 0.2%	x	x	x
	SY	Piperonyl butoxide* 0.5%	-	-	o
	SY	MGK 264 2%	x	x	o
		Di-n-propyl isocinchomeronate 1%	-	-	-

* Piperonyl butoxide causes cancer and birth
defects in rats (see pages 114-115).

Table 6.2
Indoor Use Pesticides - 1995

Brand Name	Use	Formulation	Inert Ingredients
A			
Alter Flea Control	IGR Ins	Spr	99.743%
B			
Baygon	Ins	Liq	85.3%
Bengal Indoor Flea and Tick Killer	Ins	Aer	99.341%
Bengal Indoor Fogger	Ins	Aer	98%
Bengal Roach and Ant Spray	Ins	Aer	98%
Bugs Beware	Ins	Liq	90%
C			
Combat Roach Killing System 1	Ins	Bai	99%
D			
Demize E.C.	Ins	Liq	23%
Dexol Ant Killer Dust II	Ins	Dus	99%
Dexol Home Pest Control Concentrate	Ins	Liq	93.3%
Dexol Termite Killer	Ins	Liq	87.4%
Drax Ant Kil Gel	Ins	Gel	95%

Label Word	Class	Active Ingredients	Tumors/Cancer	Repro. Damage	Genetic Damage
C		Methoprene 0.007%	o	o	o
	SP	Permethrin 0.25%	x	x	o
D	CB	Propoxur 14.7%	x	x	o
C	SP	Pyrethrins 0.025%	x	x	x
	SY	Piperonyl butoxide* 0.05%	-	-	o
	SY	MGK 264 0.084%	x	x	o
	OP	Chlorpyrifos 0.5%	o	o	x
C	SP	Phenothrin 0.1%	x	-	o
	SY	Piperonyl butoxide* 0.4%	-	-	o
C	SP	Phenothrin 1.5%	x	-	o
	PY	Pyrethroid 0.1%	-	-	-
	SY	Piperonyl butoxide* 0.4%	-	x	x
C	OP	Chlorpyrifos 10%	o	o	x
C		Hydramethylnon 1.%	o	x	o
D		Linalool 37%	o	o	o
	SY	Piperonyl butoxide* 40.%	-	-	o
C	OP	Chlorpyrifos 15%	o	o	x
C	OP	Chlorpyrifos 6.7%	o	o	x
W	OP	Chlorpyrifos 12.6%	o	o	x
C	OP	Orthoboric acid 5%	-	x	x

Table 6.2
Indoor Use Pesticides - 1995

Brand Name	Use	Formulation	Inert Ingredients
E			
Echols Roach Tablet 40% Boric Acid	Ins	Tab	60%
Enforcer 7 Month Flea Spray for Homes	IGR Ins	Spr	99.73%
Enforcer Flea Fogger with Vigren	IGR Ins	Aer	99.33%
Enforcer Flea Kill for Carpets II	Ins	Gra	99.5%
Enforcer Home Pest Control XI	Ins	Spr	99.8%
Enforcer FGR (Flea Growth Regulator) Concentrate	Ins	Liq	99%
Enforcer Rat Kill II with Bitrex	Rod	Bai	97%
F			
Ficam Plus+	Ins	Dus	59.83%
Ficam W	Ins	Pow	24%
Flee Insecticide	Ins	Liq	63.2%
G			
Green Charm Indoor Insect Fogger	Ins	Fog	99.875%
Green Light Home Pest & Carpet Dust	Ins	Dus	99%
H			
Hi-Yield Roach Blaster	Ins	Aer	97.993%
Home Pest Control Concentrate	Ins	Liq	94%
Hot Shot Indoor Flea Fogger	Ins	Fog	99.1%
Hot Shot Rid-a-Bug	Ins	Liq	99.99%
Hot Shot Rid-a-Bug Flea and Tick Killer	Ins	Liq	99.75%

Label Word	Class	Active Ingredients	Tumors/Cancer	Repro. Damage	Genetic Damage
C		Boric acid 40%	-	x	x
C		Methoprene 0.007%	o	o	o
	SP	Permethrin 0.25%	x	x	o
C		Methoprene 0.09%	o	o	o
	SP	Permethrin 0.58%	x	x	o
C	PY	Pyrethroid 0.5%	-	-	-
C	OP	Chlorpyrifos 0.2%	o	o	x
C	PY	Pyrethrins 0.1%	x	x	x
		Piperonyl butoxide* 1%	-	-	o
C		Soap 3%	o	o	o
W	CB	Bendiocarb 29.45%	-	x	x
	PY	Pyrethrins 3.06%	x	x	x
	SY	Piperonyl butoxide* 7.66%	-	-	o
W	CB	Bendiocarb 76%	-	x	x
C	SP	Permethrin 36.8%	x	x	o
C	PY	Pyrethrins 0.05%	x	x	x
	SY	MGK 264 0.04%	x	x	o
	SP	Permethrin 0.435%	x	x	o
C	CB	Bendiocarb 1%	-	x	x
C	PY	Pyrethroid 2.007%	-	-	-
C	OP	Chlorpyrifos 6%	o	o	x
C	SP	Tralomethrin 0.09%	-	-	-
C	SP	Tralomethrin 0.01%	-	-	-
C	SP	Tralomethrin 0.025%	-	-	-

Table 6.2

Indoor Use Pesticides - 1995

Brand Name	Use	Formulation	Inert Ingredients
Hot Shot Roach & Ant Killer	Ins	Aer	99.45%
Hot Shot Roach and Ant Killer 2	Ins	Aer	98.94%
Hot Shot Roach and Ant Killer 2 Unscented	Ins	Aer	98.94%
Hot Shot Sudden Death Brand Mouse Killer	Rod	Bai	99.99%
Hot Shot Sudden Death Mouse Killer	Rod	Bai	99.99%
Hot Spot Roach Preventer with Boric Acid	Ins	Dus	1%
I			
Invader - Residual Insecticide with Baygon	Ins	Spr	99%
K			
KGro Ant Flea and Tick Control	Ins	Gra	99.5%
KGro Home Pest Insect Control 2	Ins	Spr	98.8%
KGro Insect Fogger	Ins	Fog	99.284%
N			
Natural Pyrethrin Concentrate	Ins	Liq	89.44%
O			
Organic Plus Household Insecticide	Ins	Dus	8.7%

Label Word	Class	Active Ingredients	Tumors/Cancer	Repro. Damage	Genetic Damage
C	OP	Chlorpyrifos 0.5%	o	o	x
	SP	Allethrin 0.05%	o	o	o
C	SP	Tralomethrin 0.01%	-	-	-
	SP	Allethrin 0.05%	o	o	o
	SY	MGK 264 1%	x	x	o
C	SP	Tralomethrin 0.01%	-	-	-
	SP	Allethrin 0.05%	o	o	o
	SY	MGK 264 1%	x	x	o
C		Bromethalin 0.01%	-	-	-
C		Bromethalin 0.01%	-	-	-
C		Orthoboric acid 99%	-	x	x
C	CB	Propoxur 1%	x	o	o
C	OP	Chlorpyrifos 0.5%	o	o	x
C	OP	Chlorpyrifos 0.2%	o	o	x
C	PY	Pyrethroid 0.4%	-	-	-
	SY	MGK 264 0.16%	x	x	o
	SY	Piperonyl butoxide* 0.1%	-	-	o
	PY	Pyrethrins 0.05%	x	x	x
C	PY	Pyrethrins 0.96%	x	x	x
	SY	Piperonyl butoxide* 9.6%	-	-	o
C		Diatomaceous earth 90%	o	o	o
	PY	Pyrethrins 0.2%	x	x	x
	SY	Piperonyl butoxide* 1.1%	-	-	o

Table 6.2
Indoor Use Pesticides - 1995

Brand Name	Use	Formulation	Inert Ingredients
Ortho Total Flea Control	IGR Ins	Aer	99.3%
Ortho Total Flea Killer Spray with Vigren	IGR Ins	Aer	99.785%
Ortho Total Flea Killer with Vigren	IGR Ins	Liq	99.743%
P Pennington Roach and Ant Killer with Dursban	Ins	Aer	99.341%
Protexall Ant Kill	Ins	Pow	94%
Protexall Screen Pruf	Ins	Liq	0%
R Raid Max Fogger II Penetrating Micro Mist	Ins	Fog	98.4%
Raid Max Plus Egg Stoppers	Ins	Bai	9%
Raid Max Plus Roach Bait IV	Ins	Bai	99.472%
Raid Max Roach and Ant Killer	Ins	Aer	97.8%
S Super DE - Not a Plant Food Product	Ins	Dus	0%
T Term Out Kills Termites Roaches Ants	Ins	Aer	99.75%

Label Word	Class	Active Ingredients	Tumors/Cancer	Repro. Damage	Genetic Damage
C		Methoprene 0.09%	o	o	o
	SP	Permethrin 0.58%	x	x	o
C		Methoprene 0.15%	o	o	o
	PY	Pyrethrins 0.2%	x	x	x
	SY	Piperonyl butoxide* 1%	-	-	o
C		Methoprene 0.007%	o	o	o
	SP	Permethrin 0.25%	x	x	o
C	PY	Pyrethrins 0.025%	x	x	x
	SY	Piperonyl butoxide* 0.05%	-	-	o
	SY	MGK 264 0.084%	x	x	o
	OP	Chlorpyrifos 0.57%	o	o	x
C		Orthoboric acid 6%	-	x	x
C		Mineral oils 97%	-	-	-
		Methoxychlor 3%	-	x	-
C	PY	Pyrethrins 0.5%	x	x	x
	SP	Cyfluthrin 0.1%	-	-	o
	SY	Piperonyl butoxide* 1%	-	-	o
C		Hydroprene 91%	-	-	-
C	OP	Chlorpyrifos 0.528%	o	o	x
C	SP	Cyfluthrin 0.1%	-	-	o
	CB	Propoxur 1%	x	o	o
	SY	Piperonyl butoxide* 1%	-	-	o
	PY	Pyrethrins 0.05%	x	x	x
		Diatomaceous earth 100%	o	o	o
C	SP	Resmethrin 0.25%	x	x	o

Table 6.2
Indoor Use Pesticides - 1995

Brand Name	Use	Formulation	Inert Ingredients
W			
Whitmire Knox-Out PT 1500 R	Ins	Aer	99.5%
Whitmire X-Clude PT1600A Timed Release Insecticide	Ins	Aer	97.16%

Label Word	Class	Active Ingredients	Tumors/Cancer	Repro. Damage	Genetic Damage
C	OP	Diazinon 0.5%	o	x	x
C	PY	Pyrethrins 0.3%	x	x	x
	SY	Piperonyl butoxide* 2.2%	-	-	o
	SY	MGK 264 0.33%	x	x	o

* Piperonyl butoxide causes cancer and birth
defects in rats (see pages 114-115).

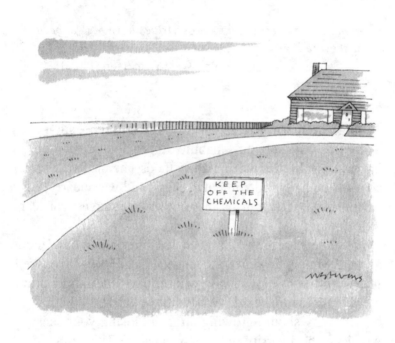

Drawing by M. Stevens; ©1992, The New Yorker Magazine, Inc.
Reprinted with permission.

7

Outdoor Use Pesticides

What is a weed? A plant whose virtues have not yet been discovered.

Ralph Waldo Emerson (1803-1882)

A homeowner wrote a letter to a newspaper question-and-answer column about his inability to get rid of dandelions in his yard. He detailed the myriad methods, chemicals, and other controls he had tried without success, and was clearly at his wit's end. The columnist's answer was "we suggest you learn to love them."

There are those of us who, as children, saw dandelions as pretty yellow flowers that changed into seeds with whiskers that were fun to blow away; whose leaves tasted good in a salad that grandma made. What did we know.

Why should growing up mean losing your sense of wonder at the diversity and variety of nature. Think of yourself as a sustainer and protector of your green patch of the planet, not a toxic avenger. As you devise ways to rid your lawn and yard of insects and weeds, remember there are old fashioned ways that are tried, true, and nontoxic. You can have a lush lawn and productive garden without using toxic pesticides and chemical fertilizers. There are ways to rid your lawn and yard of dandelions and other pests by methods that do not pose a threat to health, wildlife, and the environment.

This chapter follows the same basic pattern as chapter six on indoor pest control. We give you some information on the types of products that are widely available, and discuss outdoor use pesticides in three sections:

◆ A brief description of the use, formulations, ingredients, and chronic toxicity of active ingredients in outdoor use pesticides found in our surveys.

◆ A general discussion of nontoxic alternatives to chemicals and least toxic chemical control methods for lawn and yard care, including fire ants, fleas, and dandelions. A discussion of garden pests is beyond the scope of this book.

◆ Tables listing brand name products with their use, label ingredients, and chronic toxicity summary for the active ingredients. Table 7.1 includes survey data from 1994, and Table 7.2 from 1995. Since the tables are long, we put them at the end of the chapter to make it easier for you to use them.

Part I: General Survey Findings

There is a greater variety of pesticides used outdoors than indoors. Figure 7.1 shows that more than half of the outdoor use products were insecticides, about one-fourth were herbicides, fungicides accounted for one-tenth, and the rest were products for controlling snails (molluscicides), vertebrates (rodenticides), and repelling birds and animals.

Type of formulations. Figure 7.2 shows that over half of the outdoor products were liquids and sprays, with granules and dusts accounting for just over one-third. Aerosols and baits made up a small percentage. Granules and pellets in general pose less hazard to humans if applied directly from the package. They can be very hazardous to birds that mistake them for seeds. For a discussion of the different types of formulations see chapter two.

Table 7.1

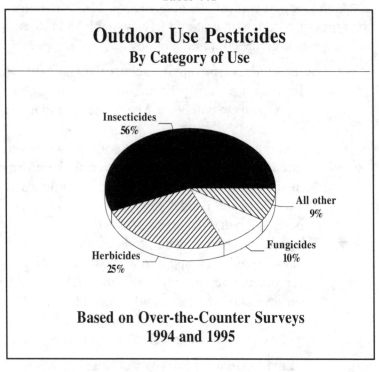

Outdoor Use Pesticides
By Category of Use

Insecticides 56%

All other 9%

Fungicides 10%

Herbicides 25%

**Based on Over-the-Counter Surveys
1994 and 1995**

Active ingredients in pesticide products. Organo-phosphate insecticides were found the most frequently, primarily chlorpyrifos, diazinon, malathion, and acephate. All of the phenoxy herbicide products contained 2,4-D with some combination of MCPA, MCPP, and dicamba. Of the seventeen different non-phenoxy herbicides, there were more products containing glyphosate (Roundup®) than any other. Most of the carbamates contained carbaryl or propoxur. The most frequently found synthetic pyrethroids were permethrin and resmethrin. All products with synergists contained piperonyl butoxide, with or without MGK 264. Only one product contained MGK 264 as the only synergist.

Table 7.2

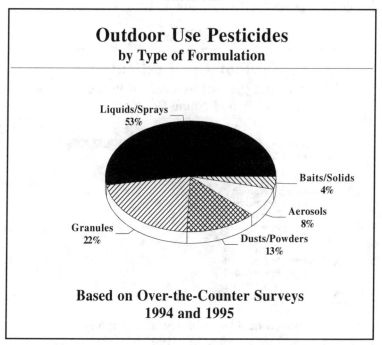

Outdoor Use Pesticides
by Type of Formulation

Liquids/Sprays
53%

Baits/Solids
4%

Aerosols
8%

Granules
22%

Dusts/Powders
13%

**Based on Over-the-Counter Surveys
1994 and 1995**

Figure 7.3 shows the actual percentages of the different classes of chemicals found in the survey. Chapters four and five discuss the acute and chronic health effects of these active ingredients.

Chronic toxicity summary. The tables at the end of this chapter list the potential for each active ingredient to cause chronic effects in laboratory animals. Figure 7.4 below summarizes the potential for ingredients in brand name products listed in the tables to cause cancer, reproductive damage and genetic damage.

As Figure 7.4 shows, almost 40% of the active ingredient pesticides are known or suspect to cause cancer or tumors in animals (x). There are data gaps for a little more than one-third of the pesticides – either no data or the available data is inadequate to determine whether the pesticide causes cancer (-). There is no apparent evidence for tumor formation for just over one-fourth of the ingredients (o).

Figure 7.3

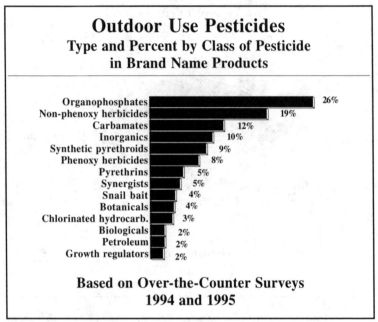

As Figure 7.4 shows, almost 40% of the active ingredient pesticides are known or suspected to cause cancer or tumors in animals (x). There are data gaps for more than one-third of the pesticides – either no data or the data available is inadequate to determine whether the pesticide causes reproductive damage. There is no apparent evidence of reproductive damage for a slightly more than one-third of the ingredients.

Finally, Figure 7.4 shows that more than one-fourth of the active ingredient pesticides are known or suspect to cause genetic damage. There are data gaps for almost one-third of the pesticides – either no data or the data available is inadequate to determine whether the pesticide causes genetic damage. There is no apparent evidence of damage for slightly less than half of the ingredients.

Figure 7.4

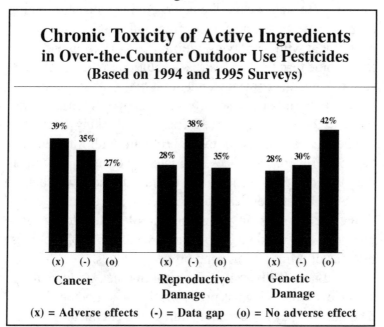

Chronic Toxicity of Active Ingredients
in Over-the-Counter Outdoor Use Pesticides
(Based on 1994 and 1995 Surveys)

Animal studies are part of determining the risk to human populations from exposure to toxic chemicals. However, because a chemical causes tumors, reproductive damage, or genetic damage in the laboratory, does not mean that it will cause that effect in those using the product or otherwise exposed to its contents.

Part II: Nontoxic alternatives and Least Toxic Chemical Methods

It is never too late to change toxic pest control practices. Your personal patch of planet earth does not have to be toxic to control insects, weeds, and plant diseases in your lawn and garden. You can solve your outdoor pest control problems without using nerve-gas types of pesticides (organophosphates and carbamates), synthetic pyrethroids, toxic herbicides, chemical fertilizers, and other harmful broadcast sprays.

Efforts to create the perfect lawn can be similar to the travails of the teen years. Teenagers coping with acne, raging hormones, self esteem, and other real and imagined problems, experiment with hair styles, tattoos, skin piercing, and other fads. Some turn to chemicals as a solution to their problems, and may even become dependent on them.

In the urban and suburban lawn, minor weed and insect problems become major crises. There is unthinking acceptance of chemical solutions for every problem, with little thought to long-term consequences. The latest in designer poisons is readily accepted and widely disseminated. Those who balk at using the latest chemical fad may be subject to gentle or not so gentle persuasion, or even ridicule. Not doing what everyone else is doing can result in accusations of that most heinous of crimes – lowering property values.

Lack of diversity. The resulting lack of diversity, in which everyone's lawn is pretty much like everyone else's, is a bonanza to pesticide manufacturers and chemical lawn care companies. Their marketing and advertising not only depends on such conformity, but encourages it.

A bonanza for pests. The lack of diversity is also a bonanza for pests. Variety and diversity are the essentials of a balanced ecosystem, which is wrecked by toxic pesticides. Most widely used outdoor pesticides kill not only the target pest, but also nontarget beneficial insects, soil organisms, and predators that keep the pests under control. Pests that were never a problem because they were being kept under control by their natural enemies, can become major pests themselves.

A threat to wildlife. Many outdoor pesticides are toxic to birds, bees, fish, and other wildlife. Pesticides can persist in the soil, get washed into storm sewers, and contaminate streams, lakes, rivers and other bodies of water.

The pesticide treadmill. Over time any semblance of a natural system is gone, and your chemical lawn and garden requires continuing inputs of toxic chemicals, often in increasing amounts. You end up on a pesticide treadmill. The more chemicals you use the more you have to use. The more you have to use the more you degrade and toxify the soil. The more you degrade and toxify the soil, the worse your pest problems become.

You can get your lawn off chemicals. How long it takes to get to a healthy and environmentally friendly lawn depends on three major factors.

(1). How toxic and exhausted the soil is from past chemical inputs and stresses.

(2). How committed and willing you are to change your thinking and your behavior.

(3). Whether you take the gradualist or kamikaze approach.

A healthy lawn in which pests are kept under control is one with healthy soil and a deep root system, with a proper balance of nutrients, including water.

Basis of a healthy lawn: There are some basic principles that must be observed as you begin your transition to a more natural lawn.

◆ Select a grass or grass mixtures that are native to your area, or that adapt well to local conditions.

◆ Do not overwater as it prevents deep root systems from developing. Daily watering encourages shallow roots.

◆ Do not cut the grass too closely since this prevents deep root systems from developing. Close mowing encourages shallow roots that are less healthy.

◆ Avoid chemical fertilizers. While they green up the lawn quickly, it is at the expense of good root development. Shallow roots mean more pest and disease problems.

- ◆ Keep the soil well aerated, and avoid compaction.
- ◆ Don't fertilize just because the neighbors are doing it; or because you are paying a lawn company on a contract basis and want to get your money's worth.
- ◆ Use organic fertilizers and increase organic matter to green up a lawn without stressing it.
- ◆ Add clover to your lawn. This past common practice is now out of favor. Mixed lawns that contain clover supply nitrogen, since clover roots can turn nitrogen in the air into a nutritional form that plants can use.
- ◆ Leave grass clippings on the lawn after mowing.
- ◆ Monitor for early signs of a potential pest problem, and take early preventive nontoxic action first.
- ◆ Use pesticides only when absolutely necessary, and only as a temporary management tool. Use only those that are least toxic, most selective, and consistent with an organic approach. The key to success is partnership with nature, not toxic domination.

Use the two cardinal rules of outdoor pest control.

- ◆ Don't panic, chemical detoxification is harder on you than on your lawn.
- ◆ Be patient, it takes time to get back in tune with nature.

How to get off the pesticide treadmill. Don't be shy about asking for help. Neighbors or friends who manage their lawns and yards using natural and organic methods are usually very willing to share their knowledge and experiences. Some of the most enthusiastic were once lawn chemical junkies themselves. They can be great hand holders during the detoxification process.

Retail outlets. If there is a *true* organic farm and garden or nursery retail outlet near your home you are in luck. Owners and proprietors of these stores are usually enthusiastic organic gardeners or farmers themselves, and usually have staff that are also knowledgeable.

Unfortunately, most stores sell predominately conventional poisons. If there is enough of a demand they will carry more organic products. Do the nose test – if the odor knocks you out when you approach the pesticide shelves the store is a long way from being organic. Do not expect sales people in stores that sell conventional pesticides (especially the large discount stores) to know much more than "what kills what". They are there to sell products, not save the planet.

Sustainability. Once you establish a chemical free lawn, it will take care of itself and require much less time, effort, and money. The grass will be slower growing, and therefore will need less mowing and watering because it has deeper roots. The lawn will be healthier because its roots are deep into nontoxic, healthy soil. It will be better able to withstand all sorts of stresses, including pests and diseases. When pest problems do arise, you can handle them in ways that are environmentally friendly, without using toxic pesticides.

Books and other resources. *Rodale's Chemical-free Yard and Garden;* and *Common Sense Pest Control* (already referred to in chapter six) are excellent sources. Other publications and resources are listed in Appendix J on page 403. You will be well served by anything from Rodale Press which has a long and stellar commitment to organic gardening.

Professional lawn care companies. You may not have the time or the inclination to "do it yourself". If you hire someone to care for your lawn or yard, make sure they are knowledgeable about nontoxic lawn and yard care. There are very few companies that manage lawns in a safe and natural way. See chapter ten for cautions and recommendations on professional lawn care services.

It is beyond the scope of this book to discuss all potential outdoor pests. We focus on lawn care and selected lawn pests, and then only in a general and brief overview. We do not address pests such as gophers and snails. Please refer to the publications recommended in Appendix J for detailed information on outdoor pest control. The discussion is in three sections: insects, weeds, and plant diseases.

Fire ants. Being severely bitten by fire ants is not an experience you forget. This pest of southern and southwestern lawns, can be a serious health threat. Many toxic chemicals have been used over the years in attempts to eradicate the fire ant, without success. You can eradicate them on your lawn without using toxic chemicals according to our experts – southern women.

During a recent visit to Florida and Louisiana, I heard about nontoxic methods for destroying fire ants, from women who had reasons for not wanting to use toxic chemicals, even minimally toxic ones, on their lawns. They had children and pets, or were chemically sensitive, or were dedicated environmentalists who wanted to do their bit for human and planetary health. Their recommendations follow.

◆ **Drowning them.** This requires hot water (most recommend that it be boiling). The biggest mistakes people make are not using enough water, or not repeating the treatment if it doesn't work the first time. If you use enough water and make sure you really flood the mound, supposedly, it works every time.

◆ **Setting them against each other.** For this method to work you have to have more than one fire ant mound on your lawn. This is not difficult. You shovel some earth from the first mound and put it on the second mound. Then you shovel some earth from the second mound and put it on the first mound. The ants destroy each others' colonies.

◆ **Overfeeding them.** This method is for those who do not like boiling water because of the scalding hazard. It involves covering the mound with dry potato flakes (directly from the carton). Here is a description of what happens: "they eat the flakes and it swells up inside their stomachs and causes them to explode which kills them." Sounds good to me.

We would like to know if you have tried any of the above methods, and whether they worked for you. We would also like to know of other nontoxic methods you may know about to share with our readers in future editions.

There is a granular product for fire ants containing the insect growth regulator, fenoxycarb. It does not kill the adult but affects the immature ones (makes them sterile). It takes time to work until there are no more ants that can reproduce. Although fenoxycarb is not highly toxic, why use it if nontoxic methods work.

Fleas. We discussed control of indoor fleas in chapter six. You may wish to look at this if you have not read it yet. Control of fleas on pets is discussed in chapter eight.

You do not have to (and should not) treat your entire lawn and yard to control fleas that your pets are bringing indoors. Use the white sock test or the white cloth test described in chapter six to find out where the flea infestation is worst and treat only that area. Use a soap solution (not detergent) to spray the infested area. You can also try diatomaceous earth. Remember these products also kill the good bugs so use them sparingly and only in the infested areas.

We just learned that lindane is being used on lawns for flea control by chemical lawn companies in Florida. This is appalling news. We oppose the use of lindane in any amount, and it should have been banned years ago with the other DDT family of pesticides. See the index for the many references to lindane in this book. See chapter ten for cautions and recommendations on professional lawn care services.

Chinch bugs. People with lawns know from chinch bugs. They smell bad and turn the lawn yellow in little round patches, and are a pest all over the country. The good news is that they are generally not a problem in a properly maintained and irrigated lawn that is not under nutritional and toxic stress. By watching for them, especially when the weather is hot and dry, you can take early corrective action, such as increasing soil moisture, which will usually prevent an outbreak. Insecticidal soaps are also an effective control. You can make your own by mixing two tablespoons liquid soap (not detergent) in a gallon of water.

Chemical lawn treatments only make the problem worse, and may be responsible for outbreaks. The insecticide chlorpyrifos (Dursban®) kills the natural enemy of the chinch bug – the big eyed bug. There is also a natural fungus in moist soil that is an enemy of the chinch bug; it secretes a toxin that kills it. Herbicides, including atrazine, kill this beneficial fungus. Another common cause of a chinch bug infestation is using too much chemical fertilizer. Certain types of grass, including St. Augustine grass, are more likely to have chinch bug problems than others. Other natural predators of chinch bugs are lacewings, lady bugs, and birds.

Mole crickets and grubs. Mole crickets tunnel under the lawn and attack grass roots causing irregular streaks of brown on the lawn. Parasitic nematodes are an effective biological control for this pest. White grubs, larvae of Japanese and other beetles, cause irregular dead patches on your lawn that turn brown. Applying milky spore disease is effective, but it may take a few seasons to eliminate them, so be patient. There are other biological controls, including B.T., beneficial nematodes, lady bugs, and other natural predators that help keep pest populations under control. Refer to the resources already mentioned for more information; use of these controls is very specific for your area.

Weed control. Keeping your lawn healthy by proper watering, feeding, and aeration can improve growing conditions for weeds as well. The goal is to keep them from taking over. Weed control is the most difficult area to transition from chemical controls to organic methods. It takes more time, commitment, and patience. There are no short cuts and quick fixes. But once you get the upper hand, as you will, the payoff is enormous – environmental sanity and a health break for all the living creatures formerly in range of the spray nozzle.

Weed seeds. They can't run away or hide, but weeds have ingenious methods of survival. They can produce hundreds of thousands of seeds, and soil contains millions of them. *Rodale's Chemical-Free Yard and Garden* cites a statistic from England of six million weed seeds from three different kinds of weeds in the top few inches of soil. If growth conditions are not right, weed seeds can lay dormant in the soil for years before germinating again. You may win an occasional battle but you cannot win the war of the weeds. Total eradication is neither possible, nor desirable. Rodale's states "... you can no more rid soil of weed seeds than sweep the sand off the beach".

Even if you maintain an organic lawn, weed seeds can blow onto it from another lawn that has been allowed to go to seed. Or weed seeds can be brought in on hay mulch, or manure, or compost.

Problems with herbicides. Herbicides are the pesticides most likely to cause a false sense of security in those who use or are otherwise exposed to them. Because many of them do not cause immediate and obvious harm, they are considered safe. As already discussed in previous chapters, there are concerns about chronic toxicity for many of the active ingredients in these products. Of the forty-seven active ingredient herbicides found in our survey, 48% are known or suspect to cause tumors or cancer, 28% caused reproductive damage, and 34% caused genetic damage. There were no data (data gaps) for about 40% of the active ingredient herbicides; we don't know what their potential is to cause tumors, and other chronic toxicity. Remember that in some of the childhood cancer studies mentioned in chapter five, if the parents used pesticides outdoors, the risk of cancer in their children was even higher than for indoor use.

The herbicide that is used in the largest amounts and is the most widely sold for outdoor home use is glyphosate (Roundup®). This pesticide contains a toxic inert ingredient, the surfactant, polyoxyethyleneamine (POEA); it also causes tumors in animals. Atrazine, another herbicide found in our survey, is widely used on lawns in the southwest where it is a groundwater and drinking water contaminant in some areas. Atrazine is also an animal carcinogen.

Herbicides are also toxic to species other than weeds, including microbes and other soil organisms that maintain ecological balance. Herbicides can destroy beneficial fungi that keep lawn and turf pests under control. Chemical herbicides have no place in an environmentally friendly and healthy yard, lawn or garden.

Orgranic herbicides. There are some organically acceptable herbicides, including soaps (potassium salts of fatty acids), some under the Safer® label. Read the labels carefully however since many of the original Safer® products are being reformulated with the toxic ingredient, piperonyl butoxide. Soap also kills other vegetation so make sure you target only the pesky weed. Organic pesticides do not cause the moon landscape created by the killing power of glyphosate, and other chemical herbicides. Vinegar and salt also kill weeds, but like the soaps will kill desirable vegetation as well. Vinegar is especially good for paved areas where weeds are breaking through, and you are not concerned about its killing surrounding vegetation.

Old fashioned ways. Confine your aggression to physical methods such as hoeing, hand pulling, and using weed whackers. Make sure you pull weeds before they set seed. As you expand your horizons beyond poisons, you may be more willing to consider replacing a weed intolerant lawn with grasses that grow more vigorously and compete better with weeds in your area . Who knows, you may even consider cover crops that out compete the weeds, or mulches, and other methods that reduce water loss and smother weeds.

About those dandelions. Dandelions go away when the roots go away. Even if you do not get the whole root the first time, if you continue to attempt to remove it, it will eventually die. Be patient, it will probably take more than one season. It really works.

Plant diseases. A healthy nontoxic lawn that is properly watered, mowed, aerated and fed is unlikely to have any serious disease problems. If you have problems with brown patch, dollar spot fungus, pythium blight or diseases, chemicals are not the answer. Find out what is making the lawn susceptible to disease. For both plant diseases and weed problems, seek assistance from organic nursery owners and local organic lawn management companies. They and cooperative extension agents can be very helpful in identifying the pest or diagnosing your particular problem. Many extension agents are devoted to conventional chemical use, so might not be as helpful in recommending nontoxic and organic solutions. Newspaper garden editors committed to natural and organic methods can be very helpful.

Part III: Brand Name Product Listing

Remember that pesticide residues from products used outdoors can be tracked into the house. The residues accumulate in house dust and can be a significant source of exposure, especially for infants and toddlers.

The following discussion is very similar to that in chapter six on indoor use. We repeat some of the information here because you might not have read that section yet.

About piperonyl butoxide (puh-PAIR-uh-nill bew-TOX-ide): As you will see in the tables, the synergist piperonyl butoxide is an active ingredient in many products containing pyrethrins and synthetic pyrethroids.

The chronic toxicity data in Table 7.1 and Table 7.2 show that there are missing data (data gaps) for piperonyl butoxide for cancer and birth defects. Two recent reports in the open literature show that piperonyl butoxide causes liver cancer and birth defects in rats. These findings are not part of the Environmental Protection Agency (EPA) assessment of piperonyl butoxide, but the agency is planning a review. This raises concerns about the potential health risks of exposure to the many products containing this ingredient. It also shows the potential risk in using products for which there are missing data. Appendix C on page 328 lists the brand name products from our surveys that contain piperonyl butoxide.

About MGK 264: Another widely used synergist is MGK 264. It may be listed on the label by its chemical name N-octylbicycloheptene dicarboximide. MGK 264, which is often used in place of, or along with piperonyl butoxide, is known or suspect to cause tumors and reproductive damage in chronic toxicity studies. As you will see in the tables, piperonyl butoxide and MGK 264 can be in products in greater amounts than other active ingredients. Brand name products containing MGK 264 are listed in Appendix C on page 328.

About chlorpyrifos (clor-PEER-ah-foss): The nerve-gas type insecticide, chlorpyrifos (Dursban®), found in many outdoor use pesticides, is the most widely used insecticide in our surveys. We are very concerned about the increasing and widespread use of this organophosphate pesticide. It persists longer in the environment and in the human body than other organophosphates.

There are also concerns about potential long-term effects on the nervous system. DowElanco chemical company, the basic producer of chlorpyrifos, knew of reports of nervous system damage to users of the pesticide, but failed to report them to the EPA as the law requires. The EPA recently fined DowElanco over $700,000, a large fine by EPA standards.

We list all the brand name products in our survey that contain chlorpyrifos and other nerve-gas type pesticides (organophosphates and carbamates) in Appendix C on page 328.

Part III: Tables Listing Brand Name Products

The products listed in Tables 7.1 and 7.2 are typical of pesticides marketed for control of common outdoor pests. The listing does not represent all of the outdoor pesticide products available throughout the country.

Table 7.1 includes products from a 1994 survey in the city and county of San Francisco. Table 7.2 includes additional products from 1995 surveys in Sarasota, Florida, in Metarie, Louisiana (near New Orleans), and in Colma, California (near San Francisco). An explanation of the abbreviations and other terms used in the tables immediately precedes them.

Key to Brand Name
Product Table

Use

Her = Herbicide
IGR = Insect Growth Regulator
Fun = Fungicide
Mol = Molluscicide

Mul = Multiple Uses
PGR = Plant Growth Regulator
Rep = Repellent
Rod = Rodenticide

Formulation

Aer = Aerosol
Bat = Bait
Bar = Barrier
Bom = Bomb
Col = Collar
Dus = Dust
Fer = Fertilizer
Fog = Fogger
Fom = Foam
Fum = Fumigant
Gas = Gas
Rep = Repellent

Gel = Gel
Grn = Granule
Liq = Liquid
Lot = Lotion
Pel = Pellet
Pow = Powder
Sld = Solid
Spr = Spray
Stp = Strip
Tap = Tape
Trp = Trap
Tab = Tablet

Label Word

D = Danger
W = Warning
C = Caution
N = Not required or not on label

Class

CB = Methyl carbamate
CH = Chlorinated hydrocarbon
OP = Organophosphate

PY = Pyrethrin
SP = Synthetic pyrethroid
SY = Synergist

Tumors/Cancer

A tumor is an abnormal growth of tissue that can be benign or malignant. Another name for a malignant tumor is cancer. Substances that cause cancer are called *carcinogens*. Substances that cause tumors are called *oncogens*.

Repro. Damage

Reproductive damage refers to effects such as death of the embryo or fetus (equivalent to spontaneous abortion and stillbirth in humans), low birth weight, sterility/infertility. It also includes birth defects such as structural defects such as missing arms or legs, or hole in the heart, spina bifida etc. Substances that cause birth defects are called *teratogens*.

Genetic Damage

Genetic damage refers to effects on genetic material including genes, chromosomes, and DNA.

(X) = Possible adverse effect

(-) = Either no data available or information available is not sufficient to make a determination

(0) = Adequate data and no adverse effect noted.

* Sources for the above chronic toxicity data are from Cal-EPA SB-950 Toxicology Summaries, U.S.EPA Factsheets, U.S.EPA R.E.Ds (Registration Eligibility Documents), and scientific journals.

Table 7.1
Outdoor Use Pesticides - 1994

Brand Name	Use	Formulation	Inert Ingredients
A			
Ace Hardware Crab Grass Killer	Her	Liq	83.40%
Ace Hardware Diazinon Spray	Ins	Liq	75.00%
Ace Hardware House & Garden Bug Killer II	Ins	Aer	99.60%
Ace Hardware Malathion 50 Multi-Purpose Insecticide	Ins	Liq	50.00%
Ace Hardware Sevin Liquid Spray	Ins	Liq	78.70%
Ace Hardware Spot Weed Killer	Her	Spr	99.45%
Ace Hardware Wasp & Hornet Killer	Ins	Aer	99.75%
B			
Bird Tanglefoot	Rep	Liq	3.00%
Black Flag House & Garden Insect Killer Fresh Scent	Ins	Aer	98.90%
Black Flag Wasp-Bee-Hornet Killer	Ins	Spr	99.50%
Black Leaf Cygon 2E Soil Drench Systemic Insecticide	Ins	Liq	76.60%
Black Leaf Eptam Weed Control	Her	Grn	97.70%
Black Leaf Home Pest Insect Killer	Ins	Liq	99.50%
Black Leaf Pruning & Tree Wound Dressing	Her	Aer	72.00%
Bug-Geta Liquid Slug & Snail Killer	Mol	Liq	96.00%
Bug-Geta Plus Snail Slug & Insect Granules	Ins Mol	Grn	93.00%
Bug-Geta Slug & Snail Pellets	Mol	Grn	96.75%
Buzz Off	Rep	Sld	

Label Word	Class	Active Ingredients	Tumors/Cancer	Repro. Damage	Genetic Damage
C		MSMA 16.6%	-	-	-
W	OP	Diazinon 25%	o	x	x
C	SP	Tetramethrin 0.2%	x	x	o
	SP	Pyrethroid 0.2%	-	-	-
C	OP	Malathion 50%	x	o	o
C	CB	Carbaryl 21.3%	x	o	x
C		2,4-D 0.26%	x	x	x
		Dicamba 0.03%	-	x	x
		MCPP 0.26%	-	x	x
C	OP	Chlorpyrifos 0.25%	o	o	x
C		Polybutene 97%	-	-	-
W	SP	Resmethrin 0.1%	x	x	o
		Pyrethrins 0.2%	x	x	x
	SY	Piperonyl butoxide* 0.8%	-	-	o
C	CB	Propoxur 0.5%	x	o	o
W	OP	Dimethoate 23.4%	o	x	x
C	CB	EPTC 2.3%	o	x	x
C	OP	Chlorpyrifos 0.5%	o	o	x
D		Asphalt solids 28%	-	-	-
C		Metaldehyde 4%	x	o	o
C	CB	Carbaryl 5%	x	o	x
		Metaldehyde 2%	x	o	o
C		Metaldehyde 3.25%	x	o	o
		Citronella scent	o	o	o

Table 7.1
Outdoor Use Pesticides - 1994

Brand Name	Use	Formulation	Inert Ingredients
C			
Chacon Animal Repellent	Rep	Grn	75.50%
Chacon Malathion Spray	Ins	Liq	50.00%
Chacon Repel Dog & Cat Repellent	Rep	Grn	75.50%
Coles Whitefly Mealybug Spray	IGR Ins	Liq	99.77%
Cooke Copper Fungicide	Fun	Dus	10.00%
Cooke Devrinol 2-G	Her	Grn	98.00%
Cooke Daconil	Fun	Liq	87.50%
Cooke Diazinon Insect Granules	Ins	Grn	95.00%
Cooke Diazinon Spray	Ins	Liq	83.25%
Cooke Dursban-Plus Lawn Insecticide	Ins	Liq	93.21%
Cooke Earwig Sowbug & Grasshopper Bait	Ins	Bat	95.00%
Cooke Fast Kill Weed & Grass Killer	Her	Liq	98.16%
Cooke Fungicide	Fun	Dus	50.00%
Cooke Garden Insect Spray Containing Thiodan	Ins	Liq	90.85%
Cooke Kop-R-Spray	Fun	Liq	92.00%
Cooke Malathion (50%) Garden Spray	Ins	Liq	50.00%
Cooke Quick Action Gopher Mix	Rod	Bat	99.50%
Cooke Ready-to-Use Spurge Oxalis & Dandelion	Her	Spr	99.06%
Cooke Rootone	PGR Rep	Pow	95.66%

Label Word	Class	Active Ingredients	Tumors/Cancer	Repro. Damage	Genetic Damage
C	CH	Paradichlorobenzene 20%	x	x	o
		Alkyl pyridines 2%	-	-	-
		Ziram 0.5%	x	x	-
		Thiram 2%	x	x	o
C	OP	Malathion 50%	x	o	o
C	CH	Paradichlorobenzene 20%	x	x	o
		Alkyl pyridines 2%	-	-	-
		Ziram 0.5%	x	x	-
		Thiram 2%	x	x	o
C		Methoprene 0.1%	o	o	o
	CH	Dienochlor 0.08%	-	-	-
	SP	Resmethrin 0.05%	x	x	o
W		Copper sulfate (basic) 90%	-	-	-
C		Napropamide 2%	x	o	x
W		Chlorothalonil 12.5%	x	o	x
C	OP	Diazinon 5%	o	x	x
W	OP	Diazinon 16.75%	o	x	x
W	OP	Chlorpyrifos 6.79%	o	o	x
C	CB	Carbaryl 5%	x	o	x
C		Diquat 1.84%	x	x	x
C	CH	PCNB 50%	x	o	x
W	CH	Endosulfan 9.15%	-	o	o
C		Copper metallic 8%	-	-	-
C	OP	Malathion 50%	x	o	o
D		Strychnine 0.5%	-	-	-
C		2,4-D 0.59%	x	x	x
		MCPP 0.28%	-	x	x
		Dicamba 0.07%	-	x	x
C		Naphthaleneacetamide 0.2%	-	-	-
		IBA 0.1%	o	o	o
		Thiram 4.04%	x	x	o

Table 7.1
Outdoor Use Pesticides - 1994

Brand Name	Use	Formulation	Inert Ingredients
Cooke Rootone Brand Rooting Hormone	PGR	Pow	95.76%
Cooke Rose & Flower Dust	Ins	Dus	60.00%
Cooke Sevin Brand (5%) Carbaryl Insecticide Dust	Ins	Dus	95.00%
Cooke Sevin Liquid Carbaryl Insecticide	Ins	Liq	77.50%
Cooke Slug-N-Snail Granules	Ins Mol	Grn	92.00%
Cooke Slug-N-Snail Spray	Mol	Liq	89.50%
Cooke Spurge Oxalis & Dandelion Killer	Her	Liq	85.01%
Cooke Sulfur Dust (wettable)	Fun	Dus	10.00%
Cooke Summer & Dormant Oil	Ins	Liq	1.00%
Cooke Tomato & Vegetable Dust	Ins	Dus	60.00%
Cooke Tomato-Plus	Her	Spr	99.99%
Corrys Liquid Slug Snail & Insect Killer	Ins Mol	Liq	93.00%
Corrys Slug & Snail Death	Mol	Grn	98.00%
Corrys Slug Snail & Insect Killer	Ins Mol	Grn	93.00%
D			
D-F-T Spray	Ins	Spr	97.50%
Daconil Lawn and Garden Fungicide	Fun	Liq	87.50%
Deadline	Mol	Liq	96.00%
Deadline 1 Last Meal for Slugs & Snails	Mol	Liq	96.00%
Dexol Gopher Gasser	Rod	Gas	10.00%
Dexol Gopher Killer Pellets	Rod	Pel	98.00%

Label Word	Class	Active Ingredients	Tumors/Cancer	Repro. Damage	Genetic Damage
C		Naphthaleneacetamide 0.2%	-	-	-
		Thiram 4.04%	x	x	o
C	OP	Malathion 5%	x	o	o
	CB	Carbaryl 5%	x	o	x
		Sulfur 30%	o	o	o
C	CB	Carbaryl 5%	x	o	x
C	CB	Carbaryl 22.5%	x	o	x
W	CB	Carbaryl 5%	x	o	x
		Metaldehyde 3%	x	o	o
W		Metaldehyde 10.5%	x	o	o
C		2,4-D 13.95%	x	x	x
		Dicamba 1.04%	-	x	x
C		Sulfur 90%	o	o	o
C		Petroleum oil 99%	x	-	-
C	OP	Malathion 5%	x	o	o
	CB	Carbaryl 5%	x	o	x
		Sulfur 30%	o	o	o
C		2,4-D 0.01%	x	x	x
C	CB	Carbaryl 5%	x	o	x
		Metaldehyde 2%	x	o	o
C		Metaldehyde 2%	x	o	o
C	CB	Carbaryl 5%	x	o	x
		Metaldehyde 2%	x	o	o
C	CB	Carbaryl 2.5%	x	o	x
W		Chlorothalonil 12.5%	x	o	x
C		Metaldehyde 4%	x	o	o
C		Metaldehyde 4%	x	o	o
W		Potassium nitrate 45%	x	-	-
		Sulfur 45%	o	o	o
C		Zinc phosphide 2%	-	-	-

Table 7.1
Outdoor Use Pesticides - 1994

Brand Name	Use	Formulation	Inert Ingredients
Dexol Tender Leaf Plant Insect Spray	Ins	Liq	99.93%
Dexol Tender Leaf Plant Insect Spray	Ins	Liq	99.28%
Dexol Tender Leaf Systemic Granules Insect. Control	Ins	Grn	99.00%
Dexol Tender Leaf Whitefly & Mealybug Spray	IGR Ins	Liq	99.77%
Diazinon 25 - KXL	Ins	Liq	75.00%
Do It Best Home Pest Insect Control	Ins	Spr	99.50%
Dowpon M Grass Killer	Her	Grn	15.50%
Dyrene Lawn Disease Control	Fun	Dus	50.00%
E			
Eatons 4 The Birds Bird Repellent	Rep	Liq	20.00%
Eatons Answer For The Control of Pocket Gophers	Rod	Bat	99.99%
Eatons Repels Mosquitoes	Ins	Sld	99.65%
Enforcer Flea Spray for Yards Concentrate	Ins	Liq	93.12%
Enforcer Wasp & Hornet Killer	Ins	Aer	99.72%
F			
Farnam Cat-Away Outdoor Cat Repellent	Rep	Aer	98.00%
Florel Brand Fruit Eliminator	PGR	Liq	96.10%
Flower & Garden Weed Preventer	Her	Grn	95.00%
G			
Garlic Barrier	Ins	Liq	00.00%
Get Off My Garden	Rep	Gel	98.10%
Grass-B-Gon Grass Killer	Her	Spr	99.50%
Green Light Amaze	Her	Pel	98.00%

Label Word	Class	Active Ingredients	Tumors/Cancer	Repro. Damage	Genetic Damage
C		Nicotine 0.07%	-	-	-
C		Petroleum oil 0.65%	x	-	-
		Nicotine 0.07%	-	-	-
W	OP	Disulfuton 1%	-	-	x
C		Methoprene 0.1%	o	o	o
	CH	Dienochlor 0.07%	-	-	-
	SP	Resmethrin 0.06%	x	x	o
W	OP	Diazinon 25%	o	x	x
C	OP	Chlorpyrifos 0.5%	o	o	x
C		Dalapon 84.5%	-	x	-
C		Anilazine 50%	o	-	x
C		Polybutene 80%	-	-	-
C		Diphacinone 0.01%	-	-	o
C	SP	Allethrin 0.35%	o	o	o
D	SP	Fenvalerate 6.88%	x	x	o
C	SP	Resmethrin 0.28%	x	x	o
C		Methyl nonyl ketone 2%	-	-	-
C		Ethephon 3.9%	-	-	x
C		DCPA 5%	x	o	o
C		Garlic 100%	o	o	o
C		Methyl nonyl ketone 1.9%	-	-	-
C		Fluazifop-butyl 0.5%	-	-	-
C		Benefin 1%	-	-	-
		Oryzalin 1%	x	o	o

Table 7.1
Outdoor Use Pesticides - 1994

Brand Name	Use	Formulation	Inert Ingredients
Green Light Fung Away	Fun	Liq	99.12%
Green Light Many Purpose Dust	Ins	Pow	95.00%
Green Light Stump Remover	Her	Pow	
Green Light Systemic Fungicide With Benomyl	Fun	Dus	50.00%
Green Light Wettable Dusting Sulfur	Fun	Pow	10.00%
Green Thumb House Plant Insect Killer	Ins	Spr	99.93%
Green Thumb White Fly & Mealy Bug Spray	Ins	Spr	99.93%
H Hot Shot Wasp & Hornet Killer III	Ins	Aer	99.70%
Hyponex Bug Spray for House Plants	Ins	Spr	99.78%
I Isotox Insect Killer	Ins	Liq	89.00%
Isotox Insect Killer Formula II	Ins	Liq	90.60%
K KXL Malathion-50	Ins	Liq	50.00%
KXL Tri-Basic Copper Fungicide	Fun	Pow	2.00%
Kleenup Grass & Weed Killer	Her	Spr	99.38%
Kleenup Spot Weed & Grass Killer	Her	Aer	99.25%
Kleenup Systemic Weed & Grass Killer	Her	Liq	95.00%
L Lambert Kay Boundary Indoor/Outdoor Dog & Cat	Rep	Aer	98.00%
Lawn Food and Crab Grass Control	Her	Dus	99.08%

Label Word	Class	Active Ingredients	Tumors/Cancer	Repro. Damage	Genetic Damage
C		Triadimefon 0.88%	x	x	o
C	OP	Diazinon 5%	o	x	x
C		Potassium nitrate	x	-	-
C		Benomyl 50%	x	x	x
C		Sulfur 90%	o	o	o
C	SP	Phenothrin 0.07%	x	-	o
C	SP	Phenothrin 0.07%	x	-	o
C	OP	Chlorpyrifos 0.25%	o	o	x
	SP	Allethrin 0.05%	o	o	o
C		Pyrethrins 0.02%	x	x	x
	SY	Piperonyl butoxide* 0.2%	-	-	o
W	SP	Acephate 8%	x	o	x
	CH	Dicofol 3%	x	x	o
W	OP	Acephate 9.4%	x	o	x
W	OP	Malathion 50%	x	o	o
C		Copper sulfate (basic) 98%	-	-	-
C		Glyphosate 0.5%	x	o	o
		Aciflurofen 0.12%	x	-	x
C		Glyphosate 0.75%	x	o	o
C		Glyphosate 5%	x	o	o
C		Methyl nonyl ketone 2%	-	-	-
C		Benefin 0.92%	-	-	-

Table 7.1
Outdoor Use Pesticides - 1994

Brand Name	Use	Formulation	Inert Ingredients
Lilly Miller Cutworm Earwig & Sowbug Bait	Ins	Bat	95.00%
Lilly Miller Diazinon Insect Dust	Ins	Dus	96.00%
Lilly Miller Diazinon Insect Granules	Ins	Grn	95.00%
Lilly Miller Granular Noxall Vegetation Killer Prevents Plant Growth for Up to One Year	Her	Grn	2.00%
Lilly Miller Grasshopper Earwig & Sowbug Bait	Ins	Bat	95.00%
Lilly Miller Hose'n Go Weed & Feed 15-0-0	Her	Liq	90.96%
Lilly Miller Malathion	Ins	Liq	50.00%
Lilly Miller Microcop Fungicide	Fun	Dus	10.00%
Lilly Miller Moss-Kil	Her	Liq	70.40%
Lilly Miller Moss-Out	Her	Liq	65.00%
Lilly Miller Ready-To-Use Bug-Off Rose & Flow	Ins	Spr	99.50%
Lilly Miller Ready-To-Use Knock Out II Weed & Grass Killer	Her	Spr	99.77%
Lilly Miller Ready-To-Use Lawn Weed Killer	Her	Spr	99.05%
Lilly Miller Ready-To-Use Moss-Kil	Her	Spr	93.80%
Lilly Miller Rootone Brand Rooting Hormone	Pgr	Pow	95.76%
Lilly Miller Sevin 5% Dust	Ins	Dus	95.00%
Lilly Miller Slug, Snai,l & Insect Killer Bait	Mol	Grn	93.00%
Lilly Miller Spurge & Oxalis Killer	Her	Liq	85.01%
Lilly Miller Superior Type Spray Oil	Ins	Liq	1.00%

Label Word	Class	Active Ingredients	Tumors/Cancer	Repro. Damage	Genetic Damage
C	CB	Carbaryl 5%	x	o	x
C	OP	Diazinon 4%	o	x	x
C	OP	Diazinon 5%	o	x	x
D		Sodium metaborate 68%	-	x	x
		Sodium chlorate 30%	-	-	-
C	CB	Carbaryl 5%	x	o	x
C		2,4-D 5.67%	x	x	x
		MCPP 2.74%	-	x	x
		Dicamba 0.63%	-	x	x
C	OP	Malathion 50%	x	o	o
W		Copper sulfate (basic) 90%	-	-	-
C		Zinc 29.60%	-	x	x
C		Ferric sulfate 35%	-	-	x
C	SP	Permethrin 0.5%	x	x	o
C		Diquat 0.23%	x	x	x
C		2,4-D 0.59%	x	x	x
		MCPP 0.29%	-	x	x
		Dicamba 0.07%	-	x	x
D		Zinc 6.2%	-	x	x
C		Naphthaleneacetamide 0.2%	-	-	-
		Thiram 4.04%	x	x	o
C	CB	Carbaryl 5%	x	o	x
C		Metaldehyde 2%	x	o	o
	CB	Carbaryl 5%	x	o	x
C		2,4-D 9.41%	x	x	x
		MCPA 4.54%	o	x	x
		Dicamba 1.04%	-	x	x
C		Petroleum oil 99%	x	-	-

Table 7.1
Outdoor Use Pesticides - 1994

Brand Name	Use	Formulation	Inert Ingredients
Lilly Miller Systemic Rose Shrub & Flower Care 6-10-4	Ins	Grn	99.00%
Lilly Miller Tomato & Vegetable Dust	Ins	Dus	60.00%
Lilly Millers Slug And Snail Line	Mol	Liq	96.00%
Lilly Millers Sta-stuk "M"	Oth	Liq	85.50%
M			
Mosquito Dunks	Ins	Sld	90.00%
Mr. Scotts Pest Control	Ins	Liq	99.50%
Multipurpose Fungicide Daconil 2787 Plant Disease Control	Fun	Liq	70.40%
O			
Orthene Systemic Insect Control	Ins	Liq	90.60%
Orthenex Rose and Flower Spray	Ins Fun	Aer	99.54%
Ortho Brush-B-Gon Brush Killer	Her	Liq	92.00%
Ortho Brush-B-Gon Poison Ivy & Poison Oak Killer	Her	Spr	99.30%
Ortho Crab Grass Killer	Her	Liq	84.00%
Ortho Diazinon Granules	Ins	Grn	98.00%
Ortho Diazinon Plus Insect Spray	Ins	Liq	75.00%
Ortho Dormant Disease Control	Fun	Liq	74.00%
Ortho Earwig Roach & Sowbug Bait	Ins	Dus	98.00%
Ortho Fruit & Vegetable Insect Control	Ins	Liq	75.00%
Ortho Funginex Rose Disease Control	Fun	Liq	93.50%

Label Word	Class	Active Ingredients	Tumors/Cancer	Repro. Damage	Genetic Damage
W	OP	Disulfuton 1%	-	-	x
C	OP	Malathion 5%	x	o	o
	CB	Carbaryl 5%	x	o	x
		Sulfur 30%	o	o	o
C		Metaldehyde 4%	x	o	o
C		Potassium resinate 12%	-	-	-
		Potassium oleate 2.5%	o	o	o
C		B.T. 10%	o	o	o
C	OP	Chlorpyrifos 0.5%	o	o	x
W		Chlorothalonil 29.6%	x	o	x
W	OP	Acephate 9.4%	x	o	x
W	OP	Acephate 0.25%	x	o	x
	SP	Resmethrin 0.11%	x	x	o
		Triforine 0.1%	x	o	o
C		Triclopyr 8%	o	o	x
C		Triclopyr 0.7%	o	o	x
D		Octyl ammonium methanearsonate 8%	-	-	-
		Dodecycloammonium methanearsonate 8%	-	-	-
C	OP	Diazinon 2%	o	x	x
W	OP	Diazinon 25%	o	x	x
D		Calcium polysulfide 26%	-	-	-
C	CB	Propoxur 2%	x	o	o
W	OP	Diazinon 25%	o	x	x
D		Triforine 6.5%	x	o	o

Table 7.1
Outdoor Use Pesticides - 1994

Brand Name	Use	Formulation	Inert Ingredients
Ortho Garden Sulfur Dust or Spray	Fun	Dus	10.00%
Ortho Garden Weed Preventer	Her	Dus	95.00%
Ortho Home & Garden Insect Killer Formula II	Ins	Aer	99.60%
Ortho Home Pest Insect Control	Ins	Liq	99.50%
Ortho Hornet & Wasp Killer	Ins	Aer	99.50%
Ortho Killer Tomato & Vegetable Dust	Fun Ins	Dus	88.50%
Ortho Lawn Insect Spray	Ins	Liq	90.00%
Ortho Lindane Borer & Leaf Miner Spray	Ins	Liq	80.00%
Ortho Liquid Sevin Brand Carbaryl Insecticide	Ins	Liq	73.00%
Ortho Malathion 50 Plus Insect Spray	Ins	Liq	50.00%
Ortho Outdoor Insect Fogger	Ins	Fog	98.72%
Ortho Poison Ivy & Poison Oak Killer Formula	Her	Aer	99.30%
Ortho Rose & Flower Insect Killer	Ins	Spr	99.78%
Ortho Rotenone Dust or Spray	Ins	Dus	98.00%
Ortho Sevin Brand Carbaryl Insecticide	Ins	Dus	95.00%
Ortho Sevin Brand Carbaryl Insecticide 5 Dust	Ins	Dus	95.00%
Ortho Systemic Rose & Flower Care 8-12-4	Ins	Dus	99.00%
Ortho Tomato & Vegetable Insect Killer	Ins	Spr	99.78%
Ortho Triox Vegetation Killer	Her	Liq	98.14%
Ortho Vegetable Disease Control	Fun	Liq	70.40%
Ortho Weed B-Gon Lawn Weed Killer	Her	Liq	77.60%

Label Word	Class	Active Ingredients	Tumors/Cancer	Repro. Damage	Genetic Damage
C		Sulfur 90%	o	o	o
C		DCPA 5%	x	o	o
C	SP	Tetramethrin 0.2%	x	x	o
	SP	Phenothrin 0.2%	x	-	o
C	OP	Chlorpyrifos 0.5%	o	o	x
W	CB	Propoxur 0.5%	x	o	o
W		Captan 5%	x	o	x
	CH	Methoxychlor 5%	-	x	-
		Rotenone 1.5%	x	x	x
C	OP	Chlorpyrifos 5.3%	o	o	x
D	CH	Lindane 20%	x	x	x
C	CB	Carbaryl 27%	x	o	x
W	OP	Malathion 50%	x	o	o
C	SP	Resmethrin 0.28%	x	x	o
		2-Hydroxyethyl-n-octyl sulfide 1%	-	-	-
C		Triclopyr 0.7%	o	o	x
C		Pyrethrins 0.02%	x	x	x
	SY	Piperonyl butoxide* 0.2%	-	-	o
C		Rotenone 2%	x	x	x
C	CB	Carbaryl 5%	x	o	x
C	CB	Carbaryl 5%	x	o	x
W	OP	Disulfuton 1%	-	-	x
C		Pyrethrins 0.02%	x	x	x
	SY	Piperonyl butoxide* 0.2%	-	-	o
W		Prometon 1.86%	o	o	o
W		Chlorothalonil 29.6%	x	o	x
D		2,4-D 10.8%	x	x	x
		MCPA 11.6%	o	x	x

Table 7.1
Outdoor Use Pesticides - 1994

Brand Name	Use	Formulation	Inert Ingredients
Ortho Weed-B-Gon Weed Killer	Her	Spr	99.60%
Ortho-Klor Soil Insect & Termite Killer	Ins	Liq	87.40%
Orthonex Insect & Disease Control Formula III	Ins Fun	Liq	92.00%
Orthonex Rose and Flower Spray	Ins Fun	Aer	99.54%
Orthorix Lime-Sulfur Spray	Fun	Liq	74.00%
P Pax Fungicide, Insecticide, Fertilizer	Ins Mol	Grn	98.96%
Payless Diazinon 25% Insect Spray	Ins	Liq	75.00%
Payless Dursban Insect Killer Yard-Soil-Home	Ins	Liq	93.30%
Payless Malathion Insect Control	Ins	Liq	50.00%
Payless Sevin Brand Carbaryl Insecticide Liquid Insect Killer	Ins	Liq	76.60%
Payless Snail and Slug Killer Pellets	Mol	Pel	98.00%
Payless Systemic Rose Care 6-10-4	Ins	Grn	99.00%
R Raid House & Garden Formula 11	Ins	Aer	98.74%
Raid Wasp & Hornet Killer IV	Ins	Aer	99.06%
Raid Wasp & Hornet Killer X	Ins	Aer	99.63%
Raid Yard Guard Outdoor Fogger Formula V	Ins	Aer	99.13%

Label Word	Class	Active Ingredients	Tumors/Cancer	Repro. Damage	Genetic Damage
C		2,4-D 0.2%	x	x	x
		MCPA 0.2%	o	x	-
W	OP	Chlorpyrifos 12.6%	o	o	x
D	OP	Acephate 4%	x	o	x
		Hexakis 0.75%	-	x	o
		Triforine 3.25%	x	o	o
W	OP	Acephate 0.25%	x	o	x
	SP	Resmethrin 0.11%	x	x	o
		Triforine 0.1%	x	o	o
D		Calcium polysulfide 26%	-	-	-
C	CB	Carbaryl 0.57%	x	o	x
		Anilazine 0.47%	o	-	x
W	OP	Diazinon 25%	o	x	x
C	OP	Chlorpyrifos 6.7%	o	o	x
C	OP	Malathion 50%	x	o	o
C	CB	Carbaryl 23.4%	x	o	x
C		Metaldehyde 2%	x	o	o
W	OP	Disulfuton 1%	-	-	x
C		Pyrethrins 0.18%	x	x	x
	SP	Tetramethrin 0.08%	x	x	o
	SY	Piperonyl butoxide* 1%	-	-	o
C	CB	Propoxur 0.48%	x	o	o
	OP	Dichlorvos 0.46%	x	o	x
C	CB	Propoxur 0.25%	x	o	o
	SP	Tetramethrin 0.12%	x	x	o
C	SP	Permethrin 0.23%	x	x	o
		2-Hydroxyethyl-n-octyl sulfide 0.5%	-	-	-
	SP	Allethrin 0.14%	o	o	o

Table 7.1
Outdoor Use Pesticides - 1994

Brand Name	Use	Formulation	Inert Ingredients
Ro-Pel Garbage Protector	Rep	Liq	99.90%
Roebic Root Killer Formula K-77	Her	Grn	1.00%
Roundup L&G Concentrate Grass & Weed Killer	Her	Liq	99.04%
Roundup L&G Ready-To-Use Fast Acting Formula Grass & Weed Killer	Her	Spr	99.04%
Roundup Quik Stik Grass & Weed Killer	Her	Tab	40.00%
Roundup Super Concentrate Grass & Weed Killer	Her	Liq	59.00%
S Safer African Violet Insect Attack For House Plants Ready-To-Use Spray	Ins	Spr	98.50%
Safer B.T. Caterpillar Attack Concentrate	Ins	Liq	98.24%
Safer Crawling Insect Attack Ready-To-Use Spray	Ins	Liq	99.56%
Safer Fruit & Vegetable Insect Attack Insecticidal Soap Ready-To-Use Spray	Ins	Spr	97.60%
Safer Garden Fungicide Ready To Use	Fun	Spr	99.60%
Safer Insecticidal Soap Concentrate	Ins	Liq	51.00%
Safer Insecticidal Soap for Houseplants Ready-To-Use	Ins	Spr	98.00%
Safer Rose & Flower Insect Attack Insecticidal Soap Ready-To-Use Spray	Ins	Spr	98.47%
Safer Sharpshooter Contact Weed Killer Ready-To-Use Spray	Her	Spr	97.00%
Safer Vegetable Insect Attack RTU Squeeze Duster	Ins	Dus	99.70%
Safer Yard & Garden Insect Attack Ready-To-Use Spray	Ins	Spr	98.99%
Schultz-Instant House Plant & Garden Insecticide Spray	Ins	Spr	99.78%

Label Word	Class	Active Ingredients	Tumors/Cancer	Repro. Damage	Genetic Damage
C		Bitrex 0.07%	-	-	-
		Thymol 0.03%	o	o	o
D		Copper pentahydrate 99%	-	-	-
C		Glyphosate 0.96%	x	o	o
C		Glyphosate 0.96%	x	o	o
C		Glyphosate 60%	x	o	o
W		Glyphosate 41%	x	o	o
C		Potassium salt of fatty acids 1.5%	o	o	o
C		B.T. 1.76%	o	o	o
C		Pyrethrins 0.04%	x	x	x
	SY	Piperonyl butoxide* 0.4%	-	-	o
C		Potassium salt of fatty acids 2%	o	o	o
		Citrus aromatics 0.4%	o	o	o
C		Sulfur 0.4%	o	o	o
C		Potassium salt of fatty acids 49%	o	o	o
C		Potassium salt of fatty acids 2%	o	o	o
C		Potassium salt of fatty acids 1.5%	o	o	o
		Citrus aromatics 0.03%	o	o	o
C		Potassium salt of fatty acids 3%	o	o	o
C		B.T. 0.3%	o	o	o
C		Pyrethrins 0.01%	x	x	x
		Potassium salt of fatty acids 1%	o	o	o
C		Pyrethrins 0.02%	x	x	x
	SY	Piperonyl butoxide*. 0.2%	-	-	o

Table 7.1
Outdoor Use Pesticides - 1994

Brand Name	Use	Formulation	Inert Ingredients
Schultz-Instant Insect Spray	Ins	Spr	99.78%
Scram Dog & Cat Repellent	Rep	Aer	98.00%
Security Brand Rootone F	PGR	Pow	95.76%
Security House Plant Insect Control	IGR Ins	Spr	99.77%
Security Systemic Granular Insecticide	Ins	Liq	99.00%
Sergeants Shoo! Dog & Cat Repellent	Rep	Aer	98.00%
Snarol Snail & Slug Killer Pellets	Mol	Pel	97.50%
Sterling Rescue Dog & Cat Repellent	Rep	Liq	98.40%
Sticker for Cooke Copper Fungicide	Oth	Liq	85.50%
Stump Remover	Her	Dus	
T Tanglefoot Tree Barrier	Rep	Bar	
The Giant Destroyer	Ins	Bom	19.00%
Timed-Release Flea Halt! Yard Spray Concentrate	Ins	Liq	98.30%
Turf Builder Plus 2 For Grass Lawns	Her	Fer	97.58%
V Vapam Soil Aid	**Her** Ins	Liq	67.30%
Volck Oil Spray	Ins	Liq	3.00%
W Walgreens House & Garden Bug Killer	Ins	Aer	99.61%

Label Word	Class	Active Ingredients	Tumors/Cancer	Repro. Damage	Genetic Damage
C	SY	Pyrethrins 0.02%	x	x	x
		Piperonyl butoxide* 0.2%	-	-	o
C		Methyl nonyl ketone 2%	-	-	-
C		Naphthaleneacetamide 0.2%	-	-	-
		Thiram 4.04%	x	x	o
C	CH	Methoprene 0.1%	o	o	o
	CH	Dienochlor 0.07%	-	-	-
	SP	Pyrethroid 0.06%	-	-	-
W	OP	Diazinon 1%	o	x	x
C		Methyl nonyl ketone 2%	-	-	-
W		Metaldehyde 2.5%	x	o	o
C		Oil of anise 1.6%	o	o	o
C		Potassium resinate 12%	-	-	-
		Potassium oleate 2.5%	o	o	o
C		Potassium nitrate	x	-	-
C		Castor oil	-	-	-
		Vegetable wax	o	o	o
W		Sodium nitrate 46.2%	x	-	-
		Sulfur 34.8%	o	o	o
C	OP	Chlorpyrifos 1.7%	o	o	x
C		2,4-D 1.21%	x	x	x
		MCPP 1.21%	-	x	x
C		Metam-sodium 32.7%	x	x	x
C		Petroleum oil 97%	x	-	-
C	SP	Resmethrin 0.23%	x	x	o
	SP	Allethrin 0.16%	o	o	o

Table 7.1
Outdoor Use Pesticides - 1994

Brand Name	Use	Formulation	Inert Ingredients
Weed-B-Gon Jet Weeder Formula III	Her	Aer	99.26%
Z Zodiac Yard & Kennel Spray	Ins	Liq	93.30%

Label Word	Class	Active Ingredients	Tumors/Cancer	Repro. Damage	Genetic Damage
C		2,4-D 0.25% MCPP 0.25% Dichlorprop 0.24%	x - -	x x -	x x -
C	OP	Chlorpyrifos 6.7%	o	o	x

* Piperonyl butoxide causes cancer and birth
  defects in rats (see pages 114-115).

Table 7.2

Outdoor Use Pesticides - 1995

Brand Name	Use	Formulation	Inert Ingredients
A			
Amdro	Ins	Pow	99.27%
Amdro Granular Insecticide Kills Fire Ants	Ins	Gra	99.27%
Amdro Insecticide	Ins	Gra	99.12%
Amdro Insecticide Bait	Ins	Gra	99.27%
Apache Fly Bait	Ins	Gra	98.975%
Apache Fly Bait	Ins	Bai	98.975%
Apache TP Fly Bait Station	Ins	Gra	98.975%
B			
BA-KIL	Ins	Liq	85.4%
BASF Poast Postemergence Grass Herbicide	Her	Liq	82%
Bait Pellets	Mol Ins	Pel	92.5%
Basagran T/O Herbicide	Her	Liq	58%
Bengal Lawn Flea and Tick Killer	Ins	Liq	99.56%
Benomyl Fungicide	Fun	Dus	50%
Black Leaf Rose & Ornamental Fungicide	Fun	Pow	50%
C			
CRC Wasp and Hornet Killer II	Ins	Aer	99.751%
Captan Fungicide	Fun	Dus	50%
Copper Sulfate Granular Crystals	Her	Gra	1%
Copper-cide Liquid Fungicide	Fun	Liq	52%
Cutworm & Cricket Bait	Ins	Gra	95%
Cygon 2E Eimethoate Systemic Insecticide	Ins	Liq	77%

Label Word	Class	Active Ingredients	Tumors/Cancer	Repro. Damage	Genetic Damage
C		Hydramethylnon 0.73%	o	x	o
C		Hydramethylnon 0.73%	o	x	o
C		Hydramethylnon 0.88%	o	x	o
C		Hydramethylnon 0.73%	o	x	o
C	CB	Methomyl 1%	o	o	o
		Z-9 Tricosene 0.025%	o	o	o
C	CB	Methomyl 1%	o	o	o
		Z-9 Tricosene 0.025%	o	o	o
C	CB	Methomyl 1%	o	o	o
		Z-9 Tricosene 0.025%	o	o	o
D	CB	Propoxur 14.6%	x	o	o
W		Sethoxydim 18%	-	-	-
C		Metaldehyde 3.25%	x	o	o
	CB	Carbaryl 4.25%	x	o	x
C		Bentazone 42%	x	x	o
C	SP	0.44%	x	x	o
C		Benomyl 50%	x	x	x
C		Thiophanate-methyl 50%	x	-	o
C	SP	Allethrin 0.129%	o	o	o
	SP	Phenothrin 0.12%	x	-	o
D		Captan 50%	x	o	x
D		Copper 25%	-	-	-
W		Copper 48%	-	-	-
C	CB	Carbaryl 5%	x	o	x
W	OP	Dimethoate 23%	o	x	x

Table 7.2

Outdoor Use Pesticides - 1995

Brand Name	Use	Formulation	Inert Ingredients
D			
Dexol Aphid Mite and Whitefly Killer	Ins	Spr	99.914%
Dexol Aphid, Mite & Whitefly Killer	Ins	Spr	99.142%
Dexol Diazinon 2% Granules	Ins	Gra	98%
Dexol Diazinon 25% Insect Spray	Ins	Liq	75%
Dexol Diazinon 5% Granules	Ins	Grn	95%
Dexol Dursban Granules Insect Control	Ins	Gra	99%
Dexol Dursban Lawn Insect Killer	Ins	Liq	93.3%
Dexol Eptam Preemergent Weed Control	Her	Gra	97.7%
Dexol Fire Ant Granules II	Ins	Gra	99.5%
Dexol Grass-Out Systemic Grass Killer	Her	Liq	98.3%
Dexol Malathion Insect Control	Ins	Liq	50%
Dexol Tender Leaf Plant Insect Spray	Ins	Liq	99.89%
Dexol Weed and Garden Killer	Her	Spr	99.77%
Dexol Weed-Out Lawn Weed Killer	Her	Liq	87.91%
Diazinon 5% Granules Ready to Use	Ins	Gra	95%
Diazinon Insecticide 25% Spray Concentrate	Ins	Liq	75%
Dithane M-45	Fun	Dus	20%
Dursban 1E Lawn Insecticide	Ins	Liq	87.4%
Dursban Lawn & Peremeter	Ins	Gra	99%
E			
Eaton's 4 the Squirrel Repellent	Rep	Pst	85%

Label Word	Class	Active Ingredients	Tumors/Cancer	Repro. Damage	Genetic Damage
C	SP	Tetramethrin 0.026%	x	x	o
	SP	Phenothrin 0.058%	x	-	o
C	SP	Tetramethrin 0.286%	x	x	o
	SP	Pyrethroid 0.549%	-	-	-
C	OP	Diazinon 2%	o	x	x
W	OP	Diazinon 25%	o	x	x
C		Methoprene 0.007%	o	o	o
	SP	Permethrin 0.25%	x	x	o
C	OP	Chlorpyrifos 1%	o	o	x
C	OP	Chlorpyrifos 6.7%	o	o	x
C		Eptam 2.3%	o	x	x
C	OP	Chlorpyrifos 0.5%	o	o	x
C		Fluazifop-butyl 1.7%	-	-	-
C	OP	Malathion 50%	x	o	o
D		Nicotine 0.07%	-	-	-
		Triethanolamine 0.04%	-	-	-
C		Diquat 0.23%	x	x	x
C		MCPA 3.66%	o	x	x
		2,4-D 7.59%	x	x	x
		Dicamba 0.84%	-	x	x
C	OP	Diazinon 5%	o	x	x
C	OP	Diazinon 25%	o	x	x
C		Manganese 16%	-	-	-
		Zinc 2%	-	x	x
		Mancozeb 62%	x	x	x
W	OP	Chlorpyrifos 12.6%	o	o	x
C	OP	Chlorpyrifos 1%	o	o	x
C		Polybutene 90%	-	-	-

Table 7.2

Outdoor Use Pesticides - 1995

Brand Name	Use	Formulation	Inert Ingredients
Enforcer Ant Kill and Barrier Treatment	Ins	Aer	99.48%
Enforcer Ant and Insect Barrier	Ins	Gra	25%
Enforcer Flea Spray for Yards III Concentrate	Ins	Spr	98.3%
Enforcer Wasp and Yellow Jacket Foam V	Ins	Aer	99.6%
Enforcer Yard and Patio Outdoor Fogger	Ins	Aer	99.716%
Eptam Granules	Her	Gra	97.7%
F			
Ferti-lone Brush Killer Stump Killer	Her	Liq	91.2%
Ferti-lone Quik-Kill for Home Garden and Pets	Ins	Spr	98.78%
Ferti-lone Triple-Action Insecticide, Miticide, & Fungicide	Mul	Liq	89.8%
Fords Diazinon	Ins	Gra	95%
G			
Golden Marlin	Ins	Gra	98.975%
Green Charm Fire Ant Granules	Ins	Gra	99.500
Green Charm Knock Out Concentrate Systemic Weed & Grass Killer	Her	Liq	95%
Green Charm Liquid Sevin Insect Spray	Ins	Liq	78.7%
Green Light Fire Ant Killer II	Ins	Gra	99%
Green Light Wasp and Hornet Spray	Ins	Aer	99.716%
Green Sweep Weed and Feed	Her	Liq	93.1%

Label Word	Class	Active Ingredients	Tumors/Cancer	Repro. Damage	Genetic Damage
C	PY	Pyrethrins 0.05%	x	x	x
	SY	MGK 264 0.25%	x	x	o
	SP	Permethrin 0.22%	x	x	o
C	OP	Acephate 75%	x	o	x
C	OP	Chlorpyrifos 1.7%	o	o	x
C	SP	Tetramethrin 0.2%	x	x	o
	SP	Phenothrin 0.2%	x	-	o
C	SP	Resmethrin 0.284%	x	x	o
C		Eptam 2.3%	o	x	x
C		Triclopyr 8.8%	o	o	x
C	PY	Pyrethrins 0.02%	x	x	x
	SY	Piperonyl butoxide* 0.2%	-	-	o
D	OP	Diazinon 4.2%	o	x	x
		Chlorothalonil 6%	x	o	x
C	OP	Diazinon 5%	o	x	x
C	CB	Methomyl 1%	o	o	o
		Z-9 Tricosene 0.025%	o	o	o
C	OP	Chlorpyrifos 0.5%	o	o	x
C		Glyphosate 5%	x	o	o
C	CB	Carbaryl 21.3%	x	o	x
C	OP	Chlorpyrifos 1%	o	o	x
C	SP	Resmethrin 0.284%	x	x	o
C		2,4-D 2.29%	x	x	x
		MCPA 2.3%	o	x	x
		2.26%	-	x	x

Table 7.2

Outdoor Use Pesticides - 1995

Brand Name	Use	Formulation	Inert Ingredients
Green Sweep Weed and Feed	Her	Liq	93.15%
Greenskote Weed and Feed	Her	Fer	98.768%
Greenview Preen	Her	Gra	98.53%

H

Brand Name	Use	Formulation	Inert Ingredients
Hawk Meal Bait Ready to Use Place Pac	Rod	Bai	99.995%
Hi-Kil	Ins	Liq	85.4%
Hi-Yield 5% Diazinon Insect Killer Granules	Ins	Dus	95%
Hi-Yield Weed Killer	Her	Liq	57%
Hi-Yield Di-Syston Systemic Granular Insecticide	Ins	Gra	98%
Hi-Yield Fire Ant Killer Country with Logic	Ins	Gra	99%
Hi-Yield Killzall Weed and Grass Killer	Her	Spr	99.5%
Hi-Yield Killzall Weed and Grass Killer Concentrate	Her	Liq	90%
Hi-Yield Male Cricket Bail	Ins	Gra	99.5%
Hi-Yield Nem-A-Cide Nematode Control	Ins	Gra	75%
Hi-Yield Rotenone Insecticide	Ins	Dus	97.7%
Hi-Yield Traimine Lawn Weed Killer	Her	Liq	86.34%
Home & Garden Home Pest Control	Ins	Liq	99.5%
Home and Garden Brush Killer	Her	Liq	66.9%
Home and Garden Dipel Dust	Ins	Dus	1%
Home and Garden Lawn Weed Killer with Trimec	Her	Liq	85.05%
Home and Garden Oftanol 1.5% Granular	Ins	Gra	98.5%

Label Word	Class	Active Ingredients	Tumors/Cancer	Repro. Damage	Genetic Damage
C		2,4-D 2.29%	x	x	x
		MCPA 2.3%	o	x	x
		DCPA 2.26%	x	o	o
C		MCPA 0.416%	o	x	x
		MCPP 0.411%	-	x	x
		2,4-D 0.405%	x	x	x
C		Trifluralin 1.47%	x	o	o
C		Bromadiolone 0.005%	-	-	-
D	CB	Propoxur 14.6%	x	o	o
C	OP	Diazinon 5%	o	x	x
C		Atrazine 43%	x	o	o
W	OP	Disulfuton 2%	-	-	x
C		Fenoxycarb 1%	-	-	-
C		Glyphosate 0.5%	x	o	o
C		Glyphosate 10%	x	o	o
C	OP	Chlorpyrifos 0.5%	o	o	x
C		Chitin protein 25%	o	o	o
C		Rotenone 2.25%	x	x	x
W		2,4-D 4.55%	x	x	x
		MCPA 4.58%	o	x	x
C	OP	Chlorpyrifos 0.5%	o	o	x
C		MCPP 16.4%	-	x	x
		2,4-D 16.7%	x	x	x
C		B.T. 0.04%	o	o	o
C		MCPA 10.6%	o	x	x
		2,4-D 3.05%	x	x	x
C		Isophenfos 1.5%	-	-	-

Table 7.2

Outdoor Use Pesticides - 1995

Brand Name	Use	Formulation	Inert Ingredients
Hot Shot House & Garden Bug Killer . Form 721	Ins	Aer	99.6%
I			
Image 1.5 LC Herbicide (in box)	Her	Liq	82.7%
J			
Jerry Baker Broadleaf Weed Killer	Her	Spr	94.57%
K			
KGro Dandelion & Broadleaf Weed Killer	Her	Spr	99.054%
KGro Dandelion Killer Formula II	Her	Spr	91.03%
KGro Diazinon Granules	Ins	Gra	98%
KGro Diazinon Insect Spray 3	Ins	Liq	75%
KGro Dog and Cat Repellent	Rep	Spr	98%
KGro Dog and Cat Repellent	Rep	Gra	98%
KGro Dursban Insect Spray Formula II	Ins	Liq	87.4%
KGro Fence and Walk Edger	Her	Liq	97.5%
KGro Fire Ant Killer Formula II	Ins	Gra	99.5%
KGro Garden Weed Preventer	Her	Gra	98.53%
KGro Malathion Insect Spray 3	Ins	Spr	50%
KGro Mole Cricket Bait	Ins	Gra	99.5%
KGro Multipurpose Rose and Flower	Ins	Dus	64.52%
	Ins		
	Fun		

Label Word	Class	Active Ingredients	Tumors/Cancer	Repro. Damage	Genetic Damage
C	SP	Tetramethrin 0.2%	x	x	o
	SP	Pyrethroid 0.2%	-	-	-
C		Imazaquin 17.3%	o	o	o
C		2,4-D 1.11%	x	x	x
		MCPA 3.85%	o	x	x
		Dicamba 0.47%	-	x	x
C		2,4-D 0.593	x	x	x
		MCPA 0.287%	o	x	x
		Dicamba 0.066	-	x	x
C		2,4-D 5.67%	x	x	x
		MCPA 2.67%	o	x	x
		Dicamba 0.63%	-	x	x
C	OP	Diazinon 2%	o	x	x
C	OP	Diazinon 2.5%	o	x	x
C		Methyl nonyl ketone 2%	-	-	-
C		Methyl nonyl ketone 2%	-	-	-
W	OP	Chlorpyrifos 12.6%	o	o	x
W		Prometon 2.5%	o	o	o
C	OP	Chlorpyrifos 0.5%	o	o	x
C		Trifluralin 1.47%	x	o	o
C	OP	Malathion 50%	x	o	o
C	OP	Chlorpyrifos 0.5%	o	o	x
C	CB	Carbaryl 5%	x	o	x
	SY	Piperonyl butoxide* 0.45%	-	-	o
	PY	Pyrethrins 0.03%	x	x	x
		Sulfur 30%	o	o	o

Table 7.2

Outdoor Use Pesticides - 1995

Brand Name	Use	Formulation	Inert Ingredients
KGro Rose and Flower Insect killer	Ins	Spr	99.78%
KGro Sevin Liquid Formula II	Ins	Liq	78.7%
KGro Snail and Slug Bait	Mol	Gra	98%
KGro Systemic Rose and Flower Care Formula II	Ins	Gra	99%
KGro Vegetation Killer Formula II	Her	Spr	99.777%
Karathane Fungicide Miticide	Fun	Dus	80.5%
Kelthane Spider Mite Spray	Ins	Spr	58%
L			
Lawn Ornamental and Vegetable Fungicide	Fun	Dus	25%
Lesco Granular Dursban Insecticide	Ins	Gra	99.03%
Lesco Horticultural Oil Insecticide	Ins	Liq	1.2%
Lesco Malathion Insecticide Concentrate	Ins	Liq	50%
Lesco Ornamental Preemergence Herbicide	Her	Gra	98.536%
Lesco Sevin Brand Carbaryl Home & Garden Insecticide	Ins	Liq	78.7%
Lesco St. Augustine Grass Weed and Feed	Her	Gra	99.2%
Lesco Touche Flowable Fungicide	Fun	Liq	8.7%
Lindane Spray Concentrate	Ins	Liq	87.2%
Liquid Copper Fungicide	Fun	Liq	52%
M			
Malathion 50% EC	Ins	Liq	50%
Malathion Dust	Ins	Dus	95%
Malathion Oil Citrus and Ornamental	Ins	Liq	20%
Monetery Liqui-Cop Fungicide Spray	Fun	Liq	92%

Label Word	Class	Active Ingredients	Tumors/Cancer	Repro. Damage	Genetic Damage
C	PY	Pyrethrins 0.02%	x	x	x
	SY	Piperonyl butoxide* 0.2%	-	-	o
C	CB	Carbaryl 21.3%	x	o	x
C		Metaldehyde 2%	x	o	o
W	OP	Disulfuton 1%	-	-	x
C		Diquat 0.23%	x	x	x
C		Dinocap 19.4%	x	x	x
C	CH	Dicofol 42%	x	x	o
D		Chlorothalonil 75%	x	o	x
C	OP	Chlorpyrifos 0.97%	o	o	x
C		Petroleum distillate 98.8%	x	-	-
C	OP	Malathion 50%	x	o	o
C		Trifluralin 1.47%	x	o	o
C	CB	Carbaryl 21.3%	x	o	x
C		Atrazine 0.80%	x	o	o
C		Vinclozolin 41.3%	x	x	x
C	CH	Lindane 12.8%	x	x	x
C		Copper 48%	-	-	-
C	OP	Malathion 50%	x	o	o
C	OP	Malathion 5%	x	o	o
C	OP	Malathion 5%	x	o	o
		Petroleum oil 75%	x	-	-
C		Copper 8%	-	-	-

Table 7.2

Outdoor Use Pesticides - 1995

Brand Name	Use	Formulation	Inert Ingredients
Monterey Vegetable Turf & Oramental Weeder	Her	Pow	25%
Monterey Weed Stopper	Her	Liq	59.6%
Monterey Weed-Hoe	Her	Liq	52.2%
N			
Natural Guard Multipurpose Neem Insecticide	Ins	Liq	99.1%
Nematrol Nematocide	Ins	Gra	0%
Neutral Copper Fungicide	Fun	Dus	2%
O			
Organic Plus Fire Ant Killer	Ins	Dus	8.7%
Orthene Turf Tree and Ornamental Spray	Ins	Pow	25%
Ortho Atrazine Plus St. Augustine Lawn Webber	Her	Liq	86.6%
Ortho Biosafe Lawn and Garden Soil Insect Concentrate	Ins	Gra	90%
Ortho Crabgrass & Nutgrass Killer	Her	Liq	99.52%
Ortho Diazinon Soil and Turf Insect Control	Ins	Gra	95%
Ortho Dormant Disease Control Lime Sulfur Spray	Fun	Spr	76%
Ortho Dursban Lawn and Garden Insect Control	Ins	Gra	99%
Ortho Fire Ant Bait	Ins	Gra	99%
Ortho Fire Ant Killer Granules	Ins	Gra	95%
Ortho Grass-B-Gon Grass Killer	Her	Spr	99.5%
Ortho Grass-B-Gon Grass Killer	Her	Liq	99.5%

Label Word	Class	Active Ingredients	Tumors/Cancer	Repro. Damage	Genetic Damage
C		DCPA 25%	x	o	o
C		Oryzalin 40.4%	x	o	o
C		Methanearsonate 47.8%	-	-	-
C		Neem 0.99%	-	-	-
C		Ground sesame plant 100%	o	o	o
W		Copper 98%	-	-	-
C		Diatomaceous earth 90%	o	o	o
	PY	Pyrethrins 0.2%	x	x	x
	SY	Piperonyl butoxide* 1.1%	-	-	o
C	OP	Acephate 75%	x	o	x
C		Atrazine 14%	x	o	o
N		Nematodes 10%	o	o	o
C		Methanearsonate 0.48%	-	-	-
C	OP	Diazinon 5%	o	x	x
C		Calcium polysulfides 26%	-	-	-
C	OP	Chlorpyrifos 1%	o	o	x
C	OP	Chlorpyrifos 1%	o	o	x
C	OP	Diazinon 5%	o	x	x
C		Fluazifop-butyl 0.48%	-	-	-
C		Fluazifop-butyl 0.5%	-	-	-

Table 7.2

Outdoor Use Pesticides - 1995

Brand Name	Use	Formulation	Inert Ingredients
Ortho Ground Clear Super Edger Grass & Weed Control	Her	Liq	99.5%
Ortho Kleeraway Systemic Weed and Grass Killer	Her	Liq	92.5%
Ortho Mole Cricket Bait Formula II	Ins	Gra	99.5%
Ortho Orthene Fire Ant Killer	Ins	Gra	25%
Ortho Sevin Brand Name Carbaryl 10 Dust	Ins	Gra	90%
Ortho Sevin Liquid	Ins	Liq	78.7%
Ortho Triox Vegetation Killer Formula A	Her	Liq	99.22%
Ortho Weed-B-Gon Ready Spray Lawn Weed Killer	Her	Spr	88.32%
Ortho Weed-B-Gone for Southern Lawns 3	Her	Liq	85.05%
P			
Pennington Penn-Organic Garden Dust	Ins	Dus	98.9%
Prentox Emulsifiable Spray Concentrate	Ins	Liq	8%
Q			
Quick Knock Down Wasp and Hornet Killer XI	Ins	Aer	99.675%
R			
Raid House and Garden Bug Killer	Ins	Aer	98.7%
Raid House and Garden Bug Killer	Ins	Aer	98.7%

Label Word	Class	Active Ingredients	Tumors/Cancer	Repro. Damage	Genetic Damage
C		Glyphosate 0.25%	x	o	o
		Oxyflurofen 0.25%	x	x	x
C		Glyphosate 7.5%	x	o	o
C	OP	Chlorpyrifos 0.5%	o	o	x
C	OP	Acephate 75%	x	o	x
C	CB	Carbaryl 10%	x	o	x
C	CB	Carbaryl 21.3%	x	o	x
D		Oxyflurofen 0.7%	x	x	x
		Imazapyr 0.08%	-	-	-
W		2,4-D 5.64%	x	x	x
		MCPA 6.04%	o	x	x
C		MCPA 10.6%	o	x	x
		2,4-D 3.05%	x	x	x
		Dicamba 1.3%	-	x	x
C	PY	Pyrethrins 0.1%	x	x	x
	SY	Piperonyl butoxide* 1%	-	-	o
C	PY	Pyrethrins 0.96%	x	x	x
	SY	Piperonyl butoxide* 9.6%	-	-	o
		Petroleum distillate 81.44%	x	-	-
C	SP	Tetramethrin 0.2%	x	x	o
	SP	Phenothrin 0.125%	x	-	o
C	PY	Pyrethrins 0.25%	x	x	x
	SY	Piperonyl butoxide* 1.05%	-	-	o
C	PY	Pyrethrins 0.25%	x	x	x
	SY	Piperonyl butoxide* 1.05%	-	-	o

Table 7.2

Outdoor Use Pesticides - 1995

Brand Name	Use	Formulation	Inert Ingredients
Raid Wasp and Hornet Killer III	Ins	Aer	99.156%
Rite Green Bahia Weed and Feed 20-4-6	Her	Gra	99.188%
Rite Green St. Augustine Weed and Feed	Her	Gra	99.08%
Rodent Pellets	Rod	Bai	98%

S

Brand Name	Use	Formulation	Inert Ingredients
Safer BioNeem Insecticide and Repellent	Ins	Liq	99.91%
Safer Flower Garden Insecticidal Soap	Ins	Liq	51%
Safer Rose & Flower Japanese Beetle Spray	Ins	Liq	99.1%
Safer Tomato and Vegetable Insect Killer	Ins	Spr	98.88%
Scotts Flower and Garden Weed Preventer	Her	Gra	98.536%
Scotts Turf Builder Plus Insect Control	Ins	Gra	97.12%
Security Fungi-Gard	Fun	Liq	88.76%
Security System Granular Insecticide for House Plants	Ins	Gra	99%
Sevin 5% Dust Brand of Carbaryl Insecticide	Ins	Dus	95%
Sevin Liquid 2F Brand of Carbaryl Insecticide	Ins	Liq	77.5%
Shoot Out Grass and Weed Killer Concentrate	Her	Spr	95%
Soluble Oil Spray Superior 70 - Second Type	Ins	Liq	2%
Spectacide Dursban Indoor & Outdoor Insect Control	Ins	Liq	94%
Spectracide Bug Stop Concentrate	Ins	Liq	97.5%

Label Word	Class	Active Ingredients	Tumors/Cancer	Repro. Damage	Genetic Damage
W	CB	Propoxur 0.475%	x	o	o
	SP	Tetramethrin 0.369%	x	x	o
C		MCPA 0.576%	o	x	x
		2,4-D 0.165%	x	x	x
		Dicamba 0.07%	-	x	x
C		Atrazine 0.928%	x	o	o
C		Magnesium phosphide 2%	-	-	-
C		Neem 0.09%	-	-	-
C		Soap 49%	o	o	o
C		Neem 0.09%	-	-	-
C	PY	Pyrethrins 0.01%	x	x	x
		Soap 1%	o	o	o
C		Trifluralin 1.47%	x	o	o
C	OP	Diazinon 2.88%	o	x	x
W		Chlorothalonil 11.24%	x	o	x
W	OP	Disulfuton 1%	-	-	x
C	CB	Carbaryl 5%	x	o	x
C	CB	Carbaryl 22.5%	x	o	x
C		Glyphosate 5%	x	o	o
C		Petroleum oil 98%	x	-	-
C	OP	Chlorpyrifos 6%	o	o	x
C	SP	Permethrin 2.5%	x	x	o

Table 7.2

Outdoor Use Pesticides - 1995

Brand Name	Use	Formulation	Inert Ingredients
Spectracide Diazinon Concentrate Lawn Garden	Ins	Liq	75%
Spectracide Dursban Indoor Outdoor Insect Concentrate	Ins	Liq	94%
Spectracide Fire Ant Killer Granules with Accelerator	Ins	Gra	95%
Spectracide Grass and Weed Killer with XLC	Her	Spr	99.77%
Spectracide Lawn & Garden Insect Control Diazinon	Ins	Liq	75%
Spectracide Lawn Weed Killer 2 WB	Her	Liq	87.91%
Spectracide Lawn and Garden Insect Control	Ins	Liq	97.5%
Spectracide Rose and Garden Insect Killer	Ins	Aer	99.96%
Spectracide Soil and Turf Insect Control 6000	Ins	Gra	95%
Spectracide Spot Weed Killer 33 Plus	Her	Spr	99.04%
Spectracide Yard Flea and Tick Killer	Ins	Spr	94%
Streptomycin Sulfate 17	Fun	Pow	78.8%
Subdue Plant Pak II	Fun	Pow	75%
Sun Spray Ultra Fine Year Round Pesticide	Ins	Liq	1.2%
Sunni Green Ironized Weed and Feed	Her	Gra	99.21%
Sunniland 25% Diazinon Liquid Concentrate	Ins	Liq	75%
Sunniland 50% Malathion Emulsifiable Concentrate	Ins	Liq	50%

Label Word	Class	Active Ingredients	Tumors/Cancer	Repro. Damage	Genetic Damage
W	OP	Diazinon 25%	o	x	x
C	OP	Chlorpyrifos 6%	o	o	x
C	OP	Diazinon 5%	o	x	x
W		Diquat 0.23%	x	x	x
W	OP	Diazinon 25%	o	x	x
C		2,4-D 7.59%	x	x	x
		MCPA 3.66%	o	x	x
		Dicamba 0.84%	-	x	x
C	SP	Permethrin 2.5%	x	x	o
C	PY	Pyrethrins 0.02%	x	x	x
	SY	Piperonyl butoxide* 0.02%	-	-	o
C	OP	Diazinon 5%	o	x	x
C		2,4-D 0.593%	x	x	x
		MCPA 0.287%	o	x	x
		Dicamba 0.066%	-	x	x
C	OP	Chlorpyrifos 6%	o	o	x
C		Streptomycin sulfate 21.2%	o	o	o
C		Metalaxyl 99%	x	o	o
C		Paraffinic oil 98.8%	-	-	-
C		Atrazine 0.79%	x	o	o
C	OP	Diazinon 25%	o	x	x
C	OP	Malathion 50%	x	o	o

Table 7.2
Outdoor Use Pesticides - 1995

Brand Name	Use	Formulation	Inert Ingredients
Sunniland Chinch Bug Spray Contains Dursban	Ins	Liq	97.65%
Sunniland Ethion and Oil Spray for Citrus	Ins	Liq	91.6%
Sunniland Liquid Lawn Edger	Her	Spr	99.77%
Sunniland Mole Cricket Bait	Ins	Bai	99.5%
Sunniland St. Augustine Lawn Weed Killer	Her	Liq	57.7%
Sunniland SuperBrand Mole Cricket Bait	Ins	Bai	99.5%
Super KGro Southern Broadleaf Weed Killer	Her	Liq	85.05%
Surflan A.S	Her	Liq	59.6%
Sweeneys Poison Peanuts Pellets	Rod	Bai	98%
T			
Terrachlor 2E Lawn Fungicide	Fun	Liq	76%
Thiodan Insect Spray	Ins	Liq	90.1%
Thiomyl Turf & Ornamental Systemic Fungicide	Fun	Dus	50%
Thuricide HPC	Ins	Liq	99.2%
Tom Cat Rat All Weather Rodent Block	Rod	Bai	99.995%
Tom Cat Rat and Mouse Bait	Rod	Bai	99.995%
Tri-basic Copper Sulfate	Fun	Dus	52%
Turf Fungicide Granule	Fun	Gra	98.5%
Two Way Miticide 25% Contains Morestan	Ins	Dus	75%
U			
Ultra-Fine Oil Year Round Pestcide Oil	Ins	Liq	1.2%

Label Word	Class	Active Ingredients	Tumors/Cancer	Repro. Damage	Genetic Damage
C	OP	Chlorpyrifos 2.35%	o	o	x
C		Ethion 8.4%	o	x	o
C		Diquat 0.23%	x	x	x
C	OP	Chlorpyrifos 0.5%	o	o	x
C		Atrazine 40.8%	x	o	o
C	OP	Diazinon 5%	o	x	x
C		MCPA 10.6%	o	x	x
		2,4-D 3.05%	x	x	x
		Dicamba 1.3%	-	x	x
C		Oryzalin 40.4%	x	o	o
C		Zinc phosphide 2%	-	-	-
C		PCNB 24%	x	o	x
W	CH	Endosulfan 9.9%	-	o	o
C		Thiophanate-methyl 50%	x	-	o
C		B.T. 0.8%	o	o	o
C		Diphacinone 0.005%	-	-	o
C		Diphacinone 0.005%	-	-	o
W		Copper 48%	-	-	-
C		Chlorophenoxy 1.5%	-	-	-
C		Oxythioquinox 25%	-	x	x
C		Paraffinic oil 98.8%	-	-	-

Table 7.2

Outdoor Use Pesticides - 1995

Brand Name	Use	Formulation	Inert Ingredients
V			
Vantage Herbicide	Her	Liq	87%
Vertagreen St. Augustine Weed and Feed	Her	Fer	98.84%
Vertagreen Weed and Feed	Her	Fer	99.663%
W			
Wettable or Dusting Sulfur	Fun	Dus	10%
Whitmire PT300 DS Orthene Directed Spray Insecticide	Ins	Aer	97%
Wilco Gopher Getter Type I Bait	Rod	Gra	99.5%

Label Word	Class	Active Ingredients	Tumors/Cancer	Repro. Damage	Genetic Damage
C		Sethoxydim 13%	-	-	-
C		Atrazine 1.16%	x	o	o
C		2,4-D 0.313%	x	x	x
		MCPA 0.314%	o	x	x
		MCPP 0.31%	-	x	x
C		Sulfur 90%	o	o	o
W	OP	Acephate 3%	x	o	x
D		Strychnine 0.5%	-	-	-

* Piperonyl butoxide causes cancer and birth defects in rats (see pages 114-115).

8

Pet Use Pesticides

So, naturalists observe, a flea
Hath smaller fleas that on him prey;
And these have smaller fleas to bite 'em,
And so proceed ad infinitum.

Jonathan Swift (1667-1745)

Kind and caring adults can be severely stressed when their personal share of the pet population becomes a walking flea factory. The response to a flea infestation is often anxiety – and reaching for a container of designer poison. This pattern, which characterizes so many human interactions with the insect world, can be very hazardous to your pet.

Pet owners would be horrified at a suggestion that they put toxic chemicals into their pet's food or water. But you are doing the equivalent of that when you use pet shampoos, dips, sprays, powders, or collars that contain toxic pesticides. The pesticides can be absorbed directly into your pet's body.

In this chapter we discuss pesticides used for fleas on cats and dogs. These products are the majority of pest control products sold over-the-counter for use on pets. Because there is a detailed discussion of nontoxic and least toxic alternative flea control methods in chapter six on indoor use pesticides, we do not repeat it here (see pages 110-114).

This chapter includes:
- ◆ A description of the use, formulations, ingredients, and acute and chronic toxicity of the ingredients in pet use pesticides found in our surveys.
- ◆ A table of brand name products from our surveys, with use, ingredients, and a chronic toxicity summary for the active ingredient. Since the tables are long, we put them at the end of the chapter to make it easier for you to use them.

Part I: Information on Pet Use Pesticides

Formulations. All of the pesticides found in our survey were insecticides or insect growth regulators. Figure 8.1 shows that slightly more than half were liquids and sprays. Pesticides in liquids and sprays are directly absorbed into your pet's body through the skin. How much is absorbed, and how readily, depends on the breed, size, length of fur, and condition of the coat. If your pet has a skin rash, irritation, or skin problems, pesticides will enter more easily and in larger amounts.

Dusts and powders were 16% of the products. Pesticides in these forms are usually poorly absorbed if they are used dry. If the pesticide is not highly toxic, dusts and powders in general pose less of a health risk to your pet than liquids and sprays. However a wet toxic dust or powder can be more hazardous than a more dilute liquid.

Aerosols were 5% of the products in our survey. Aerosols are the most likely to cause contamination beyond the treatment area. They are more likely to contain a higher percentage of toxic inert ingredients, and formulated with petroleum based solvents. We recommend you do not use any aerosol products.

Flea collars were 21% of the products in our survey. A collar may be a matter of convenience for you, but it is a source of continuing toxic exposure to your pet. Children who play with, groom, and otherwise handle the pet have exposure to toxic pesticides as well.

Figure 8.1

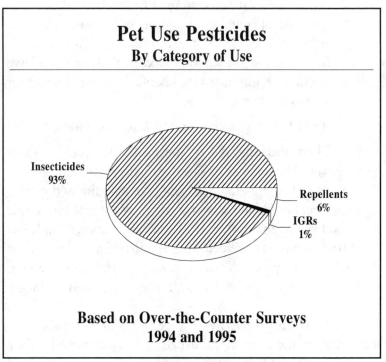

Pet Use Pesticides
By Category of Use

Insecticides 93%

Repellents 6%

IGRs 1%

**Based on Over-the-Counter Surveys
1994 and 1995**

Classes of Pesticides

Pyrethrin was the pesticide found the most often in pet products in our survey. Pyrethrins, made from flowers (a type of chrysanthemum), are usually formulated (mixed) with the synergists piperonyl butoxide or MGK 264 to increase their killing power. Figure 8.2 shows that 42% of the brand name products contained pyrethrins, and a similar percent, piperonyl butoxide. Synthetic pyrethroids, which are chemical imitations of the natural pyrethrins, were in 13% of the products.

Nerve-gas type: The pesticides second in frequency in our survey were the organophosphates. These nerve-gas type insecticides were found in 30% of the products, including the following active ingredients: chlorpyrifos, diazinon, malathion, naled, phosmet, and tetrachlorvinphos. Carbamates, also nerve-gas pesticides, were found in 17% of the products, specifically carbaryl and propoxur.

Botanicals and inorganics. Natural products from citrus, herbs, and flower and plant oils were in one-fifth of the products.

Figure 8.2

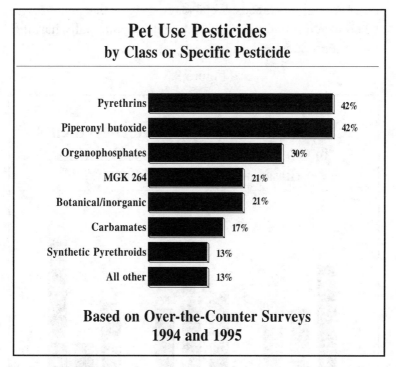

Acute Toxicity

Pets face the same risk of poisoning from toxic pesticides as humans do. Pets cannot tell you their symptoms. If you are treating your pet with pesticide products, do not assume that if they are not showing striking and obvious effects, they are not being poisoned. You should be very alert to mild treatment related effects that may only show up as subtle changes in behavior, or any unusual pattern of behavior in your pet.

The acute health effects of the active ingredient pesticides in pet products are described in detail in chapter four. This chapter has relevance since both you and your pet can be poisoned by the active ingredients in these products.

You should also be aware that just because a pet product contains "natural" ingredients does not mean that it is trouble-free for your pet. Your pet may react to some ingredients in products made from roots, flowers, plants and other natural substances. We also remind you that pennyroyal, a herb often found in natural products is potentially harmful to the reproductive system.

Figure 8.3

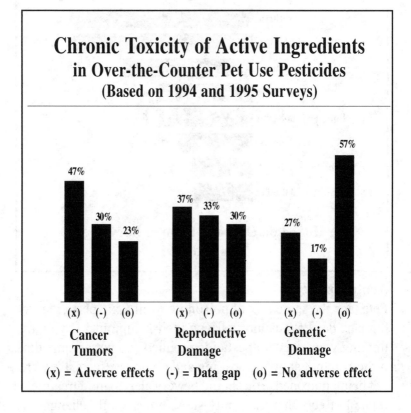

Chronic Toxicity

Table 8.1 at the end of this chapter includes the chronic toxicity potential for each active ingredient pesticide found in the brand name products from our survey. Figure 8.3 below is a summary of this information.

Cancer/tumors. Figure 8.4 shows that almost half the active ingredient pesticides in these pet use products are known or suspected to cause tumors or cancer in animals (x). There are data gaps for almost two-thirds of the pesticides – either no data or inadequate data to determine whether the pesticide causes cancer (-). There is no apparent evidence for tumor formation for about one-fourth (o).

Reproductive damage. The figure also shows that close to forty percent of the active ingredients are known or suspected to cause reproductive damage (x). There are data gaps for one-third of the pesticides. There is no apparent evidence of reproductive damage for almost one-third of the ingredients.

Genetic damage. Finally, Figure 8.3 shows that about just over one-fourth of the active ingredient pesticides are known or suspected to cause genetic damage. There are data gaps for close to twenty percent. There is no apparent evidence of direct genetic damage for close to sixty percent of the ingredients.

Animal studies are part of determining the risk to human populations from exposure to toxic chemicals. However, because a chemical causes tumors, reproductive damage, or genetic damage in the laboratory, does not mean that it will cause that effect in everyone using the product or otherwise exposed to its contents.

Cancer in dogs. A recent study found that dogs were more likely to have lymphoma (cancer of the lymphatic system) if their owners used chemical lawn treatments, compared to dogs whose owners did not. This raises concerns about long-term effects of chronic low-level exposures, especially since many products sold for use on dogs contain ingredients known or suspected to cause tumors and cancer in laboratory animals.

Cancer in children. A study done in Missouri found that children were six times more likely to get brain cancer if their parents use flea collars on their pets (see page 77 in chapter five.)

Nontoxic and Least Toxic Alternatives

At this point in our discussion, we usually provide you with our recommendations for nontoxic and least toxic alternative for flea control that do not involve the use of toxic pesticides. We have already done this in detail in chapter six on indoor use pesticides. Please refer to the discussion of fleas on page 110 -114 for this information.

Part III Brand Name Product Listing

The table that follows lists pet use brand name products found in our surveys.

About piperonyl butoxide (puh-PAIR-uh-nill bew-TOX-ide).You will see in the tables that many of the pet products contain the synergist piperonyl butoxide. The chronic toxicity data in table 8.1 show data gaps for piperonyl butoxide for cancer and birth defects. Two recent reports in the open literature show that piperonyl butoxide causes liver cancer and birth defects in rats. The EPA (Environmental Protection Agency) has not included these findings in assessing piperonyl butoxide. We think you should know this since this ingredient is in so many products. See Appendix C on page 328 for other brand name products that contain it.

About MGK-264. You will also see another synergist, MGK-264, which may be listed on the label by its chemical name – bicycloheptene dicarboximide. MGK-264, often used in place of, or along with piperonyl butoxide, causes chronic toxic effects as well. You will see in the tables, both synergists can be in the product at a higher percentage than the other active ingredients. All the surveyed brand name products containing MGK-264 are listed in Appendix C on page 328.

Key to Brand Name
Product Table

Use

Her = Herbicide   **Mul** = Multiple Uses
IGR = Insect Growth Regulator **PGR** = Plant Growth Regulator
Fun = Fungicide   **Rep** = Repellent
Mol = Molluscicide   **Rod** = Rodenticide

Formulation

Aer = Aerosol	**Gel** = Gel
Bat = Bait	**Grn** = Granule
Bar = Barrier	**Liq** = Liquid
Bom = Bomb	**Lot** = Lotion
Col = Collar	**Pel** = Pellet
Dus = Dust	**Pow** = Powder
Fer = Fertilizer	**Sld** = Solid
Fog = Fogger	**Spr** = Spray
Fom = Foam	**Stp** = Strip
Fum = Fumigant	**Tap** = Tape
Gas = Gas	**Trp** = Trap
Rep = Repellent	**Tab** = Tablet

Label Word

D = Danger
W = Warning
C = Caution
N = Not required or not on label

Class

CB = Methyl carbamate   **PY** = Pyrethrin
CH = Chlorinated hydrocarbon **SP** = Synthetic pyrethroid
OP = Organophosphate   **SY** = Synergist

Tumors/Cancer

A tumor is an abnormal growth of tissue that can be benign or malignant. Another name for a malignant tumor is cancer. Substances that cause cancer are called *carcinogens*. Substances that cause tumors are called *oncogens*.

Repro. Damage

Reproductive damage refers to effects such as death of the embryo or fetus (equivalent to spontaneous abortion and stillbirth in humans), low birth weight, sterility/infertility. It also includes birth defects such as structural defects such as missing arms or legs, or hole in the heart, spina bifida etc. Substances that cause birth defects are called *teratogens*.

Genetic Damage

Genetic damage refers to effects on genetic material including genes, chromosomes, and DNA.

(**X**) = Possible adverse effect

(**-**) = Either no data available or information available is not sufficient to make a determination

(**0**) = Adequate data and no adverse effect noted.

* Sources for the above chronic toxicity data are from Cal-EPA SB-950 Toxicology Summaries, U.S.EPA Factsheets, U.S.EPA R.E.Ds (Registration Eligibility Documents), and scientific journals.

Table 8.1
Pet Use Pesticides - 1994

Brand Name	Use	Formulation	Inert Ingredients
A			
Adams 14 Day Residual Flea & Tick Mist	Ins	Spr	97.48%
Adams Flea & Tick Dip With Dursban	Ins	Liq	96.16%
Adams Flea And Tick Dip	Ins	Liq	47.00%
Adams Flea And Tick Dust II	Ins	Dus	76.40%
Adams Flea And Tick Mist	Ins	Spr	97.35%
Adams Pyrethrin Dip	Ins	Liq	87.65%
B			
Bansect Flea & Tick Collar for Cats	Ins	Col	90.00%
Bansect Flea & Tick Collar for Dogs	Ins	Col	85.00%
C			
Cardinal Rid Flea & Tick Shampoo Concentrate	Ins	Liq	97.80%
Cardinal Rid Flea & Tick Spray	Ins	Spr	99.40%
Cardinal Rid Yard and Kennel Flea & Tick Spray	Ins	Liq	93.3%
Citrus Dip for Dogs	Ins	Liq	22.00%

Label Word	Class	Active Ingredients	Tumors/Cancer	Repro. Damage	Genetic Damage
W		Pyrethrins 0.15%	x	x	x
	SY	Piperonyl butoxide* 0.37%	-	-	o
	SY	MGK 264 1%	x	x	o
		Di-n-propyl isocinchomeronate 1%	-	-	-
C	OP	Chlorpyrifos 3.84%	o	o	x
C	OP	Malathion 53%	x	o	o
C		Pyrethrins 0.1%	x	x	x
	SY	Piperonyl butoxide* 1.0%	-	-	o
	CB	Carbaryl 12.5%	x	o	x
		Silica gel 10%	o	o	o
C		Pyrethrins 0.15%	x	x	x
	SY	Piperonyl butoxide* 1.5%	-	-	o
	SY	MGK 264 0.5%	x	x	o
		Di-n-propyl isocinchomerate 0.5%	-	-	-
C		Pyrethrins 97%	x	x	x
	SY	Piperonyl butoxide* 3.74%	-	-	o
	SY	MGK 264 5.7%	x	x	o
		Di-n-propylisocinchomerate 1.94%	-	-	-
C	OP	Naled 10%	x	x	o
C	OP	Naled 15%	x	x	o
C	SY	Piperonyl butoxide* 2%	-	-	o
		Pyrethrins 0.2%	x	x	x
C		Pyrethrins 0.05%	x	x	x
	SY	Piperonyl butoxide* 0.5%	-	-	o
	SP	Permethrin 0.05%	x	x	o
C	OP	Chlorpyrifos 6.7%	o	o	x
		D-Limonene 78%	o	o	o

Table 8.1
Pet Use Pesticides - 1994

Brand Name	Use	Formulation	Inert Ingredients
Citrus Shampoo for Dogs & Cats	Ins	Liq	
Citrus Spray for Cats	Ins	Spr	95.00%
Citrus Spray for Dogs	Ins	Spr	90.00%
Color & Herbal Dog Collar	Ins	Col	
Color & Herbal Cat Collar	Ins	Col	
Color & Herbal Renewal Oil	Ins	Liq	
Color Guard Cat Collar	Ins	Col	97.00%
Color Guard Dog Collar	Ins	Col	92.00%
ColorGuard Neon-Colored Collar for Cats	Ins	Col	97.00%
ColorGuard Neon-Colored Collar for Dogs	Ins	Col	92.00%
D			
Defend Exspot Insecticide For Dogs	Ins	Liq	35.00%
Defend Just-For-Cats	Ins	Spr	97.35%
E			
Enforcer Flea & Tick Shampoo for Pets	Ins	Liq	99.37%
F			
Farnum Flys-Off Insect Repellent For Dogs	Ins	Aer	99.24%

Label Word	Class	Active Ingredients	Tumors/Cancer	Repro. Damage	Genetic Damage
C		D-Limonene	o	o	o
		D-Limonene 5%	o	o	o
		D-Limonene 10%	o	o	o
		Chamomile	o	o	o
		Pennyroyal	-	x	-
		Eucalyptus	o	o	o
		Natural oils	o	o	o
		Citronella	o	o	o
		Chamomile	o	o	o
		Pennyroyal	-	x	-
		Eucalyptus	o	o	o
		Natural oils	o	o	o
		Citronella	o	o	o
		Natural oils	o	o	o
C	OP	Chlorpyrifos 3%	o	o	x
C	OP	Chlorpyrifos 8%	o	o	x
C	OP	Chlorpyrifos 3%	o	o	x
C	OP	Chlorpyrifos 8%	o	o	x
C	SP	Permethrin 65%	x	x	o
W		Pyrethrins 0.15%	x	x	x
	SY	Piperonyl butoxide* 1.5%	-	-	o
	SY	MGK 264 1%	x	x	o
C		Pyrethrins 0.1%	x	x	x
	SY	Piperonyl butoxide* 0.2%	-	-	o
	SY	MGK 264 0.33%	x	x	o
W		Pyrethrins 0.14%	x	x	x
		Rotenone 0.25%	x	x	x
	SY	Piperonyl butoxide* 0.37%	-	-	o

Table 8.1

Pet Use Pesticides - 1994

Brand Name	Use	Formulation	Inert Ingredients
Farnum Timed Release 8-Day Dermatological Flea Foam	Ins	Fom	98.81%
Flea Halt Collar For Dogs	Ins	Col	85.00%
Flea Stop Fly Repellent Ointment	Rep	Liq	21.80%
Flea Stop Zone Control For Home Home Zone Total Release Fogger	Ins	Fog	99.28%
Flea Stop Zone Control For Pets Pet Zone Concentrated Citrus Scent Shampoo for Cats & Kittens	Ins	Liq	96.30%
Flea Stop Zone Control for Pets, Pet Zone Pet Spray for Cats & Kittens	Ins	Spr	87.65%
G			
Grants Dog & Cat Repellent	Rep	Grn	98.00%
Grants Dog Repellent	Rep Ins	Sld	15%
H			
Hartz 2 In 1 Dog Flea Soap	Ins	Sld	10.84%
Hartz 2 In 1 Flea & Tick Collar for Cats	Ins	Col	86.30%
Hartz 2 In 1 Flea & Tick Collar for Dogs	Ins	Col	86.30%
Hartz 2 In 1 Flea & Tick Killer for Cats Fine Mist	Ins	Spr	99.62%
Hartz 2 In 1 Flea & Tick Powder For Cats	Ins	Pow	97.00%

Label Word	Class	Active Ingredients	Tumors/Cancer	Repro. Damage	Genetic Damage
C		Pyrethrins 0.15%	x	x	x
	SY	Piperonyl butoxide* 0.7%	-	-	o
	SY	MGK 264 0.34%	x	x	o
C	OP	Diazinon 15%	o	x	x
W		D-Limonene 78.2%	o	o	o
C	SP	Fenvalerate 0.4%	x	x	o
	SY	MGK 264 0.17%	x	x	o
	SY	Piperonyl butoxide* 0.1%	-	-	o
		Pyrethrins 0.05%	x	x	x
W		Linalool 3.7%	o	o	o
C		D-Limonene 0.92%	o	o	o
		Linalool 0.93%	o	o	o
	SY	Piperonyl butoxide* 0.5%	-	-	o
		Propylene Glycol 10.00%	-	-	-
C		Methyl nonyl ketone 2%	-	-	-
C		Naphthalene 78%	-	-	o
		Oil of mustard 5%	o	o	o
	CH	Paradichlorobenzene 2%	x	x	o
C		Pyrethrins 0.03%	x	x	x
	SY	Piperonyl butoxide* 0.05%	x	x	o
	SY	MGK 264 0.08%	x	x	o
		Anhydrous soap 89%	-	-	-
C	OP	Tetrachlorvinphos 13.7%	x	-	x
C	OP	Tetrachlorvinphos 13.7%	x	-	x
C		Pyrethrins. 0.06%	x	x	x
	SY	Piperonyl butoxide* 0.12%	-	-	o
	SY	MGK 264 0.2%	x	x	o
C	OP	Tetrachlorvinphos 3%	x	-	x

Table 8.1

Pet Use Pesticides - 1994

Brand Name	Use	Formulation	Inert Ingredients
Hartz 2 In 1 Flea & Tick Powder For Dogs	Ins	Pow	97.00%
Hartz 2 In 1 Flea & Tick Spray	Ins	Spr	98.92%
Hartz 2 In 1 Flea & Tick Spray For Cats	Ins	Spr	99.01%
Hartz 2 In 1 Flea & Tick Spray For Dogs	Ins	Spr	99.01%
Hartz 2 In 1 Luster Bath for Cats	Ins	Liq	99.68%
Hartz 2 In 1 Rid Flea Shampoo for Dogs	Ins	Liq	99.74%
Hartz 2 in 1 Flea & Tick Dip	Ins	Dip	97.89%
Hartz Blockade For Cats	Rep Ins	Spr	90.91%
Hills Flea Stop Zone Control for Pets, Pet Zone, Flea Spray for Dogs & Cats	Ins	Aer	95.00%
Hills Flea Stop Zone Control for Pets, Pet. Zone, Flea & Tick Powder for Dogs, Cats, Puppies, & Kittens	Ins	Pow	90.40%
Hills Flea Stop Zone Control for Pets, Pet Zone, Shampoo for Dogs, Cats, Puppies & Kittens	Ins	Liq	95.00%
Hills Flea Stop Zone Control for Pets, Pet Zone Pet Spray for Cats & Kittens	Ins	Spr	97.65%
Hills VIP Veterinarian Insecticide Products Yard Zone Control for Yard Concentrated Yard Spray	Ins	Liq	93.12%
L			
Lassie Flea & Tick Powder for Cats	Ins	Pow	97.00%

Label Word	Class	Active Ingredients	Tumors/Cancer	Repro. Damage	Genetic Damage
C	OP	Tetrachlorvinphos 3%	x	-	x
C	OP	Tetrachlorvinphos 1.08%	x	-	x
C	OP	Tetrachlorvinphos 0.99%	x	-	x
C	OP	Tetrachlorvinphos 0.99%	x	-	x
C		Pyrethrins 0.05%	x	x	x
	SY	Piperonyl butoxide* 0.1%	-	-	o
C		Pyrethrins 0.04%	x	x	x
	SY	Piperonyl butoxide* 0.08%	-	-	o
	SY	MGK 264 0.14%	x	x	o
C		Pyrethrins 0.33%	x	x	x
	SY	Piperonyl butoxide* 0.67%	-	-	o
	SY	MGK 264 1.11%	x	x	o
C		Deet 9%	-	x	o
	SP	Fenvalerate 0.09%	x	x	o
C		D-Limonene 5%	o	o	o
C	CB	Carbaryl 5%	x	o	x
		Butoxypolypropylene 4%	-	-	-
	SY	Piperonyl butoxide*. 0.5%	-	-	o
		Pyrethrins 0.1%	x	x	x
W		D-Limonene 5%	o	o	o
C		D-Limonene 0.92%	o	o	o
	SY	Piperonyl butoxide* 0.5%	-	-	o
		Linalool 0.93%	o	o	o
W	SP	Fenvalerate 6.88%	x	x	o
C	OP	Tetrachlorvinphos 3%	x	-	x

Table 8.1
Pet Use Pesticides - 1994

Brand Name	Use	Formulation	Inert Ingredients
Lassie Flea & Tick Powder for Dogs	Ins	Pow	97.00%
Lassie Flea & Tick Pump Spray for Dogs	Ins	Spr	99.34%
Lassie Flea & Tick Spray for Dogs	Ins	Aer	99.89%
Longlife 90 Day Brand Collar For Cats	Ins	Col	86.3%
Longlife 90 Day Brand Collar For Dogs	Ins	Col	86.3%
M			
Mycodex Pet Shampoo With 3X Pyrethrins	Ins	Liq	98.35%
Mycodex Pet Shampoo With Carbaryl	Ins	Liq	99.50%
P			
Pet Gold 14 Day Flea & Tick Spray	Ins	Spr	99.89%
Pet Gold Carpet Treatment #1	Ins	Pow	
Pet Gold Extra Strength Flea & Tick Powder	Ins	Pow	76.40%
Pet Gold Flea & Tick Dip	Ins	Liq	97.89%
Pet Gold Flea & Tick Shampoo	Ins	Liq	97.85%
Pet Gold Flea & Tick Spray	Ins	Spr	97.85%

Label Word	Class	Active Ingredients	Tumors/Cancer	Repro. Damage	Genetic Damage
C	OP	Tetrachlorvinphos 3%	x	-	x
C		Pyrethrins 0.06%	x	x	x
	SY	Piperonyl butoxide* 0.6%	-	-	o
C		Pyrethrins 0.06%	x	x	x
	SP	Permethrin 0.05%	x	x	o
C	OP	Tetrachlorvinphos 13.7%	x	o	x
C	OP	Tetrachlorvinphos 13.7%	x	-	x
C		Pyrethrins 0.15%	x	x	x
	SY	Piperonyl butoxide* 1.5%	-	-	o
C	CB	Carbaryl 0.5%	x	o	x
C		Pyrethrins 0.06%	x	x	x
	SP	Permethrin 0.05%	x	x	o
C		Boric acid	-	x	x
		Bitrex	-	-	-
C		Pyrethrins 0.1%	x	x	x
	SY	Piperonyl butoxide* 1%	-	-	o
	CB	Carbaryl 12.5%	x	o	x
		Silica gel 10%	o	o	o
C		Pyrethrin 0.33%	x	x	x
	SY	Piperonyl butoxide* 0.67%	-	-	o
	SY	MGK 264 0.11%	x	x	o
W		Pyrethrins 0.15%	x	x	x
	SY	Piperonyl butoxide* 1%	-	-	o
	SY	MGK 264 0.5%	x	x	o
		Di-n-propyl isocinchomeronate 0.5%	-	-	-
W		Pyrethrins 0.15%	x	x	x
	SY	Piperonyl butoxide* 1%	-	-	o
	SY	MGK 264 0.5%	x	x	o
		Di-n-propyl isocinchomeronate 0.5%	-	-	-

Table 8.1
Pet Use Pesticides - 1994

Brand Name	Use	Formulation	Inert Ingredients
Pet Gold Flea And Tick Carpet Powder	Ins	Pow	98.35%
Pet Gold Herbal Pet Powder For Dogs	Rep	Pow	
Pet Gold Pennyroyal Flea & Tick Shampoo	Ins	Liq	99.17%
Pet Gold Repellent Ointment	Ins	Sld	97.35%
S			
Safer Flea & Tick Attack for Pets Ready-To-Use Spray	Ins	Spr	98.99%
Safer Flea Soap for Cats	Ins	Liq	75.00%
Safer Flea Soap for Dogs	Ins	Liq	75.00%
Scratchex Flea & Tick Collar for Cats	Ins	Col	97.00%
Scratchex Flea & Tick Collar for Dogs	Ins	Col	92.00%
Sergeants 11 Month Flea Collar for Cats	Ins	Col	97.00%
Sergeants Dual Action Flea & Tick Collar (with Sendran)	Ins	Col	80.80%
Sergeants Dual Action Flea & Tick Collar (with Sendran) specially developed for Cats	Ins	Col	90.60%
Sergeants Flea & Tick Dip	Ins	Liq	96.80%
Sergeants Flea & Tick Powder for Cats	Ins	Pow	95.00%
Sergeants Flea & Tick Powder for Dogs	Ins	Pow	95.00%
Sergeants Flea & Tick Spray With Coat Conditioner for Dogs	Ins	Spr	99.75%
Sergeants Pump Dog Flea & Tick Spray	Ins	Spr	99.50%
Sergeants Skip Flea & Tick Spray Plus Shampoo	Ins	Spr	99.40%

Label Word	Class	Active Ingredients	Tumors/Cancer	Repro. Damage	Genetic Damage
C		Pyrethrins 0.15%	x	x	x
	SY	Piperonyl butoxide* 1.5%	-	-	o
N		Silica gel	o	o	o
		Pennyroyal	-	x	-
		Eucalyptus	o	o	o
		Pyrethrum leaf powder	-	-	-
C	SY	Piperonyl butoxide* 0.75%	-	-	o
		Pyrethrins 0.08%	x	x	x
C		Pyrethrins 0.15%	x	x	x
	SY	Piperonyl butoxide* 1%	-	-	o
	SY	MGK 264 0.5%	x	x	o
		Di-n-propyl isocinchomeronate 1%	-	-	-
C		Pyrethrins 0.01%	x	x	x
		Potassium salts of fatty acids 1%	o	o	o
C		Potassium salts of fatty acids 25%	o	o	o
C		Potassium salts of fatty acids 25%	o	o	o
C	OP	Chlorpyrifos 3%	o	o	x
C	OP	Chlorpyrifos 8%	o	o	x
C	OP	Chlorpyrifos 3%	o	o	x
C	OP	Naled 15%	x	x	o
	CB	Propoxur 4.2%	x	o	o
C	OP	Naled 7%	x	x	o
	CB	Propoxur 2.4%	x	o	o
C	SP	Permethrin 3.2%	x	x	o
C	CB	Carbaryl 5%	x	o	x
C	CB	Carbaryl 5%	x	o	x
C	CB	Propoxur 0.25%	x	o	o
C	CB	Carbaryl 0.5%	x	o	x
C	SP	Permethrin 0.1%	x	x	o
	SY	Piperonyl butoxide* 0.5%	-	-	o

Table 8.1

Pet Use Pesticides - 1994

Brand Name	Use	Formulation	Inert Ingredients
Sergeants Skip-Flea & Tick Shampoo	Ins	Liq	99.40%
Sergeants Skip-Flea Soap (with D-Phenothrin)	Ins	Sld	99.62%
Shield Flea & Tick Control for Dogs	Ins	Liq	99.75%
Shield Flea & Tick Control Spray for Dogs	Ins	Aer	99.75%
Sulfodene Scratchex Flea & Tick Shampoo for Dogs & Cats	Ins	Liq	99.54%
Sulfodene Scratchex Flea & Tick Spray for Dogs	Ins	Aer	99.89%
Sulfodene Scratchex Power Dip	Ins	Liq	96.58%
Sulfodene Scratchex Power Dust	Ins	Pow	94.58%
T			
Timed-Release Flea Halt Flea & Tick Dip for Dogs	Ins	Liq	97.50%
Tomlyn Flea Tick And Lice Shampoo	Ins	Liq	99.66%
V			
Victory Flea Soap For Dogs	Ins	Sld	99.84%
Victory 11 Guaranteed Full Season Saf-T-Stretch Cat Collar	Ins	Col	97.00%

Label Word	Class	Active Ingredients	Tumors/Cancer	Repro. Damage	Genetic Damage
C	SP	Permethrin 0.1%	x	x	o
	SY	Piperonyl butoxide* 0.5%	-	-	o
W	SP	Phenothrin 0.08%	x	o	o
W	OP	Chlorpyrifos 0.25%	o	o	x
C	OP	Chlorpyrifos 0.25%	o	o	x
W		Pyrethrins 0.07%	x	x	x
	SY	Piperonyl butoxide* 0.15%	-	-	o
	SY	MGK 264 0.24%	x	x	o
C		Pyrethrins 0.06%	x	x	x
	SP	Permethrin 0.05%	x	x	o
C		Pyrethrins 0.54%	x	x	x
	SY	Piperonyl butoxide* 1.08%	-	-	o
	SY	MGK 264 1.8%	x	x	o
C	CB	Carbaryl 5%	x	o	x
	SY	Piperonyl butoxide* 0.13%	-	-	o
	SY	0.22%	-	x	o
		Pyrethrins 0.07%	x	x	x
C	OP	Chlorpyrifos 2.5%	o	o	x
C		Pyrethrins. 0.05%	x	x	x
	SY	Piperonyl butoxide* 0.11%	-	-	o
	SY	MGK 264 0.18%	x	x	o
C		Pyrethrins 0.03%	x	x	x
C	OP	Chlorpyrifos 3%	o	o	x
	SY	Piperonyl butoxide* 0.05%	-	-	o
	SY	MGK 264 0.08%	x	x	o

Table 8.1

Pet Use Pesticides - 1994

Brand Name	Use	Formulation	Inert Ingredients
X			
X-O-Trol Flea & Tick Spray For Dogs	Ins IGR	Spr	99.19%
Z			
Z3 Flea & Tick Powder For Cats	Ins	Pow	95.00%
Zema Dip 3.84% Dursban Concentrate	Ins	Liq	96.16%
Zema Pyrethrin Dip	Ins	Liq	96.70%
Zema Super Flea & Tick Spray For Dogs, Fast Acting	Ins	Spr	99.07%
Zodiac 11 Month Flea Collar For Dogs	Ins	Col	92.00%
Zodiac 11 Month Flea Collar For Dogs	Ins	Col	84.00%
Zodiac 21 Day Flea Dust For Dogs	Ins	Dus	95.00%
Zodiac 5 Month Flea & Tick Collar For Cats	Ins	Col	90.60%
Zodiac 5 Month Flea & Tick Collar For Dogs	Ins	Col	90.60%
Zodiac 5 Month Flea & Tick Collar For Large Dogs	Ins	Col	90.60%
Zodiac 5 Month Flea & Tick Collar For Small Dogs	Ins	Col	90.60%
Zodiac 5 Month Flea & Tick Collar With One Piece Buckle for Dogs	Ins	Col	90.60%
Zodiac 7 Month Flea & Tick Collar For Dogs	Ins	Col	85.00%
Zodiac Breakaway Flea & Tick Collar For Cats	Ins	Col	90.60%

Label Word	Class	Active Ingredients	Tumors/Cancer	Repro. Damage	Genetic Damage
C		Pyrethrins 0.05%	x	x	x
	SY	Piperonyl butoxide* 0.5%	-	-	o
	SP	Permethrins 0.2%	x	x	o
		0.06%	-	-	-
C	CB	Carbaryl 5%	x	o	x
C	OP	Chlorpyrifos 3.84%	o	o	x
C		Pyrethrins 0.3%	x	x	x
	SY	Piperonyl butoxide* 3%	-	-	o
C	OP	Chlorpyrifos 0.23%	o	o	x
		Pyrethrins 0.05%	x	x	x
	SY	Piperonyl butoxide* 0.1%	-	-	o
	SY	MGK 264 0.17%	x	x	o
		Petroleum distillate 0.38%	x	-	-
C	OP	Chlorpyrifos 8%	o	o	x
C	CB	Carbaryl 16%	x	o	x
C	OP	Phosmet 5%	x	x	x
C	CB	Propoxur 9.4%	x	o	o
C	CB	Propoxur 9.4%	x	o	o
C	CB	Propoxur 9.4%	x	o	o
C	CB	Propoxur 9.4%	x	o	o
C	CB	Propoxur 9.4%	x	o	o
C	OP	Phosmet 15%	x	x	x
C	CB	Propoxur 9.4%	x	o	o

Table 8.1

Pet Use Pesticides - 1994

Brand Name	Use	Formulation	Inert Ingredients
Zodiac Flea & Tick Powder For Cats	Ins	Pow	95.00%
Zodiac Flea & Tick Powder For Dogs	Ins	Pow	95.00%
Zodiac Flea & Tick Shampoo For Dogs & Cats	Ins	Liq	99.45%
Zodiac Flea Collar For Cats	Ins	Col	91.50%
Zodiac Flea Collar For Dogs	IGR	Col	99.00%
Zodiac Pro Dip II	Ins	Liq	88.40%
Zodiac Pyrethrin Dip For Cats & Kittens	Ins	Liq	96.70%
Zodiac Pyrethrin Dip For Dogs & Puppies	Ins	Liq	96.70%
Zodiac Triple-Action Conditioning Flea &Tick Shampoo	Ins	Liq	97.85%
Zodiac Water-Based Flea & Tick Pump Spray for Cats & Dogs	Ins	Spr	98.02%

Label Word	Class	Active Ingredients	Tumors/Cancer	Repro. Damage	Genetic Damage
C	CB	Carbaryl 5%	x	o	x
C	CB	Carbaryl 5%	x	o	x
C	SY	Piperonyl butoxide* 0.5%	-	-	o
		Pyrethrins 0.05%	x	x	x
C	CB	Carbaryl 8.5%	x	o	x
C		Methoprene 1%	o	o	o
W	OP	Phosmet 11.6%	x	x	x
C		Pyrethrins 0.3%	x	x	x
	SY	Piperonyl butoxide* 3%	-	-	o
C		Pyrethrins 0.3%	x	x	x
	SY	Piperonyl butoxide* 3%	-	-	o
W		Pyrethrins 0.15%	x	x	x
	SY	Piperonyl butoxide* 1%	-	-	o
	SY	MGK 264 0.5%	x	x	o
		Di-n-propyl isocinchomeronate 0.5%	-	-	-
C		Pyrethrins 0.15%	x	x	x
	SY	Piperonyl butoxide* 1.5%	-	-	o
	SY	MGK 264 0.34%	x	x	o

* Piperonyl butoxide causes cancer and birth
defects in rats (see pages 114-115).

9

Human Use Pesticides

*Sir, there is no settling the point of precedency between a
louse and a flea.*

Samuel Johnson (1709-1784)

Tiny bloodsucking lice can decide the fate of nations.
Napoleon's defeat has been attributed to decimation of his
troops by outbreaks of epidemic typhus from infected body
lice. The lives of thousands of British soldiers in Scutari were
saved by scrupulous hygienic measures implemented by
Florence Nightingale, which stopped the transmission of
disease-spreading vermin. During the second world war, the
dusting of allied troops with DDT killed their body lice, thus
averting a typhus epidemic. This made World War II the first
war in history in which more soldiers died of their wounds
than from disease.

Modern sanitation, the universal availability of hot
water, along with profound changes in personal hygiene, has
not made lice infestation a thing of the past. It is very likely
that many reading this book, (definitely the one writing it),
shocked their mother into fits of shampooing, combing, and
nit-picking, when they came home from school one day with
more than their homework.

Head lice. Head lice infestation is common in schools,
day care centers, and other place where young children
congregate – even in the best neighborhoods. Unfortunately

many parents feel humiliated and ashamed if their children become infested. The good news is that you do not have to use pesticides to get rid of head lice. The bad news is discussed under lindane.

Nontoxic treatment. There is absolutely no need to expose children to *any* pesticide to treat head lice. Safe, nontoxic alternatives are available and effective. Shampooing and then thoroughly and methodically combing out the nits with a metal fine-tooth comb, and repeating the treatment if necessary is all that is required. Except of course for patience, sufficient time to do the job properly, and ways to distract your child as you carry out the procedure.

Soap shampoo. Soap is insecticidal, so you may wish to use a soap shampoo. But any shampoo is suitable – except lice shampoos, which are not necessary. You should thoroughly shampoo and rinse the child's hair, and then shampoo it again but do not rinse out the shampoo. Wrap a towel around the child's head for a few minutes and then begin combing. Use hot water since heat kills lice. But little ones do not tolerate hot water as well so be careful.

Metal fine tooth comb. Make sure you use a metal fine tooth comb. Separate the child's hair in one-inch sections and while it is wet and soapy, methodically comb from the scalp outward until you have combed out the nits. Long and curly hair can be difficult to comb and might have to be cut. Monitor the child carefully and repeat the procedure within the week if you see nits. If the problem continues at the school you may have to repeat the procedure every week or ten days until the problem is under control. But repeating the procedure is not a toxic threat to the child since you are only using soap and water and a comb.

No nits policy. Keeping children out of school until they are nit free is an important preventive measure in getting an outbreak under control. Some school districts have this as a matter of policy.

Separation of hats and coats. Children can easily get infested from a school mate by sharing combs, hats and other clothing. Besides trying to get the children not to share, a physical barrier separating the hooks where the children hang their hats and coats can be an effective preventive measures. Simple open partitions that extend from the wall are sufficient.

Reinfestation may be used to justify more draconian policies regarding a school lice outbreak. Everybody is starting to relax thinking the problem is solved and then another child, or more children, are found to be infested. It may not be a reinfestation at all but a failure to properly control the initial outbreak. It is crucial not to treat it as a reinfestation if it is not. Otherwise safe, sane, and healthy policies may be abandoned, and pressures build to use toxic chemicals.

The biggest reason for failure is that treatments and preventive measures were not clearly discussed and explained to *all* affected parties – the parents and the children, the school officials and the teachers. Make sure parents understand exactly how to do the shampooing and combing. It is very important to apply the Jimmy Durante principle – everybody has to get into the act!

Dealing with parents' fears. Competent, intelligent, and otherwise reasonable school officials can become irrational when confronted with a lice outbreak. They are dealing with parents whose reactions can range from slight loss of decorum to near hysteria; from petitions to fire the principal, to demands to fumigate the school from top to bottom. Sometimes, the pressure is so intense that the school authorizes spraying the school with toxic pesticides to show that they are doing something.

It is very important that everyone understand that lice like to stay on warm bodies, and cannot fly. Applying toxic pesticides from roof to basement will do nothing to solve the problem, since lice are not lurking in corners and reproducing like crazy. They are reproducing nits that are sticking to the children's hair. It is useful to remember that Florence Nightingale saved the entire British Army with soap and water, preventive measures, and common sense.

And now the bad news. Besides the application of toxic pesticides in the school, there is another toxic assault the children may have to endure – treatment with a lice shampoo containing lindane, a pesticide in the DDT family.

Lindane was formerly available over-the-counter as a shampoo and creme under the brand name Kwell®. It is now available only by doctor's prescription as a 1% shampoo or creme, under the generic name lindane. The brand name Kwell® is no longer in use. The acute and chronic health effects of lindane are discussed in chapters four and five. Some adverse human health effects attributed to the use of lindane to treat lice and scabies include:

◆ Brain and nervous system damage resulting in death in infants and children after application to the skin (see chapter four).

◆ Convulsions and other illness in children from application to the skin (see chapter four).

◆ Many reports of aplastic anemia, two recent cases being a child and a young man (see chapter five).

◆ Associated with brain cancer in children (see chapter five).

We discuss lindane in almost ever chapter of this book and always make the same recommendation. Lindane should be banned; it should not be allowed for any use whatsoever. We cannot recommend its use under any circumstances.

Other lice pesticides. There are several products available over-the-counter for treatment of lice. Most contain either pyrethrins or the synthetic pyrethroid, permethrin. Pyrethrins are made from flowers (a type of chrysanthemum). As you will see from the table at the end of this chapter, the pyrethrins are formulated (mixed) with the synergist piperonyl butoxide. There are recent reports that piperonyl butoxide causes cancer and birth defects in rats. We cannot recommend any product that contains it for use on children.

Pyrethroids are synthetic chemical imitations of pyrethrins. As Table 9.2 at the end of this chapter shows, the permethrin products listed do not contain the synergist piperonyl butoxide. However you should make sure you look at the label carefully because pesticide companies continue to reformulate their products. A product that looks familiar may have been reformulated and contain other ingredients than those in the table.

There is no reason to use these neurotoxic pesticides on children when safe nontoxic alternatives are available.

Allergies, asthma, and lice pesticides. Pyrethrins cross react with ragweed and other plant pollens. Synthetic pyrethroids can also cause allergic reactions (do not let your doctor tell you the synthetic pyrethroids do not cause allergies). These products can be very problematic for people with allergies, asthma, and chemical sensitivity – additional reasons to avoid them.

A word about scabies. Lindane, pyrethrins, and synthetic pyrethroids are also used for the treatment of scabies. We do not recommend them for the reasons discussed above. Sulfur is an effective treatment for scabies. Ask your pharmacist to make a creme of 10% precipitated sulfur in an aquasol creme base. They will know what this means. In some states you may have to get a prescription from your doctor since it has to be compounded. Sulfur can irritate the skin so make sure you use it only as directed.

Further resources. There is an excellent organization in Boston called the National Pediculosis Association. They have an 800 number to report problems, and some excellent publications you can send for. See Appendix J on page 403 for how to reach them.

Insect repellents

There is only one pesticide registered for use as an insect repellent; its common name is deet. Estimates are that 30% of the U.S. population has used this product.

Deet is applied directly to the skin. It does not kill insects but repels them; they find your skin unpalatable and seek their next blood meal elsewhere. It is used against mosquitoes, ticks, fleas, gnats, biting flies, chiggers, and other insects. It is widely used by the military for troops in the field.

Deet poisoning. As already discussed in chapter four, deet is very toxic to the brain and nervous system. Mild poisoning can cause headache, restlessness, irritability. Children might have crying spells or other changes in behavior. Severe poisoning can cause slurring of speech, tremor (shakiness), convulsions, and coma. There is a report of a five year old child at a day camp who had a major seizure (convulsion) without any other symptoms shortly after deet was applied to his skin. Deet has caused death in children from absorption through the skin when it was applied repeatedly or in a high concentration (see Appendix H).

Allergic reactions. Deet can cause a severe allergic reaction, called anaphylactic shock, which can lead to death if not treated promptly. It is very rare, however.

High concentrations. Some products contain a very high concentration of deet. We found a product in San Francisco with 100% deet — Deep Woods Off!®. Adults should not use products over 25%. There is a product for children that contains 7.125% deet, which would seem to be an improvement over higher concentrations. However, there are concerns about the ability of young children to follow directions and cooperate in the use of a toxic product.

Adhering to label directions can be a problem for adults who apply the product to children. For example OFF!®Skintastic®Insect Repellent for Children, has conflicting statements on the label as you can see on the facing page. It is an intriguing concept that somehow there will be no contamination of the hands from the deet used elsewhere on the child's body, or from contact with other children and adults who have also been treated. Neurotoxic insect repellents have no place on the skin of small children no matter what the concentration.

Nontoxic alternatives. Deet is often used in fear of ticks that carry Lyme disease. Covering the skin with clothing is more protective; ticks are after a blood meal and attach to bare skin. Wear dark clothing (ticks are attracted to white and light colors); tuck pants legs into boots when in a tick-infested area. Thoroughly check your body and your child's whether a repellent was used or not immediately after leaving the area. Use tweezers to grasp firmly and remove the entire body if you find a tick. There is probably a grace period of a few hours after biting before the tick transmits the organism that causes Lyme disease, so do not panic.

There is some evidence that deet is less effective against ticks than other insects. Beware a false sense of security that because an insect repellent was applied, there is no need to take precautions to avoid tick bites, or to be rigorous in searching for and removing them.

There is an Avon product called Skin-so-Soft® that contains mineral oil; it is widely used as an insect repellent by those who want to avoid toxic chemicals. It can apparently be effective in some cases, but must be applied more frequently and in larger amounts than deet. It is not an insect repellent and the company makes no such claims.

Brand Name Product Tables

Table 9.1 which follows lists the over-the-counter products for human use from our surveys in California and Florida. You will see that deet can cause adverse reproductive effects in laboratory animals. It would be prudent for pregnant women to avoid the use of any product containing deet.

OFF!® SKINTASTIC® INSECT REPELLENT FOR CHILDREN is a pleasant smelling lotion specially formulated to repel mosquitoes, biting flies, gnats and no-see-ums for up to two hours. It also moisturizes your skin. It contains aloe vera to leave skin feeling smooth and natural, never sticky or greasy. Keeping insects away never felt so good.

DIRECTIONS FOR USE: it is a violation of federal law to use this product in a manner inconsistent with its labeling. **Read all directions before using this product.** For best results, spread evenly and completely over all exposed skin. Apply to hand for application to face and neck and rub on. Use just enough repellent to cover exposed skin. Avoid overexposure. Frequent reapplication and saturation are unnecessary. Do not apply to eyes and mouth and <u>do not apply to hands of young children</u>. DO NOT APPLY ON OR NEAR: ACETATE, RAYON, SPANDEX, DYNEL FABRICS OR OTHER SYNTHETICS (OTHER THAN NYLON). MAY DAMAGE FURNITURE FINISHES, PLASTICS, LEATHER, WATCH CRYSTALS AND PAINTED OR VARNISHED SURFACES INCLUDING AUTOMOBILES. Do not keep product on any longer than necessary. After returning indoors, wash treated skin with soap and water. Do not use under clothing.

PRECAUTIONARY STATEMENTS: HAZARDS TO HUMANS- WARNING: Harmful if swallowed. May cause eye injury. Use sparingly on small children. <u>Do not allow children to rub eyes if hands have been treated</u>. Do not allow use by small children without close adult supervision. Do not apply to excessively sunburned or damaged skin. May cause skin reaction in rare cases.

STATEMENT OF PRACTICAL TREATMENT: IF IN EYES-flush with plenty of water. If irritation persists, get medical treatment. **IF SWALLOWED:** call a physician or poison control center. Get medical attention. If you suspect that you or your child is reacting to this product, wash treated skin and call your doctor. **STORAGE:** Store away from heat or flame in an area inaccessible to children. **DISPOSAL:** Do not reuse empty container. Wrap container and put in trash.

So
which
is it
?

Key to Brand Name
Product Table

Use

Her = Herbicide   **Mul** = Multiple Uses
IGR = Insect Growth Regulator   **PGR** = Plant Growth Regulator
Fun = Fungicide   **Rep** = Repellent
Mol = Molluscicide   **Rod** = Rodenticide

Formulation

Aer = Aerosol   **Gel** = Gel
Bat = Bait   **Grn** = Granule
Bar = Barrier   **Liq** = Liquid
Bom = Bomb   **Lot** = Lotion
Col = Collar   **Pel** = Pellet
Dus = Dust   **Pow** = Powder
Fer = Fertilizer   **Sld** = Solid
Fog = Fogger   **Spr** = Spray
Fom = Foam   **Stp** = Strip
Fum = Fumigant   **Tap** = Tape
Gas = Gas   **Trp** = Trap
Rep = Repellent   **Tab** = Tablet

Label Word

D = Danger
W = Warning
C = Caution
N = Not required or not on label

Class

CB = Methyl carbamate   **PY** = Pyrethrin
CH = Chlorinated hydrocarbon   **SP** = Synthetic pyrethroid
OP = Organophosphate   **SY** = Synergist

Tumors/Cancer

A tumor is an abnormal growth of tissue that can be benign or malignant. Another name for a malignant tumor is cancer. Substances that cause cancer are called *carcinogens*. Substances that cause tumors are called *oncogens*.

Repro. Damage

Reproductive damage refers to effects such as death of the embryo or fetus (equivalent to spontaneous abortion and stillbirth in humans), low birth weight, sterility/infertility. It also includes birth defects such as structural defects such as missing arms or legs, or hole in the heart, spina bifida etc. Substances that cause birth defects are called *teratogens*.

Genetic Damage

Genetic damage refers to effects on genetic material including genes, chromosomes, and DNA.

(x) = Possible adverse effect

(-) = Either no data available or information available is not sufficient to make a determination

(o) = Adequate data and no adverse effect noted.

* Sources for the above chronic toxicity data are from Cal-EPA SB-950 Toxicology Summaries, U.S.EPA Factsheets, U.S.EPA R.E.Ds (Registration Eligibility Documents), and scientific journals.

Table 8.1
Human Use Pesticides - 1994 & 1995

Brand Name	Use	Formulation	Inert Ingredients
Backwoods Cutter Insect Repellent	Rep	Aer	77.00%
Backwoods Cutter Insect Repellent Cream	Rep	Liq	65.00%
Backwoods Cutter Insect Repellent Pump Spray	Rep	Spr	77.00%
Backyard Cutter Insect Repellant II	Rep	Aer	85.00%
Backyard Cutter Insect Repellent	Rep	Aer	90.00%
Cutter Evergreen Insect Repellent Spray Formula MMI	Rep	Aer	85.00%
Cutter Pleasant Protection Insect Repellent	Rep	Gel	90%
Cutter Pleasant Protection Insect Repellent	Rep	Spr	90%
Deep Woods Off!	Rep	Spr	-
Deep Woods Off! For Sportsmen	Rep	Spr	75.00%
Deep Woods Off! Insect Repellent II	Rep	Aer	70.00%
Goldline Lice Treatment Liquid	Ped	Liq	96.70%
Hot Shot No-Pest Insect Repellant	Rep	Aer	98.975%
Nix Family Pak Permethrin Lice RX Creme Rinse	Ped	Liq	99.00%
Off! Insect Repellent	Rep	Aer	85.00%
Off! Skintastic Insect Repellent for Children	Rep	Lot	92.50%
Off! Skintastic II	Rep	Lot	92.50%
Off Skintastic Spray with Aloe Vera	Rep	Liq	93%
Pump Spray Off Insect Repellent	Rep	Spr	85.00%
Rid Lice Control Spray for Bedding & Furniture	Ped	Spr	99.50%
Rid Lice Killing Shampoo	Ped	Liq	95.67%
Rid Lice Elimination Kit	Ped	Liq	95.67%
Skedaddle Insect Protection For Children Fragrance Free	Rep	Lot	93.50%

Label Word	Class	Active Ingredients	Tumors/Cancer	Repro. Damage	Genetic Damage
W		Deet 23%	-	x	o
W		Deet 35%	-	x	o
W		Deet 23%	-	x	o
C		Deet 15%	-	x	o
C		Deet 10%	-	x	o
W		Deet 15%	-	x	o
W		Deet 10%	-	x	o
W		Deet 10%	-	x	o
W		Deet 100%	-	x	o
C		Deet 25%	-	x	o
W		Deet 30%	-	x	o
	SY	Pyrethrins 0.3%	x	x	x
		Piperonyl butoxide* 3.0%	-	-	o
C		Deet 15%	-	x	o
	SP	Permethrin 1%	x	x	o
C		Deet 15%	-	x	o
W		Deet 7.5%	-	x	o
W		Deet 7.5%	-	x	o
C		Deet 6.685%	-	x	o
C		Deet 15%	-	x	o
	SP	Permethrin	x	x	o
	SY	Pyrethrins 0.33%	x	x	x
		Piperonyl butoxide* 4.0%	-	-	o
	SY	Pyrethrins 0.33%	x	x	x
		Piperonyl butoxide* 4.0%	-	-	o
C		Deet 6.5%	-	x	o

* Piperonyl butoxide causes cancer and birth
defects in rats (see pages 114-115).

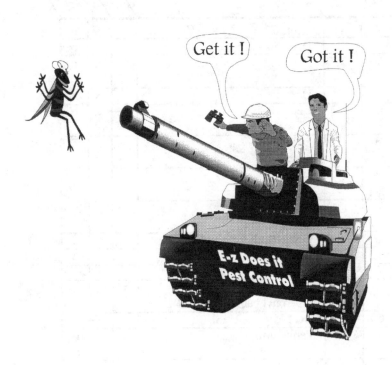

Got it?

Original drawing by George Kormendi 1995. Computer art by Russell Furbush.

Chapter 10

Commercial Use Pesticides

Results! Why, man, I have gotten a lot of results. I know several thousand things that won't work.

Thomas A. Edison (1847-1931)

If you are worried your house might fall down from a termite infestation, your hostility toward insects is probably at a peak. Anxiety, helplessness, and revulsion are common reactions to pest problems, even minor ones. These strong emotional reactions can interfere with clear thinking when hiring a pest control company, even in the most cautious of consumers. You are not thinking about health or environmental consequences of toxic pesticides applied in you home or on your property. You want the problem solved – now.

Manufacturers and providers of toxic pest control products and services understand these fears and anxieties. They promote toxic chemicals as the best solution to real or perceived threats to happiness and well being. Their definition of a pest problem is often whatever their product or service will solve.

Pest control companies may recommend preventive treatments as security to insure total control – scheduling pesticide applications over a period of several months or longer, with a renewal option. Scheduled treatments are a major source of income for the companies. In some neighborhoods, especially where chemical lawn treatment is almost a fetish, this can mean that some poison is being applied by some company on some property almost every day.

Most consumers know very little about commercial use pesticides. They can have mistaken assumptions about pest control. Some common misconceptions are:

◆ The more pests you kill, and the deader you kill them, the better. *(Remember that beneficial organisms, and natural enemies that keep pests in check are also harmed or killed).*

◆ Applying strong pesticides as a preventive measure will avert future problems. *(Such treatments can put you on the pesticide treadmill — chemical dependency that results in an ecologically unbalanced system that requires continuing toxic inputs to maintain).*

◆ Applying pesticide treatments regularly is good insurance. It does no harm and is worth it for peace of mind. *(This ignores potential health and environmental effects; it encourages overuse and misuse of toxic chemicals).*

◆ Pesticides are safe if used properly; the only problems are from misuse, and failure to follow label directions. *(This ignores known problems from legal, accepted use. It ignores the notoriously weak regulation of home use pesticides, and potential long-term effects on health and the environment).*

◆ Toxic chemicals are superior to slower, more natural methods that use pesticides rarely, or only as a last resort. *(They are not).*

This chapter focuses on commercial pesticides for home use. We are aware of community residents' concerns about toxic sprays applied by pest control companies outside the home — including schools, day care centers, restaurants, supermarkets, office buildings, hospitals and nursing homes, golf courses, parks and recreation areas, along roads and highways, and other locations.

We are concerned about these uses as well, and are currently gathering information for a publication on such involuntary exposures. Please feel free to contact us about any experiences or concerns in your community that might be helpful in this regard.

We discuss commercial use pesticides in four sections:

♦ A brief description of the pest control industry, and a general discussion of our survey findings for commercial use pesticides in San Francisco and Florida.

♦ How commercial use pesticides differ from over-the-counter products. A description of how the Environmental Protection Agency assesses acute toxicity of pesticides, the classification of pesticides into four acute toxicity categories.

♦ Making the decision to hire a pest control company. A discussion of nontoxic alternatives, and least toxic pesticides, with special attention to termite control. A brief discussion of fleas and cockroaches.

♦ A table listing active ingredient pesticides in commercial use pesticides found in our surveys. The table includes trade names, LD_{50}s, Environmental Protection Agency (EPA) toxicity categories, signal words on the label, and a summary of chronic toxicity.

Part I: General Information and Survey Findings

Nineteen million households — 20% of all the households in the country — use the services of a pest control company every year according to the EPA. The agency estimates there are 350,000 certified commercial applicators in the non-agricultural sector in the U.S..

Certification. Commercial pest control operators (PCOs, exterminators) must be certified by the state to apply restricted use pesticides. (Restricted use pesticides are discussed in Part II below). Certification requirements are not very demanding; pest control is not a difficult business to enter. Serious weaknesses in certification and training of pesticide applicators are briefly discussed in chapter eleven.

"Under the supervision of." There is a big loophole in the law that allows those who have not been fully trained and certified to apply restricted use pesticides. They can legally mix and apply restricted use pesticides if they are working "under the supervision of" a certified applicator. This does not mean they have to be in the same place at the same time. Many pest control companies have only one certified applicator, and several uncertified applicators who do most of the work. There are many more uncertified applicators than certified ones. Requirements for entry into these jobs are not rigorous, and turnover is high.

San Francisco survey summary. California is the only state that requires commercial pest control companies to report all the pesticides they apply. These "Pesticide Use Reports" are due monthly; they must include the name of the company, the trade name of the pesticide, with the amount, type, and number of applications. The reports are available to the public. This mandatory reporting system is discussed further in chapter eleven.

We summarized the information from July 1992 through July 1993 for the 157 companies licensed to apply pesticides in the City and County of San Francisco. Figure 10.1 shows that more than three-fourths of the applications were insecticides, and about one-fifth rodenticides. Figure 10.2 show the pounds of use for the different uses. Rodenticides, which are 17% of the applications, are only 5% of the amount used. This is because most formulations are baits containing a small amount of the active ingredient.

Figure 10.1

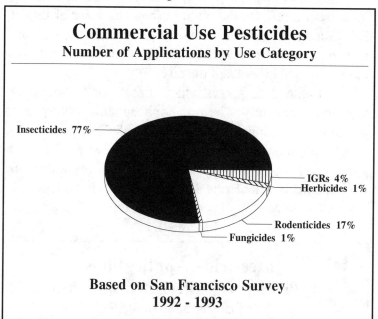

Commercial Use Pesticides
Number of Applications by Use Category

Insecticides 77%

IGRs 4%
Herbicides 1%

Rodenticides 17%

Fungicides 1%

Based on San Francisco Survey
1992 - 1993

Figure 10.2

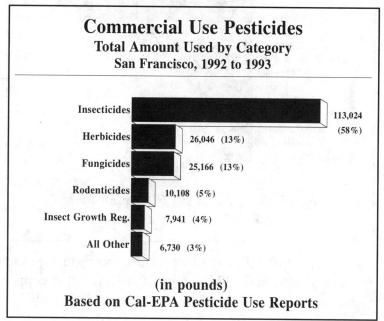

Commercial Use Pesticides
Total Amount Used by Category
San Francisco, 1992 to 1993

Insecticides — 113,024 (58%)

Herbicides — 26,046 (13%)

Fungicides — 25,166 (13%)

Rodenticides — 10,108 (5%)

Insect Growth Reg. — 7,941 (4%)

All Other — 6,730 (3%)

(in pounds)
Based on Cal-EPA Pesticide Use Reports

The large number of applications of insecticides and rodenticides reflects the highly urban character of the city. San Francisco has a large number of attached housing units and apartments. Front yards and extensive lawns are unusual in most neighborhoods of the city.

Figure 10.3 shows which insecticides were applied the most frequently. The organophosphates (chlorpyrifos, diazinon and acephate) accounted for 35% of the total. The flower-based pyrethrums and pyrethrins were 25% of the applications, and the synthetic pyrethroids (cyfluthrin and cypermethrin) 16%. Boric acid and silica gel, the least toxic pesticides, were a small percent of the total.

Figure 10.3

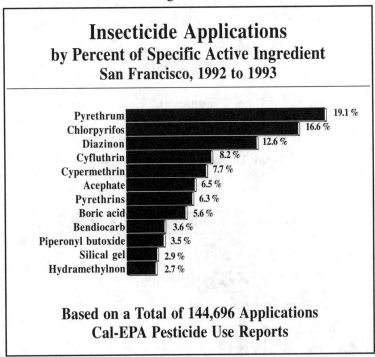

Figure 10.4 shows that glyphosate was by far the most frequently used herbicide. Figure 10.5 shows that copper compounds were the fungicides applied most frequently.

Figure 10.4

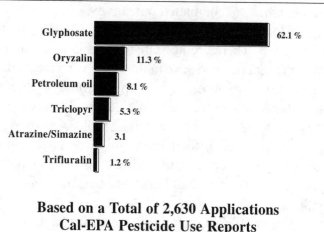

Herbicide Applications
by Percent of Specific Active Ingredient
San Francisco, 1992 to 1993

Glyphosate — 62.1 %
Oryzalin — 11.3 %
Petroleum oil — 8.1 %
Triclopyr — 5.3 %
Atrazine/Simazine — 3.1
Trifluralin — 1.2 %

Based on a Total of 2,630 Applications
Cal-EPA Pesticide Use Reports

Figure 10.5

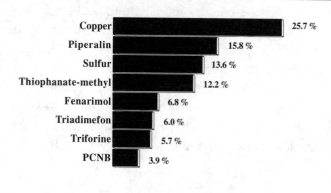

Fungicide Applications
by Percent of Specific Active Ingredient
San Francisco, 1992 to 1993

Copper — 25.7 %
Piperalin — 15.8 %
Sulfur — 13.6 %
Thiophanate-methyl — 12.2 %
Fenarimol — 6.8 %
Triadimefon — 6.0 %
Triforine — 5.7 %
PCNB — 3.9 %

Based on a Total of 647 Applications
Cal-EPA Pesticide Use Reports

California is the only state that has its own pesticide registration division; it is more stringent than the federal EPA's. Pesticides available for commercial use in other states may not be registered for use in California. Some pesticides might be available over-the-counter now in California that were not when we completed our survey.

Florida survey. Florida does not have a pesticide reporting law. There are no statistics available to the public on commercial pesticide use in the state. We have no data on amounts used or number of applications. We obtained information about home use pesticides from interviews with pest control operators, and with householders who use their services. We used information provided by chemically sensitive people (on a state notification list), of pesticide applications in their neighborhoods over the past several months.

Figure 10.6 shows the use classification for active ingredient pesticides from both California and Florida. The higher percentage of herbicides and fungicides than seen in the San Francisco data alone, reflects much greater use of outdoor pesticides in Sarasota, where many homes have yards and lawns. During our survey in Florida we found some pesticides labeled for sale only to certified professionals, available over-the-counter for sale to the public.

Chronic toxicity summary. A summary of the chronic toxicity potential of commercial use pesticides found in our surveys is shown in Figure 10.7.

You can see in the figure that 41% of commercial use pesticide ingredients in our survey are known or suspected to cause tumors or cancer; 29% cause reproductive damage; and 28% cause genetic damage in laboratory animals.

Figure 10.6

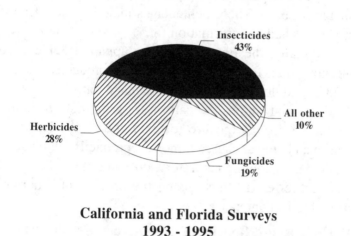

Commercial Use Pesticides
Active Ingredients by Category of Use

Insecticides
43%

All other
10%

Herbicides
28%

Fungicides
19%

California and Florida Surveys
1993 - 1995

Figure 10.7

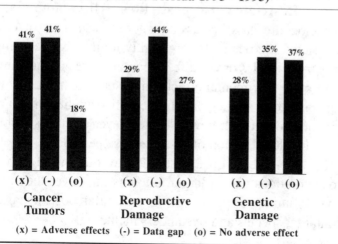

Chronic Toxicity of Active Ingredient Pesticides
In Commercial Use Pest Control Products
(San Francisco & Florida 1993 - 1995)

41% 41%

44%

35% 37%

29%

27%

28%

18%

(x) (-) (o)   (x) (-) (o)   (x) (-) (o)
Cancer   Reproductive   Genetic
Tumors   Damage   Damage

(x) = Adverse effects   (-) = Data gap   (o) = No adverse effect

For many pesticides the chronic toxicity studies are missing (data gaps). Required studies were not done, or were not done properly. Figure 10.7 shows that data on cancer are missing or not available for 41%, and for reproductive damage in 44% of the pesticides. There are data gaps on genetic damage for 35%. These percentages include pesticides that our sources had no information for.

Finally, the figure shows no apparent evidence of cancer or tumors for 18%, no evidence of reproductive damage for 28%, and no apparent genetic damage for 37%.

Animal studies are part of assessing risks to human populations from exposure to toxic chemicals. However, because a chemical causes tumors, reproductive damage, or genetic damage in the laboratory, does not mean that it will cause that effect in those using the product or otherwise exposed to its contents.

Part II: Acute Toxicity of Commercial Use Pesticides

Pest control companies use products that are very different from those you purchase over-the-counter. Commercial use pesticides are sold in bulk, and in much higher concentrations. Most are diluted and mixed by the pest control operator before applying them. Many are restricted use pesticides.

Restricted use pesticides. All commercial use pesticides are classified as either general use or restricted use. Restricted use pesticides are highly toxic, adversely impact nontarget species or wildlife, or contaminate groundwater, or have other detrimental effects on the environment. They are supposed to be applied only by a certified applicator, but most are not, as discussed above. Chapter eleven discusses problems with the classification of restricted use pesticides.

Commercial use pesticides are often used in higher concentrations and in larger amounts than over-the-counter ones. Outdoor applications in particular pose hazards to nontarget species and bystanders including:

- ◆ Beneficial species and natural predators that keep pests in check.
- ◆ Earthworms, microbes, and other organisms in the soil that keep it healthy, balanced, and aerated.
- ◆ Birds, bees, fish, and other wildlife that share or are passing through residential areas.
- ◆ Humans and pets.

Long-term health effects. You should not rely on commercial pest control operators (PCOs, exterminators) as a source of information regarding the potential long-term health effects of poisons they apply to your home or property. The most that applicators (certified or not) are likely to know is what is on the product label. The label information only refers to acute toxicity, and short term hazards. Commercial use pesticides are tested for acute toxicity before they are marketed.

Measuring acute toxicity. The ultimate acute toxic effect is death. To measure acute toxicity, pesticides are fed to laboratory rats to see how much it takes to kill half of the animals. The result is called the LD_{50} (ell dee 50) — the lethal dose for 50% of the animals. The LD_{50} is reported in milligrams per kilogram of body weight of the rat — abbreviated as mg/kg. The lower the LD_{50} (the smaller the number) the more toxic the pesticide. The LD_{50} is not a measure of chronic long-term toxicity.

EPA Categories. The EPA uses the LD_{50} to rank pesticides into four toxicity categories. The most acutely toxic pesticides are in category one (I), and the least toxic in category four (IV). A signal word – Danger, Warning, or Caution – is required to be on the label. Table 10.1 shows how the signal word relates to the toxicity category.

The LD_{50} is not the only criterion for classifying pesticides. If the product contains an active or inert ingredient that is caustic or corrosive to the skin or the eyes, it is put into toxicity category I, irrespective of the LD_{50}.

Table 10.1

EPA Acute Toxicity Categories
for Commercial Use Pesticides

EPA Toxicity Category and Label Word	Oral LD_{50}* (in mg/kg)	Fatal Dose in Humans (adult)
I Highly Toxic **DANGER**	Less than 50	It only takes a few drops to kill you.
II Very Toxic **WARNING**	50 to 500	It takes up to an ounce to kill you.
III Moderately Toxic **CAUTION**	500 to 5,000	It takes up to a pint to kill you.
IV Least Toxic **CAUTION**	>5,000	It takes up to a quart to kill you

* LD_{50} , or lethal dose 50 is the amount it takes to kill 50% of the animals it is administered to (usually rats, but rabbits and guinea pigs are also used). The pesticide can be fed to the animal (oral LD_{50}), put on the skin, (dermal LD_{50}), or breathed in (inhalation LD_{50}). The LD_{50}s in this table are oral. The lower the LD_{50} the more toxic the chemical — because it only takes a very small amount of the chemical to kill the animal. LD_{50} *is not* a measure of chronic or long-term toxicity.

Figure 10.8 shows the acute toxicity categories for the active ingredients in commercial pesticides used in California and Florida. You will see that the percentage of the most highly toxic pesticides (category I) was greater than that of the least toxic (category IV).

Figure 10.8

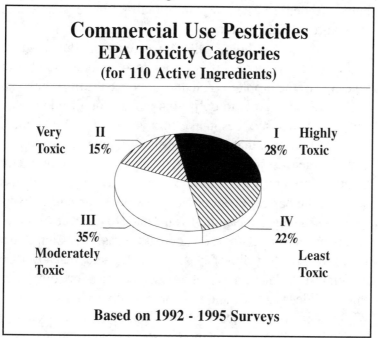

Commercial Use Pesticides
EPA Toxicity Categories
(for 110 Active Ingredients)

Based on 1992 - 1995 Surveys

Table 10.2 at the end of this chapter lists the LD_{50}, label signal words, and toxicity categories for the active ingredient pesticides in commercial use pesticides from our survey. You will see that some active ingredients have more than one toxicity category listed. This is because the toxicity category applies to a specific trade name product. Some formulations are more concentrated, are mixed with a more toxic active or inert ingredient, or are more hazardous for some uses than others.

Part III: Nontoxic alternatives and Least Toxic Chemical Methods

Professional assistance is often needed to find out what pest is causing damage and to assess the extent and severity of an infestation. A serious problem such as termites is not a do-it-yourself project, and you will need to hire a pest control company. We discuss your options in the section on termites below. Rodent infestations can sometimes be severe enough to require professional help.

Most householders hire a pest control company as a matter of convenience. It is easier to pay someone else to take care of the problem. You may not have the time, interest, ability, or inclination to do it yourself. If you decide to pay for pest control services, make sure you really need them.

Make sure that failure to follow simple housekeeping or other measures is not causing or aggravating the problem. Chapters six and seven on indoor and outdoor pests discuss some of the basics. Be sure to explore nontoxic alternatives.

Making a decision. If you decide to hire a pest control company, be very choosy; do not make a hasty decision. Most people rely on the yellow pages, or on companies that advertise on television. These may not be good sources for companies that provide least toxic and environmentally friendly services.

Limited choices. Most consumers would choose nontoxic and least toxic methods instead of conventional toxic treatments if they knew about them, and if the methods were widely available. We discuss some of these nontoxic and least toxic methods below. We encourage you to seek out pest control companies that are competent in using these methods. Try to get a company in your area to use them if none are doing so. Only when more consumer dollars support nontoxic and least toxic methods, not toxic sprays, will the industry change to meet the demand.

The current situation in pest control is reminiscent of Henry Ford's first cars. When asked what colors the buyer could choose from, he replied, "They can have any color they want as long as its black."

Chemical mindset. Commercial home pest control is a long-established industry, and most pest control operators (exterminators) have a chemical mindset. Certified applicators are essentially in the chemical business. They were trained in chemicals and most do not question their use. They may know very little about nontoxic and least toxic methods. Finding a company that does not rely on toxic broadcast sprays as the major part of its business is not going to be easy.

Resistance to change. Many companies doing conventional pest control are resistant to change. They may resist including the newer nontoxic and least toxic methods among the services they provide. The best you are likely to find in some areas is a company whose major business is conventional chemical control methods, that may also offer nontoxic and least toxic methods upon customer request. It is a rarity to find pest control companies that provide only environmentally friendly services. If there is such a company in your area, please let us know so we can share the information with others.

Be a good comparison shopper and interview several companies before making your decision. It is very important to find out if they provide nontoxic and least toxic services. Do not be surprised if the pest control company representative tries to convince you of the advantages of conventional chemical treatments.

Inspection versus treatment. When you hire a professional to assess the nature, extent and severity of a pest problem in you home, it is best to pay for the service. Many companies offer "free" inspections, expecting that you will hire them for whatever treatment is recommended. In this situation there is the risk of being given an incorrect report about the nature, extent, or even the fact of an infestation. Some unscrupulous companies may recommend treatment for nonexistent problems, overtreat, or recommend scheduled follow-up treatments that are not necessary. Separating the inspection from the treatment will help avoid such problems.

Special requests. Make it clear that you do not want foggers or bombs used, that you do not want any pesticides applied directly to furnishings, carpets, baseboards or other areas in your home. If you are pregnant, or have children and pets, or have allergies or asthma, you must be very firm with the company about any special dos and don'ts. Remember you are paying for the service; you are the ultimate one who decides what is allowed into your home.

Make sure that you read chapter two on exposure. It contains information you should know about the different types of formulations and methods of application. Other chapters also contain information that will help you to make healthier pest control decisions. We encourage you to be persistent in trying to find a company that provides benign, healthy, and environmentally friendly methods of control that do not pose potential risks to your family, pets, neighbors, and community.

There are some things you should know about a company that has the potential to put your family at risk by their methods of pest control in your home.

◆ Does the company provide nontoxic services. If they do get the specifics.

◆ Does the company answer your questions in a clear and straightforward way.

◆ Is the company willing to work with you to comply with any special requests.

◆ Is the company willing to avoid the use of specific products or pesticides that you request.

◆ Does the company provide a written estimate and description of the proposed services – including the names, concentration, and method of application of any pesticides they plan to use (before any treatment).

◆ Will the company respect a request to avoid the use of foggers, bombs, or aerosols. If so make sure this is written into the service estimate.

◆ Will the company respect a request to avoid any

spraying of furniture, carpets, and other home furnishings. If so make sure it is written into the service estimate.

◆ Is the company willing to provide you with a copy of the label and the Material Safety Data Sheet (discussed below) for all of the pesticides they propose to use in your home, if you request them.

There are other responses from the company that may suggest the company is more likely to favor toxic chemical controls over nontoxic and least toxic methods.

◆ Trying to persuade you to use chemical sprays when you request otherwise.

◆ Assuring you that the pesticides they use are registered by the EPA. (This is meaningless since all pesticides are registered).

◆ Saying that they have been working with chemicals for years and do not have any health problems.

◆ Saying they do not use anything they would not use in their own home.

◆ Saying they have a wife and kids and do you think they would use anything that might not be good for them.

Another indicator of dependence on toxic chemicals is whether or not a company is committed to a system of pest control called Integrated Pest Management, or IPM. This system is based on careful and frequent monitoring of pests to determine when treatments are necessary. Physical, biological, and other nonchemical controls are the primary treatments, and least toxic chemicals are only used as a last resort.

You might think that asking a company if they use IPM would help you decide about their suitability for work in your home. If they say no, you scratch them off your list of possibilities. But if they say yes, you really do not know what it means. The term IPM is often misused; it is applied to so many methods that are not in the spirit of what it stands for, that it can be meaningless. Some companies that use toxic sprays will call it IPM if they do some inspections and follow-up monitoring before they spray toxic chemicals again. They know that IPM is considered a good thing and that they should be using it even if they do not understand it.

It is better to get specific information about the methods and chemicals they propose to use. Telling you they use IPM does not really give you any idea what they will actually do in your home. We discuss true IPM methods for termite control later in this chapter.

Before we begin the discussion of termite control, we want to briefly mention cockroaches, fleas, and lawn pesticides.

Cockroaches. If you read chapter six on indoor pest control, you know that we are big fans of boric acid. We want to let you know about a product called Stapleton's Magnetic Roach Food. It is a paste containing 33% boric acid that comes in a tube. The advantage of this product over powders and baits is that it does not have to be spread around using a spoon or dispenser, or placed in areas potentially accessible to children and pets. It is applied in cracks and crevices and can be put into areas accessible only to cockroaches. The product has been marketed only to pest control companies in the past but is now available for retail sale. If it is not yet available in your areas, you can obtain this product by calling the 800 number listed under Blue Diamond in Appendix J on page 403.

Fleas in the carpet. Orthoboric acid and sodium metaborate are forms of boric acid. There is a carpet treatment called "Fleabusters™" in which borates are applied directly to carpet for flea control. According to the company the product stays in the fiber and remains effective at killing fleas for at least a year. The company claims that the pesticide is not released from the carpet fiber in a way that is potentially hazardous to children and pets. California is requiring testing of borates for this use because of reproductive toxicity concerns from exposure to residues released from the carpet. In chapter six on indoor pest control we described the use of diatomaceous earth to treat your carpet. This nontoxic method can last for a year or more.

Fleas in the yard. We were appalled to learn that in Florida, lindane is being applied outdoors on lawns and yards to control fleas. We discuss lindane in almost every chapter of this book and always make the same recommendation. Lindane should be banned; it should not be used for any reason whatsoever. We do not recommend its use under any circumstances. See chapters four and five for a discussion of acute and chronic health effects of lindane and other pesticides in the DDT family. Both chapter six and seven discuss nontoxic methods for controlling fleas.

Lawn and yard pesticides. We are very concerned about the health and environmental implications of the widespread use of toxic pesticides in yards and on lawns. We discuss this in detail in chapter seven on outdoor use pesticides.

Recent History of Termite Control

Before describing current termite control pesticides and methods, we present some background on the recent history of termite control in the U.S.. If this does not interest you, feel free to skip to the next section on termite control.

Chlordane. Termites are a very serious problem and cause significant structural and economic damage. About four decades ago, the discovery that chlordane, a pesticide in the DDT family, was effective in controlling termites, revolutionized home pest control. The new chemical cure fit in with prevalent attitudes of "better living through chemistry" and its use spread rapidly throughout the land.

The new treatment worked wonders. Only one application was usually needed because chlordane is so persistent. Home owners were pleased with the results, and so were pest control companies. Here was a product that made everybody happy. Estimates are that chlordane was applied in 30 million homes in the U.S. as a termiticide. If the homes are still there, so is the chlordane. Chlordane was banned in 1988 in the U.S..

So who ruined the party? Was it the environmentalists, beginning with Rachel Carson, who kept pointing out unpalatable facts about the DDT family of chemicals: bioaccumulation in, and adverse effects on, wildlife (especially birds and fish) – contamination of and persistence in soil and water (including groundwater) – enormous ecological disruptions from continuing input of such persistent toxics into the environment.

Or was it the public health fundamentalists who warned of the health implications from long-term storage and accumulation of the DDT family of chemicals in human fat and other tissue. They pointed out more unpalatable facts. These pesticides pass through the placenta to the developing fetus; there are high levels in breast milk. They raised concerns about the potential for long-term chronic health effects such as cancer, reproductive damage, and adverse effects on the brain and nervous system.

Or was it the regulators and legislators who finally had to listen to the environmentalists and public health fundamentalists. Pesticide manufacturers and major users lobbied intensively, and often successfully, over the years to keep DDT, chlordane, and related pesticides on the market. Their arguments fell in two areas, costs vs. benefits, and expertise.

Cost vs. benefits. The cost vs. benefit argument was (and still is) a variation on the theme that the pesticide is solving more problems than it is causing. In the case of termite control, pesticide interests argued that a valuable pest control agent would be denied to consumers. They could not only lose their homes, but be forced to pay more for less effective treatments. The cost of adverse health effects, and environmental contamination and degradation was not part of the equation.

The experts. The expertise argument is a variation on the theme that the company is the expert on their own products – they researched, developed, and marketed them. For this argument to have any value, potential adverse health and environmental effects must be ignored, downplayed, or discredited. This meant the pesticide interests focused on discrediting the public health and environmental experts. An important difference between these experts is that manufacturers and major users have an economic interest in the product — the environmentalists and public health fundamentalists do not.

Good-bye and good riddance. We will all be winners when the DDT era and all that it represents finally go the way of the dinosaur. The current transition period has its own dangers and relapses. A chemical is not better just because it is not DDT or another banned pesticide, as some pest control companies would like you to believe. Throughout this book we discuss pesticides in current use that future generations will no doubt look upon the same way we look at our more reckless chemical past.

Termite Control

Ironically, termite control, historically linked to some of the most toxic pesticides ever used in the home, is currently on the verge of some exciting breakthroughs. Least toxic methods and nontoxic methods that do not put your family and potential future residents of your home at risk are, in the testing or early marketing stages.

This is a response to increasing public awareness of flawed toxic technologies, and the demand for safer products that do not pose risks to health and the environment.

Termite control is not a do-it-yourself project. You will need a professional to find out if the infestation really is from termites, whether they are drywood or subterranean, and to assess the seriousness and extent of the infestation. Remember to have inspection done independently of the treatment as discussed above under inspection versus treatment.

Nontoxic method for drywood termites. Temperatures above 120° F will kill drywood termites. There is a nontoxic method called Thermal Pest Eradication (TPE) which uses specially designed heaters, blowers and ducts to blow hot air throughout an entire structure. The treatment is applied room by room, and can be completed in a day. This is a completely safe and highly effective nontoxic technology.

After completion of the treatment, the family can immediately reoccupy the house. The structure does not have to be tented. The temperature in a car parked out in the sun with both windows rolled up on a very hot day gets hotter than that used for this treatment. For chemically sensitive people it has the special advantage that volatile chemicals in glues, solvents, resins and other substances in the house will off-gas as a consequence of the treatment.

Highly recommended. The company that markets this technology is called Isothermics; and it is available throughout the country. There is an 800 number you can call to find out which pest control company in your area is licensed to use this method (see Isothermics in Appendix J on page 403). If there is no licensed company in your area, see what you can do to get one licensed. Unfortunately many companies resist making the investment in this healthy and environmentally friendly technology. The thermal method is the best method by far for treating an entire structure, and we highly recommend it.

Fumigation for drywood termites. Unfortunately many householders do not know about the TPE method described above and are not offered this as an option. To treat an entire structure, conventional treatment uses the toxic fumigants (gases), methyl bromide and sulfuryl fluoride (Vikane®).

Fumigants are among the most toxic pesticides in commercial use (chapter four discusses the acute health effects of these pesticides). These toxic gases permeate the entire structure. Houses or other structures treated with fumigants are tented during the treatment to keep the gas in and people out. Depending on State regulations, two to four days must elapse after the tarp is removed before anyone is allowed back inside. This is to allow the remaining fumigant to off-gas (dissipate) into the atmosphere. If the fumigant is methyl bromide, it is off-gassing its way to the ozone later, about which see below.

Deaths from methyl bromide. Fumigants pose a great risk of poisoning, and applicators have lost their lives to this pesticide. They also pose a risk to the public. There are several known instances of people who entered tented structures and died before they could get back out. Death has occurred even *after waiting until after it was supposed to be legally safe to go back inside.* This happened to a man in California in 1992. Within hours of going back into his apartment two days after fumigation with methyl bromide, he became ill, lapsed into a coma and died two and a half weeks later. State investigators found that methyl bromide can persist in furnishing and other areas of the home and continue to off-gas after the "safe" reentry time. See chapter four for information on acute health effects of fumigants.

Ozone depletion. Methyl bromide is a more potent depleter of the ozone layer than chlorofluorocarbons (CFCs). It has a shorter half-life however, about eighteen months. Methyl bromide is on the list of ozone-depleting chemicals to be phased out by 2001.

Spot treatments for drywood termites. Spot treatments are used to treat areas of known termite infestation, and not the entire structure. Spot treatment only works for termite infestations that are detected. Detection is not an exact science; it can be very difficult to find all the areas of termite activity throughout a structure. There are dogs (beagles) trained to detect termites which can be used for this purpose. Spot treatments include freezing (liquid nitrogen), microwaves, electricity (Electrogun), and chemical treatments (pesticides).

Liquid nitrogen. Nitrogen gas compressed into liquid form has a very low temperature. When the liquid nitrogen is released onto the drywall covering wooden beams, any termites infesting the wood are frozen to death. If the infestation is severe and widespread throughout the structure, the freezing technique is not appropriate. Freezing is not effective on exposed wooden beams in attics or basements.

Since nitrogen comprises 78% of the air we breathe (the rest is 21% oxygen and 1% carbon dioxide), there is no need to tent the structure, and no danger of contamination of food, clothing or other household furnishings as there is with methyl bromide and sulfuryl fluoride.

Liquid nitrogen can pose a risk to the applicator however. In California, a pest control operator died while applying it in an enclosed wall space where there was no ventilation. Instead of normal air, he was breathing 100% nitrogen and suffocated from lack of oxygen.

Microwaves. Microwaves can kill termites, and are used to spot treat infestations that are already detected. While microwaves are effective, the workers using the equipment may be at risk for long-term health effects. It has been reported to burn or scorch the treated wood.

Electricity. Also know as ElectroGun, this is another spot treatment which is used only on known infested areas.

Preventive treatments. Borates such as Tim-Bor® when injected into wood will prevent an infestation since termites avoid it. It will not kill termites already there. If infested wood is damp, the problem causing the dampness should be corrected. The infested wood should be removed and replaced with borate treated wood.

Subterranean termites

Subterranean termites are much harder to control than drywood. They invade your home from their nests near your home. The reason they invade the wood is because it is moist. Dry wood does not rot; the lumber used to build your house was dry when first nailed into place.

A source that we have mentioned often in this book, *Common Sense Pest Control*, discusses the conditions that lead to moisture build up, and ways to cure and prevent the wood decay that makes your home a target for invasion by termites and other pests. We especially recommend reading the chapters on structural pests if you are planning to build a house. There is an excellent discussion about sound construction techniques that will help assure the structural integrity of the wood.

We focus our discussion on the current chemicals being used and the nontoxic and least toxic alternatives to conventional toxic sprays.

Chemical treatments. The conventional method for treating subterranean termites is to create a chemical barrier between the termites and the house or other structure.

Chlordane was the chemical barrier used for many years until its ban in 1988. The most widely used pesticides in current use include the nerve-gas pesticide chlorpyrifos (Dursban ®), and the synthetic pyrethroids, permethrin (Torpedo®) and cypermethrin (Demon®).

They are mixed into the soil as a chemical barrier to keep the termites from entering the house. The soil the house is built on is treated in the crawl space, or by drilling holes into the concrete slab to inject it into the soil beneath the house. The soil around the foundation and perimeter of the house is also treated. Termites that come to forage on the wood in your house have to pass through the treated soil. They are killed or repelled by the toxic soil, if the pesticide is evenly distributed.

There can be serious problems from the application of chemical barrier pesticides. There are many reports of these toxic pesticides being injected into heating system ducts. When the heat is turned on, the pesticide volatilizes and blows throughout the house. Pesticides have also been improperly injected into water and sewer lines. There are instances in which continuing contamination of the home occurs because the drill holes in the slab were not plugged up properly.

The toxic pesticides contaminating the soil around the house is a health threat to children and pets, and can be tracked inside the house. Such treatment methods are out of the question for the chemically sensitive. Chapters four and five discuss the health effects of these chemicals.

Nontoxic nonchemical barrier. Termites cannot penetrate sand particles of a certain size. Sand put into a crawl space or inside the foundation of the house where it cannot blow or wash away, is an excellent nontoxic way to prevent subterranean termites from invading a house. See the listing under Live Oak Structural and Therm-Trol Exterminating in Appendix J on page 403 for information about this method.

Biological controls. Parasitic nematodes are not yet a dependable control for subterranean termites, except under certain soil conditions. It does work in some soils in some areas however, and since it is a nontoxic method you may wish to find out what the experience is in your area.

A green fungus that occurs naturally in soil (M. anisopliae) is fatal to termites (and cockroaches), and is being tested throughout the country for commercial development. It is applied as a conventional spray; and the infected termites take it back to the colony where it is spread by grooming and feeding behaviors.

Although this fungus is not a threat to human health (it will not grow in the high temperatures of the human body), it is apparently highly allergenic. Its use could be problematic for those with asthma, allergies, and chemical sensitivity. The method, called Bioblast, is being tested throughout the U.S.. For further information see EcoScience in the resource listing in Appendix J on page 403.

Baits. We are great fans of baits for pest control. They are designed to attract the pest, they do not give off harmful vapors, mists, sprays, or residues that contaminate the entire treated area. The pesticide stays in the container it comes in, relying on the pest coming to the bait. The amount of active ingredient pesticide is usually very low. For termite control, they are placed in inaccessible areas that are not a threat to children and pets.

At long last there are baits under commercial development and testing for subterranean termite control. They are an excellent part of a true IPM system, which relies on monitoring and preventive measures such as food and moisture reduction. Baits and a true IPM approach have the potential to replace most conventional chemical barrier methods, and significantly decrease the use of toxic pesticides in termite control.

Ask for the baiting methods. A baiting system called Sentricon® is already registered with the EPA, but is not yet widely available as of this writing. Several other baiting systems are under commercial development and may be available by the time you read this. Ask the pest control company you are considering about the new baiting systems.

Under development and testing. There is a method called trap-treat-release that shows great promise for subterranean termite control. The termites are treated with a groomable coating material that contains the insecticide sulfluramid. Termites that may avoid food bait (as they learn to do) will ingest the pesticide when grooming each other.

Traps are placed at the corners of the structure and monitored. When the termites are found they are taken from the trap, treated with the coating and then released back into the soil. They find their way back to the colony from a pheromone trail, and spread the poison.

Carpenter ants. You may have a carpenter ant infestation and not termites. You can hire a professional to find out, or take the insects to a Cooperative Extension office for identification. Carpenter ants do not destroy wood they way termites do; they show up where there is already decay, which is an excellent source of food and moisture for them.

A carpenter ant infestation is an indication of moisture and decay problems with the wood. You should not panic since the ants are not going to cause your house to fall down. An infestation can be treated with baits and do not require fumigants and chemical barrier methods to control. Again, *Common Sense Pest Control* is an excellent source if you want to learn more about wood pests before you talk to a pest control company.

Part IV: Commercial Product Listing

Table 10.2 that follows, lists the active ingredients used by pest control companies in San Francisco and Florida from our surveys. We have combined the acute and chronic toxicity data in the same table for your convenience.

Material Safety Data Sheets. There is another source of information about pesticides called a Material Safety Data Sheet or MSDS (em-ess-dee-ess). The MSDS contains additional information than that on the pesticide label. It fills the requirements of worker "Right to Know" laws (legal name is Hazard Communication Standard). The law requires the MSDS to be available to anyone exposed to chemicals in the workplace. This includes those who sell, stock, or transport it. All pesticides used by commercial pest control operators have an MSDS. You can request the company to give you a copy for the products the company proposes to use in your home. Once you read them you may decide you would prefer a safer alternative. MSDSs are not available for pesticide products you buy over-the-counter.

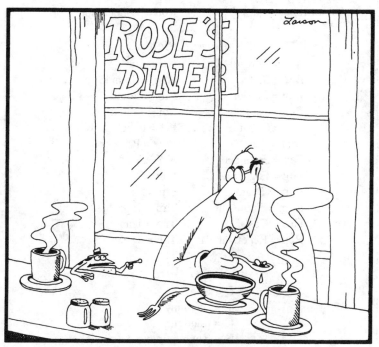

"I beg your pardon, but you're not planning just to throw that fly away, are you?"

Key to Brand Name
Product Table

Use

Her = Herbicide

IGR = Insect Growth Regulator

Fun = Fungicide

Mol = Molluscicide

Mul = Multiple Uses

PGR = Plant Growth Regulator

Rep = Repellent

Rod = Rodenticide

Formulation

Aer = Aerosol

Bat = Bait

Bar = Barrier

Bom = Bomb

Col = Collar

Dus = Dust

Fer = Fertilizer

Fog = Fogger

Fom = Foam

Fum = Fumigant

Gas = Gas

Rep = Repellent

Gel = Gel

Grn = Granule

Liq = Liquid

Lot = Lotion

Pel = Pellet

Pow = Powder

Sld = Solid

Spr = Spray

Stp = Strip

Tap = Tape

Trp = Trap

Tab = Tablet

Label Word

D = Danger

W = Warning

C = Caution

N = Not required or not on label

Class

CB = Methyl carbamate

CH = Chlorinated hydrocarbon

OP = Organophosphate

PY = Pyrethrin

SP = Synthetic pyrethroid

SY = Synergist

Tumors/Cancer

A tumor is an abnormal growth of tissue that can be benign or malignant. Another name for a malignant tumor is cancer. Substances that cause cancer are called *carcinogens*. Substances that cause tumors are called *oncogens*.

Repro. Damage

Reproductive damage refers to effects such as death of the embryo or fetus (equivalent to spontaneous abortion and stillbirth in humans), low birth weight, sterility/infertility. It also includes birth defects such as structural defects such as missing arms or legs, or hole in the heart, spina bifida etc. Substances that cause birth defects are called *teratogens*.

Genetic Damage

Genetic damage refers to effects on genetic material including genes, chromosomes, and DNA.

$(\mathbf{X})$ = Possible adverse effect

$(\mathbf{-})$ = Either no data available or information available is not sufficient to make a determination

$(\mathbf{0})$ = Adequate data and no adverse effect noted.

* Sources for the above chronic toxicity data are from Cal-EPA SB-950 Toxicology Summaries, U.S.EPA Factsheets, U.S.EPA R.E.Ds (Registration Eligibility Documents), and scientific journals.

Table 10.2

Commercial Use Pesticides

Active Ingredients by Common Name The names in parentheses are brand names or common names. Some brands contain only the ingredient listed; others contain additional ones. There are other brand name products than those listed here.	Use	Type
A		
Abamectin (Avid)	Ins	
Acephate (Orthene, Orthenex	Ins	OP
Aliette	Fun	
Allethrin (PT 515 Wasp Freeze)	Ins	SP
Aluminum phosphide (Fumitoxin, Phostoxin)	Rod	
Asulam sodium (Asulox)	Her	
Atrazine (Aatrex)	Her	
B		
B.T. (Bactospeine, Dipel, Gnatrol)	Ins	
Bendiocarb (Ficam, Turcam)	Ins	
Benomyl (Benlate)	Fun	
Boric acid (Drax Ant Kill, Borid, PT-240)	Ins	
Brodifacoum (Talon)	Rod	
Bromacil (Hyvar)	Her	
Bromadiolone (Maki)	Rod	
C		
Cacodylic acid (Montar)	Her	
Carbaryl (Sevimol, Sevin)	Ins	
Chlorfenethol (Qikron, DMC)	Ins	
Chlormequat (Cyocel)	Pgr	
Chloropicrin (Chlor-O-Pic)	Fum	
Chlorothalonil (Daconil)	Fun	
Chlorpyrifos (Dursban, Empire, Equity, PT-270)	Ins	
Chlorsulfuron (Telar)	Her	
Copper (Bordeaux Mixture)	Fun	

LD$_{50}$ mg/kg	EPA Toxicity Category	Label Word	Tumors/Cancer	Repro. Damage	Genetic Damage
5,000	III	C	o	x	x
1,030	III	C	x	o	x
5,000	III	C	x	x	o
685	III	C	o	o	o
>1	I	D	-	-	-
>5,000	IV	C	-	-	-
1,780	III	C	x	o	o
-	III	C	o	o	o
179	II	W	-	x	x
>10,000	IV	C	x	x	x
3,500	III	C	x	x	x
>1	I	D	-	-	-
5,200	II, III, IV	C	x	o	x
1.75	I	D	-	-	-
2,756	III	C	x	x	x
246	I, II, III, IV	W	x	o	x
926	III	C	-	-	-
883	III	C	-	-	-
250	I	W	-	x	x
>10,000	I, II	C	x	o	x
96	II, III	W	o	o	x
3,053	IV	C	o	o	o
1,000	I, II	C	-	-	-

Commercial Use Pesticides

Active Ingredients by Common Name The names in parentheses are brand names or common names. Some brands contain only the ingredient listed; others contain additional ones. There are other brand name products than those listed here.	Use	Type
Copper chelated (Cutrine)	Fun	
Copper hydroxide (Kocide)	Fun	
Cyfluthrin (Tempo, Optem, PT-600)	Ins	SP
Cypermethrin (Demon, Cynoff)	Ins	SP
D		
2,4-D (Weed-B-Gon)	Her	
Daminozide (B-Nine, Alar)	Pgr	
Dazomet (Basamid)	Fum	
Diatomaceous earth	Ins	
Diazinon (Knox-Out 2FM, Knox-Out 1500A)	Ins	OP
Dicamba (Banvel)	Her	
Diclofop-methyl (Illoxan, Hoelon)	Her	
Dicloran (DCNA, Botran)	Fun	
Dicofol (Kelthane)	Ins	CH
Dicrotophos (Insecticide B, Maoget)	Ins	OP
Dienochlor (Pentac)	Ins	CH
Dikegulac sodium (Atrimmec)	Pgr	
Dimethoate (Cygon)	Ins	OP
Diphacinone (Answer Gopher Bait, Di-Block)	Rod	
Diquat	Her	
Dithiopyr (Dimension)	Fun	
Diuron (Direx, Karmex)	Her	
Duosan (Thiophanate-methyl & maneb)	Fun	
E		
Endosulfan (Thiodan)	Ins	CH
Etridiazole w/T-M (Banrot)	Fun	

LD_{50} mg/kg	EPA Toxicity Category	Label Word	Tumors/Cancer	Repro. Damage	Genetic Damage
0.50-2	I	C	-	-	-
1,000	I	D	-	-	-
500	I, II	**D**	-	x	o
250	II	W	x	x	-
699	III	C	x	x	x
8,400	III	C	x	o	o
519	III	C	-	-	-
-	-	-	o	o	o
1,250	II, III	W	o	x	x
2,629	II	C	-	x	x
512	III	C	x	x	o
>5,000	IV	C	-	-	-
570	II, III	W,C	x	x	o
17	I	D	-	-	-
3,160	III	C	-	-	-
18,000	IV	C	-	-	-
235	II	W	o	x	x
1.86	I, II, III	W	-	-	o
215	II	W	x	x	x
3,600	II	W	-	o	o
>5,000	III	C	x	o	x
10,200	III	C	x	x	x
22.7	I	W	-	o	o
5,000	I, III	D, C	-	-	-

Commercial Use Pesticides

Active Ingredients by Common Name The names in parentheses are brand names or common names. Some brands contain only the ingredient listed; others contain additional ones. There are other brand name products than those listed here.	Use	Type
F		
Fenamiphos (Nemacur)	Ins	OP
Fenarimol (Rubigan)	Fun	
Fenoxycarb (Torus, Logic)	Igr	
Fenvalerate (Tribute, Pyrid, FVS Fogger)	Ins	SP
Fluazifop-butyl (Fusilade, Namec)	Her	
Fluvalinate (Mavrik)	Ins	
G		
Glyphosate (Roundup, Kleenup, Expedite)	Her	
H		
Hydramethylnon (Amdro)	Ins	
Hydroprene (Precor, Gencor)	Igr	
I		
IBA (Indole butyric acid)	Pgr	
Isazofos (Triumph)	Ins	OP
Isoxaben (Gallery)	Her	
K		
Kinoprene (Enstar)	Igr	
L		
Lambda-cyhalothrin (Scimitar, Karate, Kung Fu)	Ins	SP
Lime sulfur (Calcium polysulfides)	Fun	
Lindane (Isotox, Gamma-Mene)	Ins	CH
Liquid nitrogen	Ins	

LD_{50} mg/kg	EPA Toxicity Category	Label Word	Tumors/Cancer	Repro. Damage	Genetic Damage
140	I	D	o	-	x
2,500	III	C	x	-	o
16,800	IV	C	-	-	o
451	II	W	x	-	o
3,328	III	C	-	-	-
261	I	W	x	x	x
4,300	II	C	x	o	o
1,131	III	C	o	x	o
>34,000	IV	C	-	-	-
-	III	C	o	o	o
40	I	W	-	o	-
>10,000	IV	C	x	x	-
4,900	II, III	C	-	-	-
79	IV	W	-	-	-
400	I	D	-	-	-
88-125	II	W	x	x	x
-	-	-	o	o	o

Commercial Use Pesticides

Active Ingredients by Common Name

The names in parentheses are brand names or common names. Some brands contain only the ingredient listed; others contain additional ones. There are other brand name products than those listed here.

	Use	Type
M		
MCPA	Her	
MCPP (Mecoprop)	Her	
Magnesium phosphide (Fumi-cel, Magtoxin)	Rod	
Malathion	Ins	OP
Maleic hydrazide (Slow-Gro)	Pgr	
Maneb (Manex)	Fun	
Mefluidide (Embark)	Pgr	
Metalaxyl (Ridomil, Subdue)	Fun	
Metaldehyde (Bug-Geta, Deadline, Snarol)	Mol	
Methiocarb (Mesurol)	Ins	CB
Methomyl (Muscalure, Musca-Cide, Stimukil)	Ins	CB
Methoprene (Precor, Fleatrol)	Igr	
Methyl bromide (Bromo-Gas, Metabrom 100)	Fum	
Metolachlor (Pennant, Dual)	Her	
Metribuzin (Sencor, Lexone)	Her	
N		
Neem (Azadirachtin, Margosan-O)	Ins	
Nicotine (Nicofume, Plant Fume 103)	Ins	
O		
Orthoboric acid (Tim-Bor)	Ins	
Oryzalin (Surflan)	Her	
Oxadiazon (Ronstar)	Her	
Oxamyl (Vydate)	Ins	CB
Oxycarboxin (Plantvax)	Her	
Oxythioquinox (Morestan)	Ins	

LD$_{50}$ mg/kg	EPA Toxicity Category	Label Word	Tumors/Cancer	Repro. Damage	Genetic Damage
1,160	I	C	o	x	x
1,166	I	W	-	x	-
1	I	D	-	-	-
2,000	III	C	x	o	o
6,950	IV	C	-	-	x
7,790	IV	C	x	x	x
>4,000	III	C	x	o	o
669	III	C	x	o	o
630	III, II	C, W	x	x	o
20	I	D	o	x	o
17	I, III	D	o	x	o
>34,600	IV	C	o	o	o
214	I	W	x	x	x
2,780	III	C	x	o	o
2,000	III	C	x	o	x
>5,000	IV	C	-	-	-
50	I	D	-	-	-
3,500	III	C	x	x	x
>10,000	IV	C	x	o	o
>5,000	I, IV	C	x	x	x
5.4	I	**D**	o	o	o
2,000	III	C	-	-	-
15,000	I, II, III	C	-	x	x

Commercial Use Pesticides

Active Ingredients by Common Name The names in parentheses are brand names or common names. Some brands contain only the ingredient listed; others contain additional ones. There are other brand name products than those listed here.	Use	Type
P		
PCNB (Proturf FF, Turfside, Pentachlor)	Fun	
Permethrin (Dragnet, Torpedo)	Ins	SP
Petroleum oil (Volck Oil, Dormant Oil)	Ins	
Phenothrin (Sumithrin)	Ins	SP
Pindone (Pivalin)	Rod	
Piperalin (Pipron)	Fun	
Piperonyl butoxide* (Pybuthrin)	Syn	
Polybutenes (For the Birds, Hot Foot)	Rep	
Potash soap (Safer Miticide)	Ins	
Prodiamine (Barricade)	Her	
Prometon (Noxal)	Her	
Pronamide (Kerb)	Her	
Propamacarb (Banol)	Fun	
Propetamphos (Safrotin, RF-256 Aerosol)	Ins	OP
Propiconazole (Banner)	Fun	
Propoxur (Baygon)	Ins	CB
Pyrethrins (Pyrenone, PT 1600A, X-Clude)	Ins	PY
Pyrethrum (Synerol, PT 565, Pyrocide)	Ins	PY
R		
Resmethrin (R300 Multipurpose Spray)	Ins	SP
S		
Sethoxydim (Poast)	Her	
Silical gel (Drione)	Ins	
Simazine (SimTrol 90)	Her	
Soap (Potassium salts of fatty acids, M-Pede)	Ins	

LD$_{50}$ mg/kg	EPA Toxicity Category	Label Word	Tumors/Cancer	Repro. Damage	Genetic Damage
1,700	III	C	x	o	x
430	II, III	W	x	x	o
-	-	-	x	-	-
>10,000	IV	C	x	-	o
-	-	-	-	-	-
2,500	IV	C	-	-	-
>7,500	IV	C	-	-	o
-	-	-	-	-	-
-	-	-	-	-	-
>5,000	IV	C	x	x	-
699	I, III	C	o	o	o
5,620	III	C	x	-	o
2,000	IV	C	-	x	o
119	II	W	o	-	-
1,517	III	C	-	-	-
50	I, II, III	D, W, C	x	o	o
1,500	III	C	x	x	x
1,500	III	C	-	-	-
2,500	III	C	x	x	o
3,200	III	C	-	-	-
>5	I	D	o	o	o
5,000	IV	C	x	o	o
-	-	-	o	o	o

Commercial Use Pesticides

Active Ingredients by Common Name The names in parentheses are brand names or common names. Some brands contain only the ingredient listed; others contain additional ones. There are other brand name products than those listed here.	Use	Type
Sodium polyborate (Borax, Terro Ant Killer)	Ins	
Streptomycin (Agri-Mycin)	Ins	
Sulfluramid (Pro-Control Ant Bait)	Ins	
Sulfometuron (Oust)	Her	
Sulfotep (Plant Fume)	Ins	OP
Sulfur	Fun	
Sulfuryl fluoride (Vikane)	Fum	
T		
Thiophanate-methyl (Fungo Flo, Pro Turf VIII)	Fun	
Triadimefon (Bayleton, Pro Turf VII)	Fun	
Triclopyr (Redeem, Turflon)	Her	
Trifluralin (Greflan, Team)	Her	
Triforine (Funginex)	Fun	
V		
Vinclozolin (Ronilan)	Fun	
Z		
Zinc phosphide	Rod	

LD$_{50}$ mg/kg	EPA Toxicity Category	Label Word	Tumors/Cancer	Repro. Damage	Genetic Damage
3,479	III	C	-	x	x
9,000	IV	C	o	o	o
-	-	-	-	-	-
>5,000	IV	C	-	-	-
10	I	D	-	-	-
5,000	III	C	o	o	o
5 ppm	I	D	o	o	o
7,500	IV	C	x	-	o
1,000	III	C	x	x	o
630	III	C	o	o	x
10,000	IV	C	x	o	o
16,000	IV	C	x	o	o
>16,000	IV	C	x	x	x
46	I	D	-	-	-

* Piperonyl butoxide causes cancer and birth
defects in rats (see pages 114-115).

11

Law, Policy, and Recommendations

This country has come to feel the same when Congress is in session as when the baby gets hold of a hammer.

Will Rogers (1879-1935)

Whoever said "there are two things you don't want to watch being made – laws and sausages", must have been trying to reform pesticide laws. There is no rational way to explain pesticide laws because they are not rational. To comprehend the notorious deficiencies of pesticide laws requires an understanding of how dinosaurs think. In legislative chambers throughout the country, outrageous statements supporting the use of toxic pesticides continue to be made with a straight face.

Federal pesticide law. The federal law that governs pesticides is called FIFRA – the Federal Insecticide Fungicide and Rodenticide Act – passed in 1947 to regulate "economic poisons". (Even though herbicides are not in the title of the law, it is incorrect to say "pesticides and herbicides" as is often done. Herbicides *are* pesticides). FIFRA was administered by the U.S. Department of Agriculture (USDA) from 1947 to 1972.

USDA and FIFRA. During its tenure, the USDA worked hand-in-glove with the pesticide industry, making it very easy to register pesticides. No chronic toxicity studies were required; it was not necessary to find out whether the pesticide caused cancer, birth defects or genetic damage. There were no requirements for testing effects on birds, bees, and fish, or for environmental fate and persistence data. Pesticides were promoted and used without knowing if they contaminated groundwater, how long they stayed in the soil, and whether they broke down into more toxic compounds. There were almost no data on the exposures and health status of workers handling the toxic pesticides.

Rachel Carson. In her 1962 book, *Silent Spring,* Rachel Carson aimed her most pointed attacks at the USDA's administration of the pesticide laws. The USDA ignored or trivialized the health and environmental hazards so eloquently described in her book. Carson discussed the USDA's strong support of pesticide industry positions on DDT and other toxic pesticides. She made it clear that unless and until the administration of FIFRA was taken away from the USDA, there would be no progress towards protecting human health and the environment from pesticides.

The EPA. The Environmental Protection Agency (EPA) was created in 1970, and the responsibility for the administration of FIFRA passed over to the agency in 1972. All pesticides must be registered by the EPA before they can be marketed or sold. In 1972, the U.S. Congress passed significant amendments to FIFRA, requiring that all pesticides be tested for their potential to adversely affect human health and the environment, before they could be registered and marketed.

Already registered pesticides. The amended law had to deal with pesticides already on the market that were registered during the lax USDA years. There were no toxicity and environmental studies for 1,200 active ingredient pesticides formulated into 45,000 different products. The new FIFRA amendments required these pesticides to be re-registered to meet the new health and safety standards, setting a deadline of 1975. Pesticide industry resistance, recalcitrance, legal maneuvers, and delaying tactics, combined with poor oversight and enforcement by the EPA, has lead to several extensions of these deadlines. The latest one is 1998. Some of the pesticides have been in commercial use for more than four decades. Estimates are that it will be well into the year 2000 before the re-registration process is complete.

Inert ingredients. The new FIFRA amendments in 1972 did not include any provision on inert ingredients. It is only recently that the EPA has begun to address this crucial issue. As already discussed in chapter two, inert ingredients can be as toxic, or even more toxic, than the active ingredient pesticides they are mixed with. There are about 2,000 inert ingredients used in pesticide products.

FIFRA considers the names of inert ingredients proprietary information – a trade secret. By law, inert ingredients cannot be revealed, even when there are health problems caused by the inert and not the active ingredient.

The EPA's recent activities involve little more than classifying inert ingredients, supposedly on the basis of toxicological significance. It is difficult to have much confidence in any classification scheme that does not provide full public disclosure.

Sacred Cow. This cloak of secrecy, a sacred cow of the pesticide industry, is an anachronism in modern law, and must be removed. If all the ingredients are listed on cosmetics, they can certainly be listed on pesticides.

Missing chronic toxicity data (data gaps). The failure to reregister older pesticides to meet current FIFRA standards, means there are a significant number of pesticides on the market that have not been fully tested. The scientific studies to determine their potential to cause cancer, birth defects, genetic damage, and other chronic, long-term toxicity have not been done, or were improperly or inadequately done. These missing studies are known as 'data gaps'.

We found that almost 40% of the active ingredient pesticides in our survey had data gaps. Table 11.1 shows the percentage of active ingredient insecticides, herbicides, and fungicides from our survey that were missing chronic toxicity data for cancer, and reproductive and genetic damage.

Table 11.1

Percentage of 149 Active Ingredient Pesticides with Data gaps – Missing Chronic Toxicity Studies
(from California and Florida Surveys)

	All Ingredients (Total = 149)	Insecticides (No.=74)	Herbicides (No.=47)	Fungicides (No.=28)
Cancer	38%	37%	38%	39%
Reproductive	40%	37%	40%	46%
Genetic	37%	35%	40%	36%

Current status. We would like to report that the EPA has mended its ways, and the pesticide industry is no longer an obstructionist in assuring that pesticides are fully tested *before* registration and marketing. Not so. The EPA is registering some new pesticides without all of the required testing under a policy called "conditional registration".

The Birth Defects Prevention Act (SB-950). The state of California has a pesticide registration division more stringent than federal EPA's. In 1984, the California legislature passed a law requiring pesticide companies to submit any missing scientific studies on their products by March, 1991. The law covered two-hundred pesticides; failure to meet the requirement would result in loss of registration in California. The law, called the Birth Defects Prevention Act, or SB-950, required the following chronic toxicity studies:cancer in rats and mice, chronic effects in rats and dogs, reproductive effects in rats, birth defects in rats and rabbits, and testing for genetic mutations, chromosome abnormalities, and effects on DNA.

Toxicological evaluation. SB-950 requires evaluation by state toxicologists of chronic toxicity studies submitted to the EPA by the pesticide companies. These toxicological summaries were among the sources for the chronic toxicity information in the brand name and commercial use products tables in chapters six through ten.

Data gaps. As you will see from the tables in chapters six through nine, there are many brand name over-the-counter products sold in California that contain active ingredient pesticides with missing studies (data gaps). Many of these active ingredients remain on the market because of delaying tactics and legal maneuvers by pesticide companies. SB-950's original March, 1991 deadline was extended to March, 1996. At the time of this writing, pesticide companies are in Sacramento lobbying for another extension.

Restricted use pesticides. All pesticides are registered by the EPA for either general use or restricted use. Restricted use pesticides include some that are highly toxic, adversely impact nontarget species or wildlife, contaminate groundwater, or have other detrimental effects on the environment. Restricted use pesticides can only be applied by a state certified applicator.

Banned pesticides. Table 11.2 shows the list of pesticides banned or severely restricted in the U.S. It took years, sometimes decades, of dogged effort and struggle by many dedicated people to get most of these pesticides off the market.

Many of the 825 pesticides currently registered with the EPA, deserve to be on this list – pesticides which are highly toxic, have a poor safety record, are known animal carcinogens or teratogens, or do not meet current health and safety requirements.

Table 11.2

Pesticides Banned, Suspended, or Severely Restricted in the U.S.		
Year	**Pesticide**	**Action**
1972	DDT	Cancellation all uses except public health emergencies.
1974	Aldrin	Cancellation all uses except termite control.
1974	Dieldrin	Cancellation most uses.
1976	Kepone	Cancellation all uses.
1977	Mirex	Cancellation all uses except pineapple in Hawaii.
1978	BHC	Cancellation all uses.
1978	Chlordane	Cancellation food and most other uses except termite control.
1978	Heptachlor	Cancellation all uses except seed treatment.
1979	DBCP	Cancellation all uses except pineapple in Hawaii.
1979	2,4,5-T/Silvex	Emergency suspension most uses.
1982	Toxaphene	Cancellation all uses except animal dip banana/pineapple P.Rico, Virgin I.
1983	EPN	Cancellation mosquito larvacide use.
1983	Nitrofen (Tok)	Voluntary cancellation all uses.
1984	EDB	Cancellation all uses.
1985	DBCP	Cancellation all uses.
1985	Endrin	Voluntary cancellation all uses.
1985	2,4,5-T / Silvex	Cancellation all uses.
1986	Diazinon	Cancellation of use on golf courses and sod farms.
1986	Lindane	Cancellation indoor fumigation use.
1986	Dinoseb	Emergency suspension, cancellation.
1988	Chlordane	Cancellation termite control use.
1989	Chlordimeform	Registration voluntarily withdrawn.
1989	Heptachlor	Intent to cancel seed treatment announced.
1990	Daminozide (Alar)	Cancellation all food uses.
1994	Phosdrin (mevinphos)	Voluntary cancellation all uses.
1995	Phosdrin (mevinphos)	Delay of cancellation for one year.

Proposition 65. On November 4, 1986, California voters passed Proposition 65 by a 63% margin. Also known as the Safe Drinking Water and Toxic Enforcement Act, the purpose of the law was to protect the public from unknowing or unwilling exposure to potentially harmful products that cause cancer or birth defects.

The law required warning labels or posting of notices if a chemical contained in a product, caused cancer or birth defects based on tests performed in laboratory animals. The decision of what chemicals got on the Proposition 65 list was decided by a committee of qualified experts appointed by the governor. We will spare you the machinations, maneuvers, and other tactics that pesticide manufacturers use to keep their products off the Proposition 65 list.

Cancer and birth defects list. There are seventeen pesticides on the Proposition 65 cancer list, shown in Table 11.3. There are four pesticides on the birth defects list, shown in Table 11.4. The pesticides in italics are ones that were found in our surveys of home use pesticides.

Table 11.3

Pesticides on the Proposition 65 Cancer List
(Those in italics found in surveys)

Acifluorfen	*Lindane*
Alachlor	*Mancozeb*
Arsenic trioxide	*Maneb*
Arsenic pentoxide	Orthophenylphenol
Captan	*Oxadiazon*
Chlorothalonil	*Paradichlorobenzene*
Creosote	Pentachlorophenol
Daminozide	*Propargite*
Dichlorvos	

Table 11.4

Pesticides on the Proposition 65 Birth defects List
(Those in italics found in surveys)
Benomyl Bromoxynil Cyanazine *Methyl bromide*

Except for paradichlorobenzene, none of the over-the-counter products in our California survey containing active ingredients from the cancer list, had a Proposition 65 warning on the label. Benomyl is sold over-the-counter in California but does not have a Proposition 65 warning on the label. Methyl bromide is a restricted use pesticide for sale only to certified pest control operators, who are obligated to warn customers about its birth defect potential. See Appendix C on page 328 for brand name over-the-counter products in our surveys that contain the italicized active ingredients.

Regulation of Home Use Pesticides

Home use pesticides sold over-the-counter and for commercial use are essentially unregulated. Many pesticides initially registered for other uses (mainly agricultural) are reformulated for the home market. There are no scientific studies required to assess potential adverse health and environmental effects when using home pesticides according to label instructions.

Children's exposure: There are no data requirements to determine how long pesticide residues remain on treated lawns, carpets, or other areas and surfaces. Yet many labels state that children can return to the treated area when the sprays are dry (see Figure 2.4 in chapter two for some examples).

There are absolutely no data to back up these label statements. See the index for the many times in this book we raise concerns about the exposures of infants and children.

Drift, the movement of pesticides away from the site of application, is a very serious problem. *All* broadcast sprays drift. Pesticides can drift a mile or more in significant concentrations, and much further in lower concentrations. Pesticide drift can contaminate children's sandboxes and play equipment, fish ponds, bird feeding stations, organic gardens, lawns, yards, swimming pools, and other outdoor spaces.

Yet pesticides are registered and labeled for home outdoor use without any data required on drift potential. The EPA seems to take the view that if enough warning statements are put on the label, the drift problem will somehow disappear. Pesticide molecules follow the laws of physics, not those on a pesticide label. If birds, bees, fish, and frolicking children would only read the label they could protect themselves. See figure 2.6 in chapter two for a list of some of these label warnings.

Regulatory flaws. Uncontrolled, unregulated, and unacknowledged problems from pesticide drift are among the most serious of many flaws and deficiencies in the regulation of home use pesticides. Anyone within drift distance of a spray nozzle can be involuntarily, unwillingly, and unknowingly exposed. And in areas where outdoor broadcast sprays are frequent and pervasive, entire neighborhoods and communities are at risk of exposure.

Those with asthma, allergies, and chemical sensitivity are vulnerable to very small amounts of pesticide residues. Drift exposures pose unacceptable potential health risks to infants, children, pregnant women, the elderly, the ill, and the immunocompromised.

Recommendations

Throughout this book we discuss ways you can protect your health and personal patch of the planet from toxic pesticides. We describe nontoxic and less toxic pest control methods that enable you to get off the pesticide treadmill.

Getting off the treadmill yourself is only part of the solution to the hazards of home pesticide use. There is an enormous infrastructure in place, built up since the 1940s, that supports and promotes the use of toxic pesticides. The commercialization and delivery of pest control services to the home, are an important and increasing contribution to this toxic infrastructure. In this section we discuss broader issues that relate to taming the toxic beast; our recommendations are in four areas:

I. Information
II. Exposure
III. Health
IV. Services

Part I. Information

Consumers cannot make appropriate decisions about buying a product if they know very little about it. Product labels hinder rather than simplify obtaining information — limiting choice even further. The possibility of an informed choice almost vanishes when advertising and marketing downplays the hazard and trivializes the risk of using a product.

Our recommendations focus on access to easily and readily available high quality information that is clear, comprehensive, and user friendly. They apply to over-the-counter brand name pesticides sold directly to the consumer, and to pest control services.

◆ All over-the-counter products should have the names of both active *and inert* ingredients on the label.

◆ There should be a standardized common name chosen for all active *and inert* ingredients. This common name should be on the label for all pesticide products containing the ingredient.

◆ There should be a consumer's product information sheet for *each* brand name product available at the point of purchase. This specific product information sheet should contain everything that is on the label plus additional information discussed below, in a standardized form that is easy to read. The information could be in a single volume, well indexed, on the model of the PDR (Physicians Desk Reference).

◆ All over-the-counter products should be labeled with what is known about the chronic toxicity potential for each active *and inert* ingredient in the product to cause cancer and tumors (C), reproductive damage (R), and genetic damage (G). All ingredients can be classified into one of four mutually exclusive categories:

1. The ingredient is *known* to cause the effect (C, R or G).
2. The ingredient is *suspected* to cause the effect (C, R or G).
3. There is *insufficient data* to make a determination (data gap) (C,R or G).
4. There is *no apparent* adverse effect (C, R or G).

Objections. We already hear the objections from pesticide producers that there is not enough room on the label. Yes there is, and here is a way to do it. Use the designated letters, C for cancer and tumors, R for reproductive damage, and G for genetic damage. Next, choose a color for each mutually exclusive chronic toxicity category: *red* for known to cause, *blue* for suspected to cause, *yellow* for missing data, and *green* for no apparent adverse effect. The colored letter can be put in a very small white box next to the name of each ingredient, or in a narrow rectangular white strip to the right of the ingredients listing. Where there's a will there's a way.

Guilty until proven innocent. We hear another objection. Pesticide producers will say the data are not sufficient, or there is no agreement among scientists how to properly categorize each active and inert ingredient. If so, then the ingredient should automatically go into the suspect or data gap category until the data *are* sufficient and agreed upon. It is the pesticide manufactures and major users who insist their pesticides are scientifically tested, and meet rigorous government rules and regulations. If their products are scientifically tested, then why not label them – unless there is something the companies do not want the public to know. The process of categorizing should not take years. It should be done *immediately* for all products, using the most current data. It is a simple matter of giving the consumer the best available current information. Pesticides are guilty until proven innocent.

Honesty and openness needed. Pesticide companies cannot have it both ways. Either their products are adequately tested or they are not. The data to support the registration and marketing of the products is complete or it is not. Whatever the truth is, put it on the product label. Let us have some honesty and openness on these issues.

◆ All pesticide labels should be in a standardized format, with key information in a single place on the label. The new nutrition label is a good model.

◆ Require mandatory use reporting by commercial pest control companies, for both restricted *and* general use pesticides. The reports should include the name of the company, the name of the product used, the formulation type, amount used, specific location of use, and number of applications. All reports should be readily available to the public at a central location at no cost, and a summary report released annually.

- All of the information described above, pesticide label information, the consumer's product information sheet, and the pesticide use reports should be available on-line.

Part II. Exposure

Throughout this book we discuss contamination problems and involuntary exposures. We recommended that you not use any pesticides that are in the form of foggers, bombs and aerosols, because of their ability to contaminate the entire area being treated. These formulations are also more likely to contain toxic inert ingredients, and petroleum based compounds. We also discussed the serious problem of drift, volatilization, and off-gassing from pesticides applications that result in involuntary, unwilling, and unknowing exposures to toxic pesticides. These problems are especially important for vulnerable populations such as the fetus, infants and children, asthmatics, and the chemically sensitive. Our recommendations to deal with these problems are:

- Nerve-gas type pesticides (organophosphates and carbamates) should be prohibited in any product formulated as a fogger, bomb, or aerosol.
- Nerve-gas type pesticides (organophosphates and carbamates) should be prohibited for use on carpet, lawns, and any areas where children and pets will contact the resulting residues.
- Pesticides that are known carcinogens, oncogens, or teratogens should be prohibited in any product formulated as a fogger, bomb, or aerosol.
- Pesticides that are known carcinogens, oncogens, or teratogens should be prohibited for use on carpet, lawns, and any areas where children and pets will contact the resulting residues.

◆ Broadcast sprays should be prohibited where there is any
   potential for drift, volatilization, or off-gassing, in any
   amount, to unwilling and unknowing persons

◆ All pesticides sold over-the-counter should be in child-
   proof containers.

◆ All pesticide containers should require a deposit and be
   returnable to the point of purchase for return of deposit.
   This will prevent the problem of improper storage and
   disposal of unused pesticides, and provide an incentive
   for proper disposal of toxic products.

Part III. Health Risks

The only way to decrease or eliminate the health risks from
pesticides is to eliminate the exposure. We are realistic and
know that pesticides with significant potential acute and
chronic health risks, are not going to disappear tomorrow.
We focus our recommendations on certain products that pose
unacceptable risks to children. These are not the only ones,
just the most egregious ones.

◆ All use of lindane should be prohibited.

◆ All use of paradichlorobenzene should be prohibited.

◆ All use of dichlorvos (DDVP) should be prohibited.

◆ All deet products should not be available by prescription
   only.

◆ All use of deet should be prohibited for use in young
   children (twelve years old or less), or any child with
   illness, disability, or other reasons they cannot
   understand or are unable to follow instructions for use
   of the product.

◆ All deet prescriptions for older children should contain
   less than 10% of the active ingredient.

◆ All deet prescriptions for adults should contain 25% or
   less of the active ingredient.

- ◆ Vulnerable populations adversely affected by pesticides should have prior notification for any pesticide use that will potentially expose them to residues resulting from drift, volatilization, or off-gassing, in any amount.
- ◆ Vulnerable populations adversely affected by pesticides, should be able to prevent any pesticide use that will potentially expose them as a result of drift, volatilization, or off-gassing, in any amount, upon certification by their physician.

Part IV. Services

In chapter ten we discuss the companies that provide commercial pest control services. There are some obvious recommendations. For example, noncertified applicators should not apply restricted use pesticides as current law allows. However, requiring better qualifications for those who apply restricted use pesticides, ignores the problem of using such toxic pesticides in the home in the first place. Improving the education and training of pesticide applicators falls under the same conundrum.

Therefore, our recommendations are not in the spirit of what we can do to see that toxic chemicals can be used more safely – this is a fool's errand, and has been going on much too long. The current chemical dominance in home use pest control is based on downplaying the hazards and trivializing the risks of their use. There must be changes in a positive direction, ways that provide the public with safer options for their pest control problems We recommend some important first steps.

- ◆ There should be a new category of pest control operator trained in nontoxic and least toxic methods.
- ◆ The new category of pest control operator should be authorized to use pesticides – but only those formulated as baits and traps that do not involve

broadcast sprays, or result in drift, volatilization, or off-gassing.

◆ The new category of pest control operator should *not* be required to be certified in conventional chemical methods, since they will not be authorized to use them.

◆ Pest control companies should be required to inform potential clients in writing of all options for treating their pest problem *before* any delivery of services, including nontoxic and least toxic methods.

◆ Pest control companies that do not provide nontoxic and least toxic methods should be required to refer potential clients to companies that do.

◆ Pest control companies should be required to provide potential clients with a copy of labels, and material safety data sheets, upon request *prior* to any delivery of services.

The Last Word

Readers who have gotten this far may be thinking "What are you going to do about all these problems you have been telling us about". We hope many are also thinking "What can I do." You can begin by changing your personal use of pest control products and services, and persuade your friends and neighbors to do the same. If you would like to get more involved with groups and organizations dedicated to making homes and communities safer from toxic pesticides, Appendix J lists some that you can contact in your area.

We will continue to do our part to educate the public about health effects of home use pesticides, and to advocate and promote nontoxic methods for home pest control. We are aware of concerns about toxic sprays applied outside the home – including schools, day care centers, restaurants, supermarkets, office buildings, hospitals and nursing homes, golf courses, parks and recreation areas, along roads and highways, and other locations. We are concerned as well, and are gathering information for a publication about these involuntary exposures.

Please feel free to contact us about any experiences in your community that might be helpful, and about any effective nontoxic methods you know about that we did not discuss in this book.

Appendix A
Pronunciation Guide

Many of our readers will not be familiar with some of the terms used in this book. Knowing how to pronounce them can make it easier for you to talk to, pest control operators, your doctor and others. This pronunciation guide is based on the author's personal system with revisions after trying it out on several people unfamiliar with medical and pesticide terminology. If you come up with a better 'sound bite' for a particular entry let us know and we will consider it for inclusion in later editions.

A
Abrasion: uh–BRAY–jun
Acephate: ASS–uh–fate
Aciflurofen: ass–uh–FLUR–oh–fen
Alkaloids: ALK–ah–loyds
Alkyl pyridines: ALK–ill PEER–ah–deens (fix)
Allethrin: ah–LEE–thrin
Ammonium thiosulfate: ah–MOAN–ee–um thigh–oh–SUL–fate
Anaphylaxis: ana–fuh–LAX–iss
Anaphylactic: ana–fuh–LACK–tic
Anhydrous: an–HI–druss
Anilazine: ah–NILL–ah–zeen
Anticoagulant: anti–co–AG–you–lant
Arsenic trioxide: ARE–suh–nick try–OX– ide
Asphyxiation: us–fix–ee–A–shun

B
Bacillus thuringiensis: bah–SILL–us thur–in– gee–ENN–sis
Bendiocarb: ben–DIE–oh–carb
Benefin: BEN–eh–fin
Benomyl: BEN–oh–mill
Bitrex: BY–trex
Brodifacoum: bro–DIFE–uh–koom
Bromadiolone: brome–uh–DIE–oh–lone
B.T.: bee–tee

C
Calcium carbonate: CAL–see–um CAR–bo–nate

Calcium polysulfide: CAL–see–um polly– SULF–ide
Captan: CAP–tan
Carbamates: car–BAM–ates
Carbaryl: CAR–buh–rill
Carcinogen: car–SIN–oh–gen
Carcinogenic: CAR–sin–oh–gen–ick
Chlorophacinone : cloro–FASS–ah–known
Chlorothalonil: cloro–THAL–ah–nill
Chlorpyrifos: clor–PEER–ah–foss
Chlorinated hydrocarbons: CLORA–nated HIE–droh–car–buns
Cholinesterase: coal–in–ESTER–ace
Choreoathetosis: core-ee-oh-ath-uh-TOE-sus
Citronella: sit–trow–NELL–uh
Conjunctivitis: con–junk–tuh–VITE–us
Cyfluthrin: sigh–FLEW–thrin

D

2,4–D: two–four–dee
Dalapon: DOWL–ah–pawn
DCPA: dee–cee–pee–ay
DDVP: dee–dee–vee–pee
Deoxy–ribonucleic acid: dee–OXY RYE–bow– new–clay–ick acid
Diatomaceous: die–ah–toe–MAY–shuss
Diazinon: die–AZZ–ah–non
Dicamba: die–CAM–buh
Dichlorprop: die–CLOR–prop
Dichlorvos: die–CLOR–voss
Dicofol: DIKE–oh–foll, or die–COH–foll
Dienochlor: die–EEN–oh–clor
Dimethoate: die–METH–oh–ate
Diphacinone: die–FASS–ah–known
Diquat: DIE–kwat
Disulfuton: die–SULF–uh–tawn
D–Limonene: dee–LIM–oh–neen

E

Encephalopathy: en–seff–ah–LOFF–ah–thhee
Endosulfan: en-doe–SULF–ann
Epidemiology: ep–uh–deem–ee–ALL–uh–gee
Epidemiological: ep–uh–deem–ee–uh–LODGE–uh–kull
EPTC: ee–pee–tee–cee
Estrogen: ESS–trow–gen
Ethephon: ETH–uh–fawn or EETH–uh–fawn

F

Fenoxycarb: fen–OX–ee–carb
Fenvalerate : fen–VAL–ur–ate
Ferric sulfate: FAIR–ick SULL–fate
FIFRA: FIFF–ra
Fluazifop–butyl: flew–AZA—fop BEW–tull
Formulation: form–you–LAY–shun
Fungicide: FUNG–uh–side or FUNGE–uh–side

G

Glyphosate: GLY–foe–sate

H

Herbicide: HERB–uh–side
Hexakis: HEX–ah–kiss
Hydramethylnon: hie–druh–METH–ul–nawn
Hydroprene: HIE–dro–preen

I

Insecticide: in–SECT–tuh–side

M

Malathion: mal–ah–THIGH–on
MCPA: em–cee–pee–ay
MCPP: em–cee–pee–pee
Metabolite: meh–TAB–oh–lite
Metaldehyde: Meh–TOWL–duh–hide
Metam sodium: MEH–tam SO–dee–um
Methoprene: METH–oh–preen
Methoxychlor: meth–OX–ee–clor
Methyl nonyl ketone: METH–ull NON–ull KEE–tone
MGK 264: em–gee–kay two sixty four
MSMA: em–ess–em–ay
Mutagen: MUTE–uh–gen
Mutagenic: mute–uh–GEN–ick
Mutation: mew–TAY–shun

N

Naled: NAY–led
Naphthalene: NAFF–thuh–leen
Naphthalene acetamide: NAFF–thuh–leen ah–SEAT-uh–mide
Napropamide: nuh–PROPE–ah–mide
Neurological: nurr–oh–LODGE–uh–kull
Neurobehavioral: nurr–oh–bee–HAYVE—yurr–ull
Neurophysiological: nurr–oh–sigh–co–LODGE– uh–kull

O

Oleate: OH–lee–ate
Oncogen: ONK–oh–gen
Oncogenic: onk–oh–GEN–ick
Organophosphate: or–gan–oh–FOSS–fate
Ortho–phenylphenol: OR–tho fen–ull–fuh– NALL
Oryzalin: oh–RIZZ–ah–lin
Oxon: OX–on
Oxonase: OX–on–ace

P

Paradichlorobenzene: para–die–cloro–BEN–zeen
Permethrin: per–METH–rin
Petroleum distillates: puh–TROLL–ee–um DIS–till–ates
Phenothrin: FEEN–oh–thrin
Piperonyl butoxide: puh–PAIR–uh–nill bew– TOX–ide
Polyaromatic hydrocarbons: polly–arrow–MAT–ick HIE–droh–
    car–buns
Polybutene: polly–BEW–teen
Polychlorinated biphenyls: polly–CHLOR–un– nated BY–fen–ulls
Potassium: po–TASS–ee–um
Prometon: PROME–uh–tawn
Propoxur: pro–POX–ur
Pyrethrin: pie–REE–thrin
Pyrethroid: pie–REE–throid
Pyrethrums: pie–REE–thrum

R

Resinate: REZ–uh–nate
Resmethrin: rezz–METH–rin
Rodenticide: row–DENT–uh–cide
Rotenone: ROTE–uh–known

S

Sequelae: Suh–KWILL–eye
Sodium chlorate: SO–dee–um CLOR–ate
Sodium metaborate: SO–dee–um met–ah– BORE–ate
Sodium nitrate: SO–dee–um NI–trate
Strychnine: STRICK–nine
Sulfluramid: sul–FLUR–ah–mid

T

Teratogen: teh–RAT–oh–gen

Teratogenic: teh–rat–oh–GEN–ick
Tetrachlorvinphos: tetra–clor–VIN–foss
Tetramethrin: tetra–METH–rin
Thiram: THIGH–ram
Thymol: THIGH–mall
Toxicity: tox–SIS–ah–tee
Toxicology: toxa–CALL–ah–gee
Toxicological: toxa–kuh–LODGE–ah–kull
Triadimefon: tria–DIME–uh–fawn
Triclopyr: TRIKE–low–peer
Triethanolamine: try–etha–NOLE–ah–meen
Triforine: TRY–for–een

U

Ulceration: ull–sir–RAY–shun

W

Warfarin: WAR–fuh–rin

Z

Zinc phosphide: zinc FOSS–fide

Appendix B

Cholinesterase Testing

1. What is a cholinesterase test?

A cholinesterase test is a blood test to determine if you were poisoned by a nerve–gas type organophosphate or carbamate pesticide. It is *not* a test for other kinds of pesticides. The test does *not* measure pesticides in your blood. It measures whether nerve-gas type pesticides are affecting a chemical in your blood called cholinesterase. Your brain and nerves need cholinesterase to function properly. Nerve–gas pesticides make the level of cholinesterase go down. This is what causes the poisoning.

You have two kinds of cholinesterase in your blood — one in your red blood cells and the other in your plasma. Therefore there are two kinds of cholinesterase tests — red blood cell (RBC) cholinesterase, and plasma cholinesterase.

2. If there are two kinds of cholinesterase tests, which one should I have done?

If only one test is going to be done it should be the red blood cell test. The red blood cell test provides more information over a longer period of time. It is more useful to the doctor in diagnosing and managing a poisoning episode than the plasma test. It is also a better indicator of the cholinesterase levels in your brain and nerves. Ideally both should be done because they tell you different things.

3. Will my cholinesterase test be abnormal if I am poisoned?

If you are very severely poisoned your cholinesterase test will be abnormal — that is, your cholinesterase activity level will be too low.

If you are mildly or moderately poisoned, your test may or may not be abnormal. It can be difficult to tell from the results of one test if you were poisoned. You can feel fine and have an abnormal cholinesterase. You can have symptoms and have a normal cholinesterase.

Doctors who do not know how to interpret cholinesterase tests may tell you that you were not poisoned because your cholinesterase test is normal. You can be poisoned and still have a normal cholinesterase test.

4. How can I be poisoned and still have a normal cholinesterase test?

What is normal for someone else may not be normal for you. The range of measurements considered normal for this test is very wide. The reference values (the highest and lowest measurements considered normal) are based on testing hundreds of people. Everyone has their own personal level of cholinesterase. This personal level, called a base–line, can be higher or lower in some people than in others.

If your doctor tells you that your level is normal, it could be that pesticides have affected your cholinesterase level, but you had a pretty high level to start off with. The only way to know if your level is too low for you is to compare it to what your personal base–line level was before you were exposed to the nerve–gas type pesticide. Unfortunately this base–line level is usually not available. A doctor who knows how to interpret the results of your test will know this. He or she will know that one cholinesterase test is not enough, that you need another test to compare it to.

If you don't have a base–line, then you may need two or more additional tests to find out if you were poisoned. Unfortunately some doctors resist doing a second test if the first one was "normal". Often by the time you get the doctor to agree to do a repeat the test it is too late to be useful. Additional tests should be done within a week of each other.

Because there are several methods that measure cholinesterase, it is very important that all tests be done at the same laboratory using the same method. To make sure that a series of cholinesterase tests are properly interpreted, you should insist that your doctor have all of the tests done at the same laboratory using the same method.

5. If I have more than one cholinesterase test done, what do the results mean?

If more than one test is done the results must be compared to each other. You need to know if your second level is higher than your first one. If the second test is at least 15% higher than the first one, it could mean that you were poisoned and your level is rising up to what is normal for you. In this case you should have a third test done no more than a week later to see if it is still rising.

If the result of the second test is lower, about the same, or less than 15% higher than the first test, it is unlikely that further testing will be useful.

Your doctor may tell you that all the tests are normal without comparing the results. This is not the proper way to explain the results. You should ask the doctor what percent difference there is between the tests. If the doctor says the difference is 15%, you should ask if it is 15% higher or 15% lower. If it is higher another test should be done.

Some laboratories can take a week or more to get the test results back to your doctor. By the time you see the doctor to get the results, it might be too late for a repeat test to be helpful. This is often the case in situations where you meet a lot of resistance from the doctor to do the test in the first place.

6. When should a cholinesterase test be done?

A cholinesterase test should be done if there is a suspicion that exposure to a nerve–gas type of pesticide is causing a health problem, and the exposure was very recent.

The test must be done soon after the exposure to the pesticide suspected of causing the problem — within minutes or hours if possible. The first test should be done within a week of exposure to be beneficial in diagnosis and management. In most situations, it is not useful to do the test if two or more weeks have passed since the last exposure. The best time to do the test is at the time of initial presentation to the emergency room or doctor's office.

Take the pesticide container with you to show the doctor. If the health warnings say "Atropine is an antidote"; or "This product contains a cholinesterase inhibiting pesticide", or similar language, then it is appropriate for the doctor to do a cholinesterase test, if the exposure was recent. However, remember that not all products containing nerve–gas pesticides will have such a warning on the label. All of the nerve–gas type pesticides in this guide are identified by and OP or CB in all of the tables where they appear — whether or not there is a cholinesterase or atropine statement on the label.

The doctor may tell you a cholinesterase test is not necessary because the only problem is a rash, or the patient is improving, or there are no significant symptoms. There are not good enough reasons to avoid doing the test. Cholinesterase activity levels can be low in the absence of symptoms under some circumstances. A cholinesterase test should be done if the following conditions are met:

♦ There has been exposure to a pesticide known to affect cholinesterase.

♦ The exposure occurred within the previous week or less.

♦ There is a known or suspected health problem related to the exposure.

7. Does emergency treatment with atropine change the results of a cholinesterase test?

No, it is O.K. for the doctor to draw blood for a cholinesterase test after atropine has been administered. In an emergency situation, the doctor should not wait for the results of a cholinesterase test before giving atropine if he or she suspects poisoning by a nerve–gas type pesticide. Atropine can be life–saving in severe poisoning by these pesticides.

However blood for a cholinesterase test must be drawn before the drug Protopam® (pralidoxime, 2–PAM) is given. This drug does interfere with the test.

Caveat: People who decide to pay for a cholinesterase test themselves tell us they have been charged as much as $200 to $300 for a single test. This is outrageous since the cost to the doctor or hospital is most likely $25 to $35 per test, or even less, depending on the laboratory.

Appendix C

Over-the-Counter Pesticides
Brand Names by Pesticide Active Ingredient

Active Ingredient	EPA Reg. No.
Acephate (Organophosphate Insecticide)	
Enforcer Ant and Insect Barrier Treatment	769-726-48849
Isotox Insect Killer	239-2470-AA
Isotox Insect Killer Formula II	239-2461-ZA
Isotox Insect Killer Formula IV	239-2595
Orthene Systemic Insect Control	239-2461-AA
Orthene Turf Tree and Ornamental Spray	59639-26
Orthenex Rose and Flower Spray	239-2476-ZA
Orthonex Rose and Flower Spray	239-2496-0947
Orthonex Insect & Disease Control Formula III	239-2594-AA
Ortho Orthene Fire Ant Killer	239-2406
Whitmire PT300 DS Orthene Directed Spray Insecticide	499-380
Aciflourfen (Herbicide)	
Kleenup Grass & Weed Killer	239-2509-AA
Alkyl Pyridines (Repellent)	
Chacon Animal Repellent	5719-86
Chacon Repel Dog & Cat Repellent	20215-1-5719
Allethrin (Synthetic Pyrethroid Insecticide)	
Ace Hardware Home Fogger	9688-63
Black Flag Liquid Roach & Ant Killer	475-290
CRC Wasp and Hornet Killer II	
Eatons Repels Mosquitoes	43917-2-56
Hot Shot Flea & Tick Killer	9688-53-8845
Hot Shot Roach & Ant Killer	9688-47-8845
Hot Shot Roach and Ant Killer 2	9688-86-8845
Hot Shot Roach and Ant Killer 2 Unscented	9688-86-8845
Hot Shot Roach & Ant Killer 4	9688-75-8845
Hot Shot Wasp & Hornet Killer III	9688-62-8845
Ortho Flying & Crawling Insect Killer Formula	239-2512
Raid Flying Insect Killer Formula 5	4822-284
Raid Multibug Killer Formula D-39	4822-186-3
Raid Yard Guard Outdoor Fogger Formual V	4822-309
Thrifty Ant & Roach Killer	10900-64-9744
Victory Carpet & Household Spray with Dursban	9688-47-8220
Victory Veterinary Formula Indoor Fogger with Dursban	9688-63-8220

Over-the-Counter Pesticides
Brand Names by Pesticide Active Ingredient

Active Ingredient	EPA Reg. No.
Allethrin [continued]	
Walgreens Ant & Roach Killer Contains Dursban	334-456-43428
Walgreens House & Garden Bug Killer	334-381-43428
Ammonium Thiosulfate (Herbicide)	
Spurge-X	9499-1
Anhydrous Soap (Insecticide)	
Hartz 2 In 1 Dog Flea Soap	2596-18
Anilazine (Fungicide)	
Dyrene Lawn Disease Control	239-2242-ZB
Pax Fungicide, Insecticide, Fertilizer	3234-50008-AA
Arsenic Trioxide (Insecticide)	
Grants Ant Control	1663-15
Asphalt Solids (Herbicide)	
Black Leaf Pruning & Tree Wound Dressing	5887-39-AA
Atrazine (Herbicide)	
Hi-Yield Atrazine Weed Killer	7401-318-34911
Lesco St. Augustine Grass Weed and Feed	10404-39
Ortho Atrazine Plus St. Augustine Lawn Webber	239-2618
Rite Green St. Augustine Weed and Feed	9404-51
Sunni Green Ironized Weed and Feed	9404-55
Sunniland St. Augustine Lawn Weed Killer	9404-72
Vertagreen St. Augustine Weed and Feed	8660-12
Bendiocarb (Carbamate Insecticide)	
Lilly Miller Ant Killer Plus	802-537
Ficam Plus+	45639-66
Ficam W	45639-1
Green Light Home Pest & Carpet Dust	869-176
Benefin (Herbicide)	
Green Light Amaze	62719-136-869
Lawn Food and Crab Grass Control	228-159-2491
Benomyl (Fungicide)	
Benomyl Fungicide	829-217
Green Light Systemic Fungicide With Benomyl	869-125
Bentazon (Herbicide)	
Basagran T/O Herbicide	7969-45

Over-the-Counter Pesticides
Brand Names by Pesticide Active Ingredient

Active Ingredient	EPA Reg. No.
Bitrex (Insecticide)	
Pet Gold Carpet Treatment #1	NIA
Ro-Pel Garbage Protector	457-35-2
Boric Acid (Insecticide)	
Antrol Ant Killer Formula II	475-237
Boric Acid Roach Killer III Pic	3095-20201
Echols Roach Tablet 40% Boric Acid	3941-17
Pet Gold Carpet Treatment #1	NIA
Pic Ant Trap	3095-24
Roach Prufe (roach prufe)	9608-2
Terro Ant Killer II	149-8
Victor Liquid Ant Killing System	9444-131-47629
Zap-A-Roach	51311-1
Brodifacoum (Rodenticide)	
d-Con Bait Pellets	3282-66
d-Con Mouse-Prufe II	3282-65
d-Con Ready Mixed Bait Bits	3282-81
Enforcer Rat & Mouse Bars	10182-48-40849
Enforcer Rat & Mouse Bars II	10182-339-40849
Enforcer Rat Kill	10182-93-40849
Ortho Pet Flea and Tick Spray Formula III	239-2536
Bromodialone (Rodenticide)	
Enforcer Mouse Kill III	7173-188-40849
Bromethalin (Rodenticide)	
Hot Shot Sudden Death Brand Mouse Killer	602-315-8845
B.T. (Insecticide)	
Home and Garden Dipel Dust	829-196
Mosquito Dunks	6218-47
Safer B.T. Caterpillar Attack Concentrate	42697-23-AA
Safer Vegetable Insect Attack RTU Squeeze Duster	36488-25-42697
Thuricide HPC	892-202
Calcium Polysulfides (Fungicide)	
Orthorix Lime-Sulfur Spray	239-309-ZA
Ortho Dormant Disease Control Lime Sulfur Spray	239-309-AA

Over-the-Counter Pesticides
Brand Names by Pesticide Active Ingredient

Active Ingredient	EPA Reg. No.
Captan (Fungicide)	
Captan Fungicide	10182-149-829
Ortho Killer Tomato & Vegetable Dust	239-565-AA
Carbaryl (Carbamate Insecticide)	
Ace Hardware Sevin Liquid Spray	9688-NIA
Adams Flea And Tick Dust II	37425-13
Bait Pellets	829-182
Bug-Geta Plus Snail Slug & Insect Granules	239-2514-AA
Cooke Earwig Sowbug & Grasshopper Bait	802-493-909
Cooke Rose & Flower Dust	49585-8-909
Cooke Sevin Brand (5%) Carbaryl Insecticide Dust	802-442-909
Cooke Sevin Liquid Carbaryl Insecticide	264-334-909
Cooke Slug-N-Snail Granules	909-83
Cooke Tomato & Vegetable Dust	49585-7-909
Corrys Liquid Slug Snail & Insect Killer	8119-3
Corrys Slug Snail & Insect Killer	8119-5
Cutworm & Cricket Bait	829-285
D-F-T Spray	2382-68
Green Charm Liquid Sevin Insect Spray	59144-6
Hills Flea Stop Zone Control for Pets, Pet Zone Flea & Tick Powder for Dogs, Cats, Puppies &Kittens	4758-32
KGro Multipurpose Rose and Flower Dust	49585-24
KGro Sevin Liquid Formula II	264-334-46515
Lesco Sevin Brand Carbaryl Home & Garden Insecticide	264-33-10404
Lilly Miller Cutworm Earwig & Sowbug Bait	802-493
Lilly Miller Grasshopper Earwig & Sowbug Bait	802-493
Lilly Miller Sevin 5% Dust	802-442
Lilly Miller Slug Snail & Insect Killer Bait	802-351
Lilly Miller Tomato & Vegetable Dust	49585-7-802
Mycodex Pet Shampoo With Carbaryl	2097-8
Ortho Liquid Sevin Brand Carbaryl Insecticide	239-2356-AA
Ortho Sevin Brand Carbaryl Insecticide	239-2181-ZB
Ortho Sevin Brand Carbaryl Insecticide 5 Dust	239-1349-ZA
Ortho Sevin Brand Name Carbaryl 10 Dust	239-1513
Ortho Sevin Liquid	264-334-239

Over-the-Counter Pesticides
Brand Names by Pesticide Active Ingredient

Active Ingredient	EPA Reg. No.
Carbaryl [continued]	
Pax Fungicide, Insecticide, Fertilizer	3234-50008-AA
Payless Sevin Brand Carbaryl Insecticide Liquid Insect Killer	33955-533-192
Pet Gold Extra Strength Flea & Tick Powder	51793-21-57286
Sergeants Flea & Tick Powder for Cats	2517-31
Sergeants Flea & Tick Powder for Dogs	2517-31
Sergeants Pump Dog Flea & Tick Spray	2517-36
Sevin 5% Dust Brand of Carbaryl Insecticide	829-128
Sevin Liquid 2F Brand of Carbaryl Insecticide	264-334-829
Sulfodene Scratchex Power Dust	4306-10
Z3 Flea & Tick Powder For Cats	45087-15
Zodiac Flea & Tick Powder For Cats	2724-75-11786
Zodiac Flea Collar For Cats	2724-272-11786
Chitin Protein (Insecticide)	
Hi-Yield Nem-A-Cide Nematode Control	58200-9-7401
Chlorophacinone (Rodenticide)	
Eatons A-C Formula 90	56-56
Enforcer Rat & Mouse Killer	7173-128-40849
Enforcer Rat Bait V Kills Rats & Mice	7173-161-40849
Chlorthalonil (Fungicide)	
Daconil Lawn and Garden Fungicide	2935-456-909
Ferti-lone Triple-Action Insec. Mitic. Fung.	7401-67-10159
Lawn Ornamental and Vegetable Fungicide	829-232
Multipurpose Fungicide Daconil 2787 Plant Disease Control	239-2522-AA
Ortho Vegetable Disease Control	239-2438-AA
Security Fungi-Gard	56644-42
Chlorpyrifos (Organophosphate Insecticide)	
Ace Hardware Dursban Insect Killer	33955-547-9688
Ace Hardware Home Fogger	9688-63
Ace Hardware Wasp & Hornet Killer	264-334-9688
Adams Flea & Tick Dip With Dursban	45087-26-622
Bengal Indoor Flea and Tick Killer	11715-139-53719
Black Flag Ant Control System	475-254
Black Flag Liquid Roach & Ant Killer	475-290
Black Leaf Home Pest Insect Killer	70-288-5887

Over-the-Counter Pesticides
Brand Names by Pesticide Active Ingredient

Active Ingredient	EPA Reg. No.
Chlorpyrifos [continued]	
Black Leaf Termite Killer Contains Dursban	70-290-5887
Bugs Beware (very poor label)	9406-67
Cardinal Rid Yard and Kennel Flea & Tick Spray	192-142-29909
Color Guard Cat Collar	8220-39
Color Guard Dog Collar	8220-38
Cooke Ant Barrier	909-93
Cooke Dursban-Plus Lawn Insecticide	909-94
d-Con d-stroy Roach Killing Station	3282-76
Dexol Ant Killer Dust II	192-171
Dexol Dursban Granules Insect Control	192-180
Dexol Dursban Lawn Insect Killer	192-142
Dexol Fire Ant Granules II	6720-131-192
Dexol Home Pest Control Concentrate	192-142
Dexol Termite Killer	192-173
Do It Best Home Pest Insect Control	9688-42
Dursban 1E Lawn Insecticide	16-146-829
Dursban Lawn & Peremeter	10370-47
Enforcer Flea Spray for Yards Concentrate III	10350-12-40849
Enforcer Home Pest Control XI	62719-90-40849
Grants Kills Ants Insect Granules	802-532-1663
Green Charm Fire Ant Granules	59144-8
Green Light Fire Ant Killer II	869-210
Hi-Yield Male Cricket Bail	7401-296
Holiday Roach Control System	475-254
Home & Garden Home Pest Control	829-250
Home Pest Control Concentrate	829-281
Hot Shot Roach & Ant Killer	9688-47-8845
Hot Shot Roach & Ant Killer 4	9688-75-8845
Hot Shot Wasp & Hornet Killer III	9688-62-8845
KGro Ant Flea and Tick Control	62719-14-49585
KGro Dursban Insect Spray Formula II	62719-56-46515
KGro Fire Ant Killer Formula II	62719-14-49585
KGro Home Pest Insect Control 2	62719-90-46515
KGro Mole Cricket Bait	49585-18
Lesco Granular Dursban Insecticide	10404-81
Mr. Scotts Pest Control	9172-7-ZB

Over-the-Counter Pesticides
Brand Names by Pesticide Active Ingredient

Active Ingredient	EPA Reg. No.
Chlorpyrifos [continued]	
Nu-MRK Nu-Method Ant & Roach Killer Made by Professionals	334-518-6911
Ortho Dursban Lawn and Garden Insect Control	239-2570
Ortho Fire Ant Bait	100-725-239
Ortho Home Pest Insect Control	239-2490-AA
Ortho-Klor Ant Killer Dust	239-2517-2A
Ortho-Klor Soil Insect & Termite Killer	239-2513-AA
Ortho Lawn Insect Spray	239-2423-AA
Ortho Mole Cricket Bait Formula II	239-2521
Payless Dursban Insect Killer Yard-Soil-Home	192-142
Pennington Roach and Ant Killer with Dursban	11715-142-59144
Power House Ant & Roach Killer	498-127-51463
Raid Ant & Roach Home Insect Killer FormulaII	4822-238
Raid Ant Baits	4822-335
Raid Liquid Roach & Ant Killer Formula I	4822-189-ZA
Raid Max Plus Roach Bait IV	4822-411
Raid Roach Baits	4822-153
Rid-A-Bug Flea & Tick Killer Brand TF5	8845-31
Scratchex Flea & Tick Collar for Cats	4306-16
Scratchex Flea & Tick Collar for Dogs	4306-15
Sergeants 11 Month Flea Collar for Cats	8220-39-2517
Shield Flea & Tick Control for Dogs	8220-37
Shield Flea & Tick Control for Dogs	8220-50
Spectacide Dursban Indoor & Outdoor Insect Control	8845-30
Spectracide Dursban Indoor Outdoor Insect Control	8845-30
Spectracide Yard Flea and Tick Killer	8845-30
Sunniland Chinch Bug Spray	6404-73
Sunniland Mole Cricket Bait	9404-71
Timed Release 120 Day Flea Halt! House &. Carpet Spray	10350-11-270
Victory 11 Guaranteed Full Season Saf-T-Stretch Collar for Cats	8220-39
Victory Carpet & Household Spray with Dursban	9688-47-8220
Victory Household Flea and Tick Killer	8220-32

Over-the-Counter Pesticides
Brand Names by Pesticide Active Ingredient

Active Ingredient	EPA Reg. No.
Chlorpyrifos [continued]	
Victory Veterinary Formula Indoor Fogger with Dursban	9688-63-8220
Walgreens Ant & Roach Killer Contains Dursban	334-456-43428
Zema Dip 3.84% Dursban Concentrate	45087-26
Zema Super Flea & Tick Spray For Dogs, Fast Acting	45087-35
Zodiac 11 Month Flea Collar For Dogs	2724-282-11786
Zodiac Yard & Kennel Spray	2724-327-11786
Copper (Fungicide)	
Cooke Kop-R-Spray	909-92
Copper-cide Liquid Fungicide	1109-25-9404
Cooke Copper Fungicide	802-12-909
Copper Sulfate Granular Crystals	829-210
KXL Tri-Basic Copper Fungicide	1109-36-58866
Lilly Miller Microcop Fungicide	802-12-61002-3
Liquid Copper Fungicide	1109-25-829
Monetery Liqui-Cop Fungicide Spray	10465-3-AA-54705
Neutral Copper Fungicide	829-258
Roebic Root Killer Formula K-77	7792-1-AA
Tri-basic Copper Sulfate	1109-13
Cyfluthrin (Synthetic Pyrethrins)	
Raid Max Fogger	121-39-4822
Raid Max Fogger II Penetrating Micro Mist	4822-578
Raid Max Roach and Ant Killer	121-40-4822
2,4-D (Herbicide)	
Ace Hardware Spot Weed Killer	478-44-9688
Cooke Ready-to-Use Spurge Oxalis & Dandelion Killer	802-568-909
Cooke Spurge Oxalis & Dandelion Killer	802-485-909
Cooke Tomato-Plus	7401-268-909
Dexol Weed-Out Lawn Weed Killer	192-118
Green Sweep Weed and Feed	524-470
Green Sweep Weed and Feed by Monsanto	228-216-524
Greenskote Weed and Feed	228-219-8660
Hi-Yield Traimine Lawn Weed Killer	228-181-7401
Home and Garden Brush Killer	264-307-829

Over-the-Counter Pesticides
Brand Names by Pesticide Active Ingredient

Active Ingredient	EPA Reg. No.
2,4-D [continued]	
Home and Garden Lawn Weed Killer with Trimec	2217-570-829
Jerry Baker Broadleaf Weed Killer	2217-716-66630
KGro Dandelion & Broadleaf Weed Killer	2217-2851
KGro Dandelion Killer Formula II	2217-540-46515
Lilly Miller Hose'n Go Weed & Feed 15-0-0	802-586
Lilly Miller Ready-To-Use Lawn Weed Killer	802-580
Lilly Miller Spurge & Oxalis Killer	802-485
Ortho Weed B-Gon Lawn Weed Killer	239-2342-AA
Ortho Weed-B-Gon Ready Spray Lawn Weed Killer	239-2851
Ortho Weed-B-Gon Weed Killer	239-2499-AA
Ortho Weed-B-Gone for Southern Lawns 3	2217-570-239
Rite Green Bahia Weed and Feed 20-4-6	2217-603-9440
Spectracide Lawn Weed Killer 2 WB	478-121-8845
Spectracide Spot Weed Killer 33 Plus	2217-537-8845
Super KGro Southern Broadleaf Weed Killer	2217-570-572
Turf Builder Plus 2 For Grass Lawns	538-28
Vertagreen Weed and Feed	228-179-8660
Weed-B-Gon Jet Weeder Formula III	239-2623
Dalapon	
Dowpon M Grass Killer	464-473-739
DCPA	
Flower & Garden Weed Preventer	538-235
Green Sweep Weed and Feed by Monsanto	228-216-524
Monterey Vegetable Turf & Oramental Weeder	50534-1-54705
Ortho Garden Weed Preventer	677-227-AA-239
Ortho Diazinon Plus Insect Spray	239-2364-ZA
Ortho Diazinon Soil and Turf Insect Control	239-2479-AA
Ortho Fire Ant Killer Granules	239-2503
Ortho Fruit & Vegetable Insect Control	239-2350-AA
Ortho Fruit & Vegetable Insect Control	239-2350-AA
Scotts Turf Builder Plus Insect Control	538-204
Security Systemic Granular Insecticide	56644-79
Spectracide Diazinon Concentrate Lawn & Garden Insect Control	8842-92

Over-the-Counter Pesticides
Brand Names by Pesticide Active Ingredient

Active Ingredient	EPA Reg. No.
DCPA [Continued]	
Spectracide Fire Ant Killer Granules with Accelerator	8845-101
Spectracide Lawn & Garden Insect Control	8845-92
Spectracide Soil and Turf Insect Control	60008845-95
Sunniland 25% Diazinon Liquid Concentrate	9404-65
Sunniland SuperBrand Mole Cricket Bait	9404-71
Whitmire Knox-Out PT 1500 R	499-248
Deet (Repellent)	
Backwoods Cutter Insect Repellent	121-33
Backwoods Cutter Insect Repellent Pump Spray	121-34
Backwoods Cutter Insect Repellent Cream	121-30
Backwoods Cutter Insect Repellent	121-31
Backyard Cutter Insect Repellant II	7056-20-121
Backyard Cutter Insect Repellent	121-50
Cutter Pleasant Protection Insect Repellent	121-53
Cutter Pleasant Protection Insect Repellent	121-75
Deep Woods Off! For Sportsmen	4822-276
Deep Woods Off! For Sportsmen Insect Repellent III	4822-206
Deep Woods Off! Insect Repellent II	4822-204
Hartz Blockade For Cats	2596-114
Hartz Blockade For Dogs	2596-115
Hot Shot No-Pest Insect Repellant	478-40-8845
Off! Insect Repellent	4822-380
Off! Insect Repellent	4822-10
Off! Skintastic	4822-362
Off! Skintastic II	4822-373
Off! Skintastic Spray with Aloe Vera	4822-368
Pump Spray Off! Insect Repellent	4822-205
Skedaddle Insect Protection For Children Fragrance Free	64583-2
Diatomaceous earth (Insecticide)	
Insectigone Ant Killer	59913-1
Organic Plus Fire Ant Killer	65462-4
Organic Plus Flea Control for Cats	65462-4
Organic Plus Flea Control for Dogs	65462-4

Over-the-Counter Pesticides
Brand Names by Pesticide Active Ingredient

Active Ingredient	EPA Reg. No.
Diatomaceous earth [continued]	
Organic Plus Household Insecticide	65462-4
Super DE - Not a Plant Food Product	
Diazinon (Organophosphate Insecticide)	
Ace Hardware Diazinon Spray	8845-92-9688
Black Leaf Ant Killer Powder	5887-104
Cooke Diazinon Insect Granules	802-556-909
Cooke Diazinon Spray	802-444-909
Dexol Diazinon 2% Granules	192-165
Dexol Diazinon 25% Insect Spray	192-145
Diazinon 5% Granules Ready to Use	16-119-829
Diazinon Insecticide 25% Spray Concentrate	829-249
Enforcer Ant Kill Granules	6720-35-40849
Ferti-lone Triple-Action Insecticide. Miticicide Fungicide	7401-67-10159
Flea Halt Collar For Dogs	2517-21-270
Fords Diazinon	10370-44
Green Light Many Purpose Dust	869-159
Hi-Yield 5% Diazinon Insect Killer Granules	34911-13
KGro Diazinon Granules	49583-3
KGro Diazinon Insect Spray 3	46515-17
KXL Diazinon 25	33955-556-58866
Lilly Miller Diazinon Insect Dust	802-360
Lilly Miller Diazinon Insect Granules	802-556
Ortho Diazinon Granules	239-2375-AA
Ortho Diazinon Plus Insect Spray	239-2364-ZA
Ortho Diazinon Soil and Turf Insect Control	239-2479-AA
Ortho Fire Ant Killer Granules	239-2503
Ortho Fruit & Vegetable Insect Control	239-2350-AA
Ortho Fruit & Vegetable Insect Control	239-2350-AA
Payless Diazinon 25% Insect Spray	192-145
Scotts Turf Builder Plus Insect Control	538-204
Security Systemic Granular Insecticide	56644-79
Spectracide Diazinon Concentrate Lawn & Garden Insect Control	8842-92
Spectracide Fire Ant Killer Granules with Accelerator	8845-101

Over-the-Counter Pesticides
Brand Names by Pesticide Active Ingredient

Active Ingredient	EPA Reg. No.
Diazinon [continued]	
Spectracide Lawn & Garden Insect Control Diazinon	8845-92
Spectracide Soil and Turf Insect Control	60008845-95
Sunniland 25% Diazinon Liquid Concentrate	9404-65
Sunniland SuperBrand Mole Cricket Bait	9404-71
Whitmire Knox-Out PT 1500 R	499-248
Dicamba (Herbicide)	
Ace Hardware Spot Weed Killer	478-44-9688
Cooke Ready-to-Use Spurge Oxalis & Dandelion	802-568-909
Cooke Spurge Oxalis & Dandelion Killer	802-485-909
Lilly Miller Hose'n Go Weed & Feed 15-0-0	802-586
Lilly Miller Ready-To-Use Lawn Weed Killer	802-580
Lilly Miller Spurge & Oxalis Killer	802-485
Dexol Weed-Out Lawn Weed Killer	192-118
Jerry Baker Broadleaf Weed Killer	2217-716-66630
KGro Dandelion & Broadleaf Weed Killer	2217-2851
KGro Dandelion Killer Formula II	2217-540-46515
Ortho Weed-B-Gone for Southern Lawns 3	2217-570-239
Rite Green Bahia Weed and Feed 20-4-6	2217-603-9440
Spectracide Lawn Weed Killer 2 WB	478-121-8845
Spectracide Spot Weed Killer 33 Plus	2217-537-8845
Super KGro Southern Broadleaf Weed Killer	2217-570-572
Dichlorprop (Herbicide)	
Weed-B-Gon Jet Weeder Formula III	239-2623
Dichlorvos (Organophosphate Insecticide)	
Holiday Indoor Fogger	4758-139
Pest Strip	5481-344-61292
Raid Wasp & Hornet Killer IV	4822-267
Dicofol (Chlorinated Hydrocarbon Insecticide)	
Isotox Insect Killer	239-2470-AA
Kelthane Spider Mite Spray	707-202-829
Dienochlor (Chlorinated Hydrocarbon Insecticide)	
Coles Whitefly Mealybug Spray	55947-127-192
Dexol Tender Leaf Whitefly & Mealybug Spray	55947-127-192

Over-the-Counter Pesticides
Brand Names by Pesticide Active Ingredient

Active Ingredient	EPA Reg. No.
Dimethoate (Organophosphate Insecticide)	
Black Leaf Cygon 2E Soil Drench Systemic Insecticide	5887-128
Cygon 2E Eimethoate Systemic Insecticide	829-251
Diphacinone (Rodenticide)	
Eatons Answer For The Control of Pocket Gophers	56-57
Tom Cat Rat All Weather Rodent Block	12455-5-3240
Tom Cat Rat and Mouse Bait	12455-81-3240
Warf With Diphacinone	12455-5-5887
Diquat (Herbicide)	
Lilly Miller Ready-To-Use Knock Out II Weed & Grass Killer	802-572
Dexol Weed and Garden Killer	192-177
KGro Vegetation Killer Formula II	46515-16
Spectracide Grass and Weed Killer with XLC	478-114-8845
Sunniland Liquid Lawn Edger	9404-75
Disulfoton (Organophosphate Insecticide)	
Dexol Tender Leaf Systemic Granules Insect Control	192-126
Lilly Miller Systemic Rose Shrub & Flower Care	802-426
Endosulfan (Chlorinated Hydrocarbon Insecticide)	
Cooke Garden Insect Spray Containing Thiodan	802-516-909
Thiodan Insect Spray	16-141-829
Eptam (Herbicide)	
Black Leaf Eptam Weed Control	476-1910-5887-AA
Dexol Eptam Preemergent Weed Control	10182-172-192
Eptam Granules	829-225
Ethephon (Plant Growth Regulator)	
Florel Brand Fruit Eliminator	264-263-AA-54705
Ethion (Organophosphate Insecticide)	
Sunniland Ethion and Oil Spray for Citrus	9404-14
Fenoxycarb (Carbamate Insecticide)	
Hi-Yield Fire Ant Killer Country with Logic	100-725-7401
X-O-Trol Flea & Tick Fogger	8220-59
X-O-Trol Flea & Tick Household Spray	8220-58
X-O-Trol Flea & Tick Spray For Dogs	8220-60

Over-the-Counter Pesticides
Brand Names by Pesticide Active Ingredient

Active Ingredient	EPA Reg. No.
Fenvalerate (Synthetic Pyrethroid Insecticide)	
Bengal Lawn Flea and Tick Killer	53719-190
Enforcer Flea Spray for Yards Concentrate	1021-1538-40849
Flea Stop Zone Control For Home, Home Zone, Total Release Fogger	11715-178-4758
Hartz Blockade For Cats	2596-114
Hartz Blockade For Dogs	2596-115
Hills VIP Veterinarian Insecticide Products, Yard Zone, Concentrated Yard Spray	1021-1538-4758
Sergeants Indoor Fogger	11715-178-2517
Ferric Sulfate (Herbicide)	
Lilly Miller Moss-Out	802-509
Fluazifop-butyl (Herbicide)	
Grass-B-Gon Grass Killer	239-2531
Dexol Grass-Out Systemic Grass Killer	2217-751-192
Ortho Grass-B-Gon Grass Killer	239-2521-AA
Ortho Grass-B-Gon Grass Killer	239-2620
Garlic (Insecticide)	
Garlic Barrier	62998-1-AA
Glyphosate (Herbicide)	
Green Charm Knock Out Concentrate Systemic Weed & Grass Killer	239-2469-59144
Hi-Yield Killzall Weed and Grass Killer	7401-401
Hi-Yield Killzall Weed and Grass Killer Concentrate	7401-405-10159
Kleenup Grass & Weed Killer	239-2509-AA
Kleenup Spot Weed & Grass Killer	239-2596
Kleenup Systemic Weed & Grass Killer	239-2469-ZB
Ortho Ground Clear Super Edger Grass & Weed Control	239-2516
Kleeraway Systemic Weed & Grass Killer	239-2629
Roundup L&G Concentrate Grass & Weed Killer	524-370
Roundup L&G Ready-To-Use Fast Acting Formula Grass & Weed Killer	524-451
Roundup Quik Stik Grass & Weed Killer	524-452

Over-the-Counter Pesticides
Brand Names by Pesticide Active Ingredient

Active Ingredient	EPA Reg. No.
Glyphosate [Continued]	
Roundup Super Concentrate Grass & Weed Killer	524-445
Shoot Out Grass and Weed Killer Concentrate	45515-5
Hexakis (Fungicide)	
Isotox Insect Killer Formula IV	239-2595
Orthonex Insect & Disease Control Formula III	239-2594-AA
Hydramethylnon (Insecticide)	
Amdro	214-357
Amdro Granular Insecticide Kills Fire Ants	241-322
Amdro Insecticide	241-260
Amdro Insecticide Bait	241-357
Combat Ant Control System	1730-68
Combat Ant Killing System	64240-3
Combat Roach Killing System	64240-2
Combat Roach Killing System 1	64240-4
Combat Superbait Brand Insecticide Patented Action Roach Control	64240-2
Combat Superbait Brand Insecticide Patented Action Roach Control	64248-2-64240
Hydroprene (Insect Growth Regulator)	
Black Flag Roach Ender Spray	475-270
Raid Max Plus Egg Stoppers	4822-400
IBA (Plant Growth Regulator)	
Cooke Rootone	264-29-909
Imazapyr (Herbicide)	
Ortho Triox Vegetation Killer Formula A	239-2622
Imazaquin (Herbicide)	
Image 1.5 LC Herbicide (in box)	241-303
Insecticidal Soap (Potassium Salts of Fatty Acids)	
Enforcer Rat Kill II with Bitrex	10182-237-40849
Safer African Violet Insect Attack For House Plants Ready-To-Use Spray	42697-16
Safer Flea & Tick Attack Premise Spray Ready-To-Use	42697-33-ZD
Safer Flea & Tick Attack for Pets Ready-To-Use Spray	42697-33-ZE

Over-the-Counter Pesticides
Brand Names by Pesticide Active Ingredient

Active Ingredient	EPA Reg. No.
Insecticidal Soap [Continued]	
Safer Flea Soap for Cats	42697-6-ZE
Safer Flower Garden Insecticidal Soap	42697-1
Safer Fruit & Vegetable Insect Attack Insecticidal Soap Ready-To-Use Spray	36488-36-42697
Safer Insecticidal Soap Concentrate	42697-1-ZA
Safer Insecticidal Soap for Houseplants Ready-To-Use	42697-2
Safer Rose & Flower Insect Attack Insecticidal Soap Ready-To-Use Spray	36488-33-42697
Safer Sharpshooter Contact Weed Killer Ready-To-Use	42697-22
Safer Tomato and Vegetable Insect Killer	42697-33
Safer Yard & Garden Insect Attack Ready-To-Use Spray	42697-33
Isofenphos (Organophosphate Insecticide)	
Home and Garden Oftanol 1.5% Granular	829-257
Karathane (Fungicide)	
Karathane Fungicide Miticide	829-230
Lethane (Chlorinated Hydrocarbon Insecticide)	
Black Flag Insect Spray	475-156-AA
D-Limonene (Insecticide)	
Flea Stop Zone Control For Pets , Pet Zone, Pest Spray for Cats & Kittens	4758-153
Hills Flea Stop Zone Control for Pets, Pet Zone, Flea Spray for Dogs & Cats	4758-146
Hills Flea Stop Zone Control for Pets , Pet Zone, Shampoo for Dogs, Cats, Puppies, & Kittens	4758-141
Hills Flea Stop Zone Control for Pets, Pet Zone Pet Spray for Dogs, Cats, Puppies, & Kittens	4758-153
Stop Fly Repellent Ointment	4758-11
Linalool (Insecticide)	
Demize E.C.	4768-161
Flea Stop Zone Control For Pets, Pet Zone, Citrus Scent Shampoo for Cats & Kittens	4758-155
Flea Stop Zone Control For Pets, Pet Zone, Pet Spray for Cats & Kittens	4758-153

Over-the-Counter Pesticides
Brand Names by Pesticide Active Ingredient

Active Ingredient	EPA Reg. No.
Linalool [continued]	
Hills Flea Stop Zone Control for Pets, Pet Zone Pet Spray for Dogs, Cats, Puppies, & Kittens	4758-153
Lindane (Chlorinated Hydrocarbon Insecticide)	
Ace Hardware Lindane Spray Concentrate	829-221
Ortho Lindane Borer & Leaf Miner Spray	239-1173-AA
Magnesium phosphide (Rodenticide)	
Rodent Pellets	12455-18-2340
Malathion (Organophosphate Insecticide)	
Adams Flea And Tick Dip	37425-9
Chacon Malathion Spray	5719-41
Cooke Malathion (50%) Garden Spray	802-123-909
Cooke Rose & Flower Dust	49585-8-909
Cooke Tomato & Vegetable Dust	49585-7-909
Dexol Malathion Insect Control	192-16-ZB
KGro Malathion Insect Spray 3	802-123-46515
KXL Malathion-50	33955-394-58866
Lesco Malathion Insecticide Concentrate	4-99-10404
Lilly Miller Malathion	802-123
Lilly Miller Tomato & Vegetable Dust	49585-7-802
Malathion Dust	829-61
Malathion 50% EC	829-282
Malathion 50 Multi-Purpose Insecticide.	33704-302-9688
Malathion Oil Citrus and Ornamental Spray	829-175
Ortho Malathion 50 Plus Insect Spray	239-739-ZF
Payless Malathion Insect Control	192-96
Sunniland 50% Malathion Emulsifiable Concentrate	9404-2
Mancozeb (Fungicide)	
Dithane M-45	829-286
MCPA (Herbicide)	
Dexol Weed-Out Lawn Weed Killer	192-118
Green Sweep Weed and Feed	524-470
Green Sweep Weed and Feed by Monsanto	228-216-524
Greenskote Weed and Feed	228-219-8660
Hi-Yield Traimine Lawn Weed Killer	228-181-7401
Home and Garden Lawn Weed Killer with Trimec	2217-570-829

Over-the-Counter Pesticides
Brand Names by Pesticide Active Ingredient

Active Ingredient	EPA Reg. No.
MCPA [continued]	
Jerry Baker Broadleaf Weed Killer	2217-716-66630
KGro Dandelion & Broadleaf Weed Killer	2217-2851
KGro Dandelion Killer Formula II	2217-540-46515
Lilly Miller Spurge & Oxalis Killer	802-485
Ortho Weed-B-Gone for Southern Lawns 3	2217-570-239
Ortho Weed B-Gon Lawn Weed Killer	239-2342-AA
Ortho Weed-B-Gon Ready Spray Lawn Weed Killer	239-2851
Ortho Weed-B-Gon Weed Killer	239-2499-AA
Rite Green Bahia Weed and Feed 20-4-6	2217-603-9440
Spectracide Lawn Weed Killer 2 WB	478-121-8845
Spectracide Spot Weed Killer 33 Plus	2217-537-8845
Super KGro Southern Broadleaf Weed Killer	2217-570-572
Vertagreen Weed and Feed	228-179-8660
MCPP (Herbicide)	
Ace Hardware Spot Weed Killer	478-44-9688
Cooke Ready-to-Use Spurge Oxalis & Dandelion Killer	802-568-909
Green Sweep Weed and Feed	524-470
Greenskote Weed and Feed	228-219-8660
Home and Garden Brush Killer	264-307-829
Lilly Miller Hose'n Go Weed & Feed 15-0-0	802-586
Lilly Miller Ready-To-Use Lawn Weed Killer	802-580
Turf Builder Plus 2 For Grass Lawns	538-28
Vertagreen Weed and Feed	228-179-8660
Weed-B-Gon Jet Weeder Formula III	239-2623
Metalaxyl (Herbicide)	
Subdue Plant Pak II	100-717
Metaldehyde (Molluscicide)	
Bait Pellets	829-182
Bug-Geta Liquid Slug & Snail Killer	8119-2-239
Bug-Geta Plus Snail Slug & Insect Granules	239-2514-AA
Bug-Geta Slug & Snail Pellets	239-2373-AA
Cooke Slug-N-Snail Granules	909-83
Cooke Slug-N-Snail Spray	802-506-909
Corrys Liquid Slug Snail & Insect Killer	8119-3

Over-the-Counter Pesticides
Brand Names by Pesticide Active Ingredient

Active Ingredient	EPA Reg. No.
Metaldehyde [continued]	
Corrys Slug & Snail Death	8119-1-AA
Corrys Slug Snail & Insect Killer	8119-5
Deadline	64864-1
Deadline 1 Last Meal for Slugs & Snails	8501-25
KGro Snail and Slug Bait	802-549-4985
Lilly Miller Slug Snail & Insect Killer Bait	802-351
Lilly Millers Slug And Snail Line	8501-25-802
Payless Snail and Slug Killer Pellets	802-549-26874
Snarol Snail & Slug Killer Pellets	475-129
Metam Sodium (Herbicide)	
Vapam Soil Aid	476-2171-192
Methanearsonate (Herbicide)	
Ace Hardware Crab Grass Killer	2217-630-9688
Monterey Weed-Hoe	2853-38-AA-54705
Ortho Crab Grass Killer	239-873-ZA
Ortho Crab grass & Nutgrass Killer	239-2572
Methomyl (Carbamate Insecticide)	
Apache Fly Bait	270-255
Apache Fly Bait	270-255
Apache TP Fly Bait Station	270-255
Golden Marlin	2724-274-11787
Methoprene (Insect Growth Regulator)	
Alter Flea Control	2724-401-10370
Black Flag Flea Ender Fogger	2724-337-475
Black Flag Flea Ender Spray	2724-338-475
Coles Whitefly Mealybug Spray	55947-127-192
Dexol Diazinon 5% Granules	192-161
Dexol Tender Leaf Whitefly & Mealybug Spray	55947-127-192
Enforcer Flea Fogger	2724-337-40849
Enforcer Flea Fogger with Vigren	2724-454-40849
Enforcer 7 Month Flea Spray For Homes	2724-401-40849
Grants Dog & Cat Repellent	572-209-1663
KGro Dog and Cat Repellent	46515-33
KGro Dog and Cat Repellent	49585-23
Lambert Kay Boundary Indoor/Outdoor Dog & Cat Repellent	8220-17

Over-the-Counter Pesticides
Brand Names by Pesticide Active Ingredient

Active Ingredient	EPA Reg. No.
Methoprene [Continued]	
Ortho Total Flea Control	2724-337-239
Ortho Total Flea Control	2724-454-239
Ortho Total Flea Killer with Vigren	2724-401-239
Raid Flea Killer Plus Egg Stop Formula	4822-273
Scram Dog & Cat Repellent	11715-13-AA-239
Security House Plant Insect Control	55947-127-56644
Sergeants Shoo! Dog & Cat Repellent	11715-13-2517
Starbar 1% Indoor Concentrate	2724-352-11787
Zodiac Flea Collar For Dogs	2724-273-11786
Zodiac Fleatrol Carpet Spray	2724-338-11786
Zodiac Fleatrol Flea Spray	2724-404-11786
Zodiac Fleatrol Fogger	2724-337-11786
Zodiac Fleatrol Fogger	2724-454-11786
Zodiac Fleatrol Indoor Spray	2724-401-11786
Zodiac Fleatrol Premise Spray	2724-339-11786
Methoxychlor (Chlorinated Hydrocarbon Insecticide)	
Black Flag Insect Spray	475-156-AA
Ortho Killer Tomato & Vegetable Dust	239-565-AA
Protexall Screen Pruf	4972-9
Methyl nonyl ketone (Repellent)	
Farnam Cat-Away Outdoor Cat Repellent	11715-13-270
Get Off My Garden	59578-1
Grants Dog & Cat Repellent	572-209-1663
KGro Dog and Cat Repellent	46515-33
KGro Dog and Cat Repellent	49585-23
Lambert Kay Boundary Indoor/Outdoor Dog & Cat Repellent	8220-17
Scram Dog & Cat Repellent	11715-13-AA-239
Sergeants Shoo! Dog & Cat Repellent	11715-13-2517
MGK 264 (Synergist)	
Adams 14 Day Residual Flea And Tick Mist	37425-16
Adams Flea And Tick Mist	37425-12
Adams Pyrethrin Dip	37425-19
Bengal Indoor Flea and Tick Killer	11715-139-53719
Black Flag Flea Ender Fogger I	475-286-99
Black Flag Flea Ender Spray	2724-338-475

Over-the-Counter Pesticides
Brand Names by Pesticide Active Ingredient

Active Ingredient	EPA Reg. No.
MGK 264 [Continued]	
Black Flag Liquid Roach & Ant Killer	475-290
Carpet Magic Household Flea & Tick Killer	10350-8-2596
Combat Ant & Roach Killer 2	8845-122-64-240
Defend Just-For-Cats	6175-38-773
Enforcer Ant Kill and Barrier Treatment	40849-33
Enforcer Flea & Tick Shampoo for Pets	40849-14
Enforcer Four Hour Fogger X	40849-35
Farnum Timed Release 8-Day Dermatological Flea Foam	499-231-270
Flea Stop Zone Control For Home Home Zone, Total Release Fogger.	11715-178-4758
Green Charm Indoor Insect Fogger	498-146-59144
Hartz 2 In 1 Dog Flea Soap	2596-18
Hartz 2 In 1 Flea & Tick Killer for Cats Fine Mist Spray	2596-93
Hartz 2 In 1 Flea & Tick Killer for Cats Fine Mist Spray	2596-94
Hartz 2 In 1 Rid Flea Shampoo for Dogs	2596-22
Hartz 2 in 1 Flea & Tick Dip	2596-86
Holiday Bug Bomb I	475-286
Hot Shot Flea & Tick Killer	9688-53-8845
Hot Shot Roach and Ant Killer 2	9688-86-8845
KGro Insect Fogger	11715-178-41515
Pennington Roach and Ant Killer with Dursban	11715-142-59144
Pet Gold Flea & Tick Dip	51793-3-57286
Pet Gold Flea & Tick Shampoo	51793-157-57286
Pet Gold Repellent Ointment	51793-156-57286
Raid Flea Killer	4822-73
Raid Flea Killer Plus Egg Stop Formula	4822-273
Raid Indoor Fogger II	4822-180
Raid Max Fogger	121-39-4822
Sergeants Indoor Fogger	11715-178-2517
Sulfodene Scratchex Flea & Tick Shampoo for Dogs & Cats	4306-7
Sulfodene Scratchex Power Dip	4306-8
Sulfodene Scratchex Power Dust	4306-10
Tomlyn Flea Tick And Lice Shampoo	50414-4

Over-the-Counter Pesticides
Brand Names by Pesticide Active Ingredient

Active Ingredient	EPA Reg. No.
MGK 264 [Continued]	
Victory Flea Soap For Dogs	8220-20
Walgreens Ant & Roach Killer Contains Dursban	334-456-43428
Walgreens Roach & Flea Fogger	334-562-43428
Whitmire X-Clude PT1600A Timed Release Insecticide	499-239
Zema Super Flea & Tick Spray For Dogs, Fast Acting	45087-35
Zodiac Fleatrol Carpet Spray	2724-338-11786
Zodiac Fleatrol Flea Spray	2724-404-11786
Zodiac Super Tick & Fly Spray	51793-91-11786
Zodiac Triple-Action Conditioning Flea & Tick Shampoo	51793-157-11786
Zodiac Water-Based Flea & Tick Pump Spray For Cats & Dogs	7056-100-11786
NAA (Plant Growth Regulator)	
Cooke Rootone	264-29-909
Cooke Rootone Brand Rooting Hormone	264-499-909
Lilly Miller Rootone Brand Rooting Hormone	264-499-802
Naled (Organophosphate Insecticide)	
Bansect Flea & Tick Collar for Cats	2517-44
Bansect Flea & Tick Collar for Dogs	2517-43
Sergeants Dual Action Flea & Tick Collar (with Sendran)	2517-45
Sergeants Dual Action Flea & Tick Collar (with Sendran) Specially Devloped for Cats	2517-46
Sergeants Dual Action Flea & Tick Collar with	2517-45
Naphthalene (Repellent)	
Cooke Rootone	264-29-909
Cooke Rootone Brand Rooting Hormone	264-499-909
Grants Dog Repellent	1663-11-ZA
Lilly Miller Rootone Brand Rooting Hormone	264-499-802
Napropamide (Herbicide)	
Cooke Devrinol 2-G	476-2205-909
Neem (Insecticide)	
Natural Guard Multipurpose Neem Insecticide	11688-6-10159
Safer BioNeem Insecticide and Repellent	11688-6-42697

Over-the-Counter Pesticides
Brand Names by Pesticide Active Ingredient

Active Ingredient	EPA Reg. No.
Neem [continued]	
Safer Rose & Flower Japanese Beetle Spray	11688-6-42697
Nematodes (Insecticide)	
Ortho Biosafe Lawn and Garden Soil Insect Concentrate	Exempt
Nicotine (Insecticide)	
Dexol Tender Leaf Plant Insect Spray	192-45-ZA
Orthoboric acid (Insecticide)	
Drax Ant Kil Gel	9444-131
Hot Spot Roach Preventer with Boric Acid	9444-130-8845
Protexall Ant Kill	4972-23
Oryzalin (Herbicide)	
Green Light Amaze	62719-136-869
Monterey Weed Stopper	62719-113-AA-54705
Surflan A.S	62719-113-829
Oxyflurofen (Herbicide)	
Ortho Ground Clear Super Edger Grass & Weed Control	239-2516
Ortho Triox Vegetation Killer Formula A	239-2622
Oxythioquinox (Insecticide)	
Two Way Miticide 25% Contains Morestan	3125-117-829
Paradichlorobenzene (Insecticide/Repellent)	
Chacon Animal Repellent	5719-86
Chacon Repel Dog & Cat Repellent	20215-1-5719
Enoz Cedar-Ize Moth Bar	475-113
Enoz Perfumed Cedar Pine Closet Freshener	1475-126
Enoz Plastic Hang-up Moth Case With Para-Cake	1475-121
Excell Moth-Tek Paper Covered Moth Ball Hangers	3884-62
Grants Dog Repellent	1663-11-ZA
Paraffinic oil (Insecticide)	
Sun Spray Ultra Fine Year Round Pesticide	862-28
Ultra-Fine Oil Year Round Pestcide Oil	862-28
PCNB (Fungicide)	
Cooke Fungicide	909-105
Terrachlor 2E Lawn Fungicide	400-404-829

Over-the-Counter Pesticides
Brand Names by Pesticide Active Ingredient

Active Ingredient	EPA Reg. No.
Permethrin (Synthetic Pyrethroid Insecticide)	
Alter Flea Control	2724-401-10370
Black Flag Ant Roach Killer Formula B Water Based	475-329
Black Flag Flea Ender Fogger	2724-337-475
Black Flag Flea Ender Fogger I	475-286-99
Black Flag Roach Ender Spray	475-270
Cardinal Rid Flea & Tick Spray	29909-34
Combat Room Fogger1	478-126-64240
Defend Exspot Insecticide For Dogs	59-231
Defend Home & Carpet Spray	59-210-773
Dexol Diazinon 5% Granules	192-161
Enforcer Ant Kill and Barrier Treatment	40849-33
Enforcer Flea and Tick Spray for Dogs II	40849-34
Enforcer Flea Fogger	2724-337-40849
Enforcer Flea Fogger with Vigren	2724-454-40849
Enforcer Flea Killer For Carpets II	40849-44
Enforcer Four Hour Fogger X	40849-35
Enforcer 7 Month Flea Spray for Homes	2724-401-40849
Enforcer 7 Month Flea Spray For Homes	2427-401-40849
Flea Insecticide	279-3092
Green Charm Indoor Insect Fogger	498-146-59144
Green Thumb Home Insect Fogger	5887-118-12140
Holiday Bug Bomb I	475-286
Hot Shot Fogger 3	478-126-8845
Lassie Flea & Tick Spray for Dogs	8220-43
Lilly Miller Ready-To-Use Bug-Off Rose & Flower Spray	802-573
Ortho Total Flea Control	2724-337-239
Ortho Total Flea Control	2724-454-239
Ortho Total Flea Killer with Vigren	2724-401-239
Pet Gold 14 Day Flea & Tick Spray	51793-47-57286
Raid Ant & Roach Killer 6	4822-323
Raid Fumigator Fumigating Fogger	4822-278
Raid Indoor Fogger II	4822-180
Raid Yard Guard Outdoor Fogger Formual V	4822-309
Sergeants Flea & Tick Dip	59-195-2517
Sergeants Skip Flea & Tick Spray Shampoo Plus	2517-66

Over-the-Counter Pesticides
Brand Names by Pesticide Active Ingredient

Active Ingredient	EPA Reg. No.
Permethrin [continued]	
Sergeants Skip-Flea & Tick Shampoo	2517-63
Spectracide Bug Stop Concentrate	9688-84-8845
Spectracide Indoor Fogger 2	478-126-8845
Spectracide Lawn and Garden Insect Control	9688-84-8845
Sulfodene Scratchex Flea & Tick Spray for Dogs	4306-11
Walgreens Roach & Flea Fogger	334-562-43428
X-O-Trol Flea & Tick Fogger	8220-59
X-O-Trol Flea & Tick Household Spray	8220-58
X-O-Trol Flea & Tick Spray For Dogs	8220-60
Zodiac Fleatrol Fogger	2724-337-11786
Zodiac Fleatrol Fogger	2724-454-11786
Zodiac Fleatrol Indoor Spray	2724-401-11786
Zodiac Fleatrol Premise Spray	2724-339-11786
Zodiac House & Kennel Fogger	2724-292-11786
Zodiac Super Tick & Fly Spray	51793-91-11786
Petroleum distillate (Herbicide/Insecticide)	
Lesco Horticultural Oil Insecticide	10404-66
Monterey Herbicide Helper	54705-50001-AA
Prentox Emulsifiable Spray Concentrate	655-587
Petroleum oil (Herbicide/Insecticide)	
Cooke Summer & Dormant Oil	802-415-909
Lilly Miller Superior Type Spray Oil	802-415
Malathion Oil Citrus and Ornamental Spray	829-175
Second Type Soluble Oil Spray Superior 70	829-83
Volck Oil Spray	239-16-AA
Phenothrin (Synthetic Pyrethroid Insecticide)	
Ace Hardware Flying Insect Killer II	478-93-9688
Bengal Indoor Fogger	53719-21
Bengal Roach and Ant Spray	53719-22
Black Flag Flying Insect Killer I	475-214
CRC Wasp and Hornet Killer II	not visible
Dexol Aphid Mite and Whitefly Killer	192-153
Enforcer Wasp and Yellow Jacket Foam V	40849-4
Green Thumb House Plant Insect Killer	5887-126-12140
Green Thumb White Fly & Mealy Bug Spray	4887-126-12140
Holiday Tick And Flea Killer	475-220

Over-the-Counter Pesticides
Brand Names by Pesticide Active Ingredient

Active Ingredient	EPA Reg. No.
Phenothrin [continued]	
Ortho Ant-Stop Ant Killer Spray	239-2524
Ortho Flea-B-Gon Flea Killer Formula II	239-2523-AA
Ortho Flying & Crawling Insect Killer Formula	239-2512
Ortho Home & Garden Insect Killer Formula II	239-2524-AA
Ortho Household Insect Killer Formula II	239-2525-AA
Quick Knock Down Wasp and Hornet Killer XI	40849-52
Sergeants Rug Patrol Carpet Insecticide and Freshener	2517-55
Sergeants Skip-Flea Soap (with D-Phenothrin)	2517-59
Thrifty Flying Insect Killer	10900-60-8744
Phosmet (Organophosphate Insecticide)	
Zodiac 21 Day Flea Dust For Dogs	2724-277-11786
Zodiac 7 Month Flea & Tick Collar For Dogs	2724-279-11786
Zodiac Pro Dip II	2727-169-11786
Piperonyl butoxide (Synergist)	
Adams 14 Day Residual Flea And Tick Mist	37425-16
Adams Flea And Tick Dust II	37425-13
Adams Flea And Tick Mist	37425-12
Adams Pyrethrin Dip	37425-19
Bengal Indoor Flea and Tick Killer	11715-139-53719
Bengal Indoor Fogger	53719-21
Bengal Roach and Ant Spray	53719-22
Black Flag Ant Roach Killer Formula B Water Based	475-329
Black Flag Flea Ender Spray	2724-338-475
Black Flag House & Garden Insect Killer Fresh Scent	75-180
Blue Lustre Flea Killer for Carpets	50697-1
Cardinal Rid Flea & Tick Shampoo Concentrate	29909-1-AA
Cardinal Rid Flea & Tick Spray	29909-34
Carpet Magic Household Flea & Tick Killer	10350-8-2596
Cooke Ant Barrier	909-93
Defend Just-For-Cats	6175-38-773
Demize E.C.	4768-161
Enforcer Flea & Tick Shampoo for Pets	40849-14
Enforcer Flea and Tick Spray for Dogs II	40849-34

Over-the-Counter Pesticides
Brand Names by Pesticide Active Ingredient

Active Ingredient	EPA Reg. No.
Piperonyl butoxide [continued]	
Enforcer IGR (Flea Growth Regulator) Concentrate	2724-352-40849
Farnum Flys-Off Insect Repellent For Dogs	270-218
Farnum Timed Release 8-Day Dermatological Flea Foam	499-231-270
Ferti-lone Quik-Kill for Home Garden and Pets	7401-319
Ficam Plus+	45639-66
Flea Stop Zone Control For Home, Home Zone, Total Release Fogger	11715-178-4758
Flea Stop Zone Control For Pets , Pet Zone, Pet Spray for Dogs, Cats, Puppies, & Kittens	4758-153
Hartz 2 In 1 Dog Flea Soap	2596-18
Hartz 2 In 1 Flea & Tick Killer for Cats Fine Mist Spray	2596-93
Hartz 2 In 1 Flea & Tick Killer for Cats Fine Mist Spray	2596-94
Hartz 2 In 1 Luster Bath for Cats	2596-23
Hartz 2 In 1 Rid Flea Shampoo for Dogs	2596-22
Hartz 2 in 1 Flea & Tick Dip	2596-86
Hills Flea Stop Zone Control for Pets, Pet Zone, Flea & Tick Powder for Dogs, Cats, Puppies, & Kittens	4758-32
Hills Flea Stop Zone Control for Pets, Pet Zone, Pest Spray for Dogs, Cats, Puppies & Kittens	4758-153
Holiday Indoor Fogger	4758-139
Hyponex Bug Spray for House Plants	88-24
KGro Insect Fogger	11715-178-41515
KGro Multipurpose Rose and Flower Dust	49585-24
KGro Rose and Flower Insect Killer	46515-9
Lassie Flea & Tick Pump Spray for Dogs	11715-115-8220
Mycodex Pet Shampoo With 3X Pyrethrins	2097-17
Natural Pyrethrin Concentrate	655-587-829
Organic Plus Fire Ant Killer	65462-4
Organic Plus Flea Control for Cats	65462-4
Organic Plus Flea Control for Dogs	65462-4
Organic Plus Household Insecticide	65462-4
Ortho Rose & Flower Insect Killer	239-2498-AA

Over-the-Counter Pesticides
Brand Names by Pesticide Active Ingredient

Active Ingredient	EPA Reg. No.
Piperonyl butoxide [continued]	
Ortho Tomato & Vegetable Insect Killer	239-2497-AA
Ortho Total Flea Killer Spray with Vigren	2724-401-239
Pennington Penn-Organic Garden Dust	28293-207-59144
Pennington Roach and Ant Killer with Dursban	11715-142-59144
Pet Gold Extra Strength Flea & Tick Powder	51793-21-57286
Pet Gold Flea & Tick Dip	51793-3-57286
Pet Gold Flea & Tick Shampoo	51793-157-57286
Pet Gold Flea And Tick Carpet Powder	51793-62-57286
Pet Gold Pennyroyal Flea And Tick Shampoo	29909-21-57286
Pet Gold Repellent Ointment	51793-156-57286
Prentox Emulsifiable Spray Concentrate	655-587
Raid Ant & Roach Killer 6	4822-323
Raid Flea Killer	4822-73
Raid Flea Killer Plus Egg Stop Formula	4822-273
Raid Flying Insect Killer Formula 5	4822-284
Raid House and Garden Bug Killer	4822-38
Raid House & Garden Formula 11	4822-279
Raid Indoor Fogger II	4822-180
Raid Liquid Roach & Ant Killer Formula I	4822-189-ZA
Raid Max Fogger	121-39-4822
Raid Max Fogger II Penetrating Micro Mist	4822-578
Raid Max Roach and Ant Killer	121-40-4822
Ringer Crawling Insect Attack	36488-37
Ringer Flea & Tick Attack "Contains Pyrethrum"	36488-41
Safer Crawling Insect Attack Ready-To-Use Spray	36488-37-42697
Schultz-Instant House Plant & Garden Insecticide Spray	39609-1
Schultz-Instant Insect Spray	39609-1
Sergeants Indoor Fogger	11715-178-2517
Sergeants Rug Patrol Carpet Insecticide and Freshener	2517-55
Sergeants Skip Flea & Tick Spray Shampoo Plus	2517-66
Sergeants Skip-Flea & Tick Shampoo	2517-63
Spectracide Rose and Garden Insect Killer	478-46-8845
Sulfodene Scratchex Flea & Tick Shampoo for Dogs & Cats	4306-7

Over-the-Counter Pesticides
Brand Names by Pesticide Active Ingredient

Active Ingredient	EPA Reg. No.
Piperonyl butoxide [continued]	
Sulfodene Scratchex Power Dip	4306-8
Sulfodene Scratchex Power Dust	4306-10
Tomlyn Flea Tick And Lice Shampoo	50414-4
Victory Carpet Powder Flea & Tick Killer	51793-42-8220
Victory Flea Soap For Dogs	8220-20
Walgreens Ant & Roach Killer Contains Dursban	334-456-43428
Whitmire X-Clude PT1600A Timed Release Insecticide	499-239
X-O-Trol Flea & Tick Fogger	8220-59
X-O-Trol Flea & Tick Household Spray	8220-58
X-O-Trol Flea & Tick Spray For Dogs	8220-60
Zema Pyrethrin Dip	45087-51
Zema Super Flea & Tick Spray For Dogs, Fast Acting.	45087-35
Zodiac Flea & Tick Shampoo for Dogs & Cats	29909-2-11786
Zodiac Fleatrol Carpet Spray	2724-338-11786
Zodiac Fleatrol Flea Spray	2724-404-11786
Zodiac Pyrethrin Dip For Cats & Kittens	4816-684-11786
Zodiac Pyrethrin Dip For Dogs & Puppies	4816-684-11786
Zodiac Super Tick & Fly Spray	51793-91-11786
Zodiac Triple-Action Conditioning Flea & Tick Shampoo	51793-157-11786
Zodiac Water-Based Flea & Tick Pump Spray For Dogs & Cats	7056-100-11786
Potassium Nitrate (Rodenticide)	
Dexol Gopher Gasser	192-49
Prometon (Herbicide)	
KGro Fence and Walk Edger	46515-16
Ortho Triox Vegetation Killer	239-2381-AA
Propoxur (Carbamate Insecticide)	
BA-KIL	422-18
Baygon	3125-214
Black Flag Ant And Roach Killer	475-258
Black Flag Wasp-Bee-Hornet Killer	475-269
Holiday Indoor Fogger	4758-139
Invader - Residual Insecticidal w/Baygon	9444-92

Over-the-Counter Pesticides
Brand Names by Pesticide Active Ingredient

Active Ingredient	EPA Reg. No.
Propoxur [continued]	
Ortho Ant Killer Bait	506-137-AA-239
Ortho Earwig Roach & Sowbug Bait	239-2426-ZA
Ortho Hornet & Wasp Killer	239-2390-ZB
Raid Max Roach and Ant Killer	121-40-4822
Raid Wasp and Hornet Killer III	4822-224
Raid Wasp & Hornet Killer IV	4822-267
Raid Wasp & Hornet Killer X	4822-333
Sergeants Dual Action Flea & Tick Collar (with Sendran)	2517-45
Sergeants Dual Action Flea & Tick Collar (with Sendran) Specially Developed for Cats	2517-46
Sergeants Flea & Tick Spray With Coat Conditioner for Dogs	2517-65
TAT Ant Trap	506-137
TAT Roach Killer VI	506-125
Walgreens Roach Control System	3095-25-43428
Zodiac 5 Month Flea & Tick Collar For Cats	2724-275-11786
Zodiac 5 Month Flea & Tick Collar For Dogs	2724-254-11786
Zodiac Breakaway Flea & Tick Collar For Cats	2724-275-11786
Pyrethrins (Insecticide)	
Adams 14 Day Residual Flea And Tick Mist	37425-16
Adams Flea And Tick Dust II	37425-13
Adams Flea And Tick Mist	37425-12
Adams Pyrethrin Dip	37425-19
Bengal Indoor Flea and Tick Killer	11715-139-53719
Black Flag Flea Ender Fogger I	475-286-99
Black Flag Flea Ender Spray	2724-338-475
Black Flag House & Garden Insect Killer - Fresh Scent.	75-180
Blue Lustre Flea Killer for Carpets	50697-1
Cardinal Rid Flea & Tick Shampoo Concentrate	29909-1-AA
Cardinal Rid Flea & Tick Spray	29909-34
Carpet Magic Household Flea & Tick Killer	10350-8-2596
Combat Ant & Roach Killer 2	8845-122-64-240
Cooke Ant Barrier	909-93
Defend Just-For-Cats	6175-38-773
Enforcer Ant Kill and Barrier Treatment	40849-33

Over-the-Counter Pesticides
Brand Names by Pesticide Active Ingredient

Active Ingredient	EPA Reg. No.
Pyrethrins [Continued]	
Enforcer Flea & Tick Shampoo for Pets	40849-14
Enforcer Flea and Tick Spray for Dogs II	40849-34
Enforcer Four Hour Fogger X	40849-35
Enforcer FGR (Flea Growth Regulator) Concentrate	2724-352-40849
Farnum Flys-Off Insect Repellent For Dogs	270-218
Farnum Timed Release 8-Day Dermatological Flea Foam	499-231-270
Ferti-lone Quik-Kill for Home Garden and Pets	7401-319
Ficam Plus+	45639-66
Flea Stop Zone Control For Home, Home Zone, Total Release Fogger	11715-178-4758
Green Charm Indoor Insect Fogger	498-146-59144
Hartz 2 In 1 Dog Flea Soap	2596-18
Hartz 2 In 1 Flea & Tick Killer for Cats Fin.	2596-93
Hartz 2 In 1 Flea & Tick Killer for Cats Fine Mist Spray	2596-94
Hartz 2 In 1 Luster Bath for Cats	2596-23
Hartz 2 In 1 Rid Flea Shampoo for Dogs	2596-22
Hartz 2 in 1 Flea & Tick Dip	2596-86
Hills Flea Stop Zone Control for Pets, Pet Zone, Flea & Tick Powder for Dogs, Cats, Puppies, & Kittens	4758-32
Holiday Bug Bomb I	475-286
Holiday Indoor Fogger	4758-139
Hyponex Bug Spray for House Plants	88-24
KGro Insect Fogger	11715-178-41515
KGro Multipurpose Rose and Flower Dust	49585-24
KGro Rose and Flower Insect killer	46515-9
Lassie Flea & Tick Pump Spray for Dogs	11715-115-8220
Lassie Flea & Tick Spray for Dogs	8220-43
Natural Pyrethrin Concentrate	655-587-829
Mycodex Pet Shampoo With 3X Pyrethrins	2097-17
Organic Plus Fire Ant Killer	65462-4
Organic Plus Flea Control for Cats	65462-4
Organic Plus Flea Control for Dogs	65462-4
Organic Plus Household Insecticide	65462-4

Over-the-Counter Pesticides
Brand Names by Pesticide Active Ingredient

Active Ingredient	EPA Reg. No.
Pyrethrins [Continued]	
Ortho Rose & Flower Insect Killer	239-2498-AA
Ortho Tomato & Vegetable Insect Killer	239-2497-AA
Ortho Total Flea Killer Spray with Vigren	2724-401-239
Pennington Penn-Organic Garden Dust	28293-207-59144
Pennington Roach and Ant Killer with Dursban	11715-142-59144
Pet Gold 14 Day Flea & Tick Spray	51793-47-57286
Pet Gold Extra Strength Flea & Tick Powder	51793-21-57286
Pet Gold Flea & Tick Dip	51793-3-57286
Pet Gold Flea & Tick Shampoo	51793-157-57286
Pet Gold Flea And Tick Carpet Powder	51793-62-57286
Pet Gold Pennyroyal Flea And Tick Shampoo	29909-21-57286
Pet Gold Repellent Ointment	51793-156-57286
Prentox Emulsifiable Spray Concentrate	655-587
Raid Ant & Roach Killer 6	4822-323
Raid Flea Killer	4822-73
Raid Flea Killer Plus Egg Stop Formula	4822-273
Raid House and Garden Bug Killer	4822-38
Raid House & Garden Formula 11	4822-279
Raid Indoor Fogger II	4822-180
Raid Liquid Roach & Ant Killer Formula I	4822-189-ZA
Raid Max Fogger	121-39-4822
Raid Max Fogger II Penetrating Micro Mist	4822-578
Raid Max Roach and Ant Killer	121-40-4822
Ringer Crawling Insect Attack	36488-37
Ringer Flea & Tick Attack "Contains Pyrethrum	36488-41
Safer Crawling Insect Attack Ready-To-Use Spray	36488-37-42697
Safer Flea & Tick Attack Premise Spray Ready-To-Use	42697-33-ZD
Safer Flea & Tick Attack for Pets Ready-To-Use Spray	42697-33-ZE
Safer Tomato and Vegetable Insect Killer	42697-33
Safer Yard & Garden Insect Attack Ready-To-Use Spray	42697-33
Schultz-Instant House Plant & Garden Insecticide Spray	39609-1

Over-the-Counter Pesticides
Brand Names by Pesticide Active Ingredient

Active Ingredient	EPA Reg. No.
Pyrethrins [Continued]	
Schultz-Instant House Plant & Garden Insecticide Spray	39609-1
Schultz-Instant Insect Spray	39609-1
Sergeants Indoor Fogger	11715-178-2517
Spectracide Rose and Garden Insect Killer	478-46-8845
Sulfodene Scratchex Flea & Tick Shampoo for Dogs & Cats	4306-7
Sulfodene Scratchex Flea & Tick Spray for Dog	4306-11
Sulfodene Scratchex Power Dip	4306-8
Sulfodene Scratchex Power Dust	4306-10
Tomlyn Flea Tick And Lice Shampoo	50414-4
Victory Carpet Powder Flea & Tick Killer	51793-42-8220
Victory Flea Soap For Dogs	8220-20
Walgreens Roach & Flea Fogger	334-562-43428
Whitmire X-Clude PT1600A Timed Release Insecticide	499-239
X-O-Trol Flea & Tick Fogger	8220-59
X-O-Trol Flea & Tick Household Spray	8220-58
X-O-Trol Flea & Tick Spray For Dogs	8220-60
Zema Pyrethrin Dip	45087-51
Zema Super Flea & Tick Spray For Dogs, Fast. Acting	5087-35
Zodiac Flea & Tick Shampoo for Dogs & Cats	29909-2-11786
Zodiac Fleatrol Carpet Spray	2724-338-11786
Zodiac Fleatrol Flea Spray	2724-404-11786
Zodiac Pyrethrin Dip For Cats & Kittens	816-684-11786
Zodiac Pyrethrin Dip For Dogs & Puppies	4816-684-11786
Zodiac Super Tick & Fly Spray	51793-91-11786
Zodiac Triple-Action Conditioning Flea & Tick Shampoo	51793-157-11786
Zodiac Water-Based Flea & Tick Pump Spray for Cats & Dogs	056-100-11786
Pyrethroids (Synthetic Pyrethroid Insecticide)	
Ace Hardware House & Garden Bug Killer II	478-101-9688
Bengal Roach and Ant Spray	53719-22
Black Flag Ant Roach Killer Formula B Water Based	475-329

Over-the-Counter Pesticides
Brand Names by Pesticide Active Ingredient

Active Ingredient	EPA Reg. No.
Pyrethroids [Continued]	
Dexol Aphid, Mite & Whitefly Killer	192-153
Dr. X Roach Killer Dry Spray Formula	51033-92
Enforcer Flea Kill for Carpets II	40489-44
Hi-Yield Roach Blaster	5693-76-7401
Hot Shot Flea & Tick Killer	9688-53-8845
Hot Shot Flying Insect Killer Formula 411	8845-63
Hot Shot House & Garden Bug Killer Formula 721	721 8845-68
KGro Insect Fogger	11715-178-41515
Raid Flying Insect Killer Formula 5	4822-284
Resmethrin (Synthetic Pyrethroid Insecticide)	
Black Flag House & Garden Insect Killer - Fresh Scent	475-180
Coles Whitefly Mealybug Spray	55947-127-192
Dexol Tender Leaf Whitefly & Mealybug Spray	55947-127-192
Enforcer Wasp & Hornet Killer	40849-1
Enforcer Yard and Patio Outdoor Fogger	11715-26-40849
Green Light Wasp and Hornet Spray	7056-51-869
Nu-MRK Nu-Method Ant & Roach Killer Made by Professionals	334-518-6911
Orthenex Rose and Flower Spray	239-2476-ZA
Ortho Outdoor Insect Fogger	239-2421-AA
Orthonex Rose and Flower Spray	239-2496-0947
Raid Multibug Killer Formula D-39	4822-186-3
Term-Out	35054-1
Term Out Kills Termites Roaches Ants	35054-2
Thrifty Ant & Roach Killer	10900-64-9744
Walgreens House & Garden Bug Killer	334-381-43428
Rotenone (Insecticide)	
Farnum Flys-Off Insect Repellent For Dogs	270-218
Hi-Yield Rotenone Insecticide	655-704-7401
Ortho Killer Tomato & Vegetable Dust	239-565-AA
Ortho Rotenone Dust or Spray	239-690
Ortho Rotenone Dust or Spray	239-690-AA
Sethoxydim (Herbicide)	
BASF Poast Postemergence Grass Herbicide	7969-58

Over-the-Counter Pesticides
Brand Names by Pesticide Active Ingredient

Active Ingredient	EPA Reg. No.
Sethoxydim [Continued]	
Vantage Herbicide	7969-88
Silica gel (Insecticide)	
Adams Flea And Tick Dust II	37425-13
Pet Gold Extra Strength Flea & Tick Powder	51793-21-57286
Sodium chlorate (Herbicide)	
Lilly Miller Granular Noxall Vegetation Killer	7001-341-802
Sodium metaborate (Insecticide)	
Lilly Miller Granular Noxall Vegetation Killer	7001-341-802
Sodium nitrate (Herbicide)	
The Giant Destroyer	10551-1
Streptomycin sulfate (Insecticide)	
Lilly Miller Granular Noxall Vegetation Killer	7001-341-802
Streptomycin Sulfate 17	1007-24-829
Strychnine (Rodenticide)	
Cooke Quick Action Gopher Mix	909-2
Wilco Gopher Getter Type I Bait	36029-1
Sulfluramid (Insecticide)	
Raid Max Ant Bait	4822-356
Raid Max Roach Bait	4822-355
Sulfur (Fungicide)	
Cooke Rose & Flower Dust	49585-8-909
Cooke Sulfur Dust (wettable)	802-16-909
Cooke Tomato & Vegetable Dust	49585-7-909
Dexol Gopher Gasser	192-49
Green Light Wettable Dusting Sulfur	839-39-AA
KGro Multipurpose Rose and Flower Dust	49585-24
Lilly Miller Tomato & Vegetable Dust	49585-7-802
Ortho Garden Sulfur Dust or Spray	239-15
Safer Garden Fungicide Ready To Use	42697-17
The Giant Destroyer	10551-1
Wettable or Dusting Sulfur	829-163
Tetrachlorvinphos (Organophosphate Insecticide)	
Hartz 2 In 1 Flea & Tick Collar for Cats	2596-63
Hartz 2 In 1 Flea & Tick Collar for Dogs	2596-62
Hartz 2 In 1 Flea & Tick Powder For Cats	2596-78

Over-the-Counter Pesticides
Brand Names by Pesticide Active Ingredient

Active Ingredient	EPA Reg. No.
Tetrachlorvinphos [continued]	
Hartz 2 In 1 Flea & Tick Powder For Dogs	2596-79
Hartz 2 In 1 Flea & Tick Spray	2596-122
Hartz 2 In 1 Flea & Tick Spray For Cats	2596-87
Hartz 2 In 1 Flea & Tick Spray For Dogs	2596-89
Lassie Flea & Tick Powder for Cats	56493-44-8220
Longlife 90 Day Brand Collar For Cats	2596-46
Longlife 90 Day Brand Collar For Dogs	2596-50
Tetramethrin (Synthetic Pyrethroid Insecticide)	
Ace Hardware Flying Insect Killer II	478-93-9688
Ace Hardware House & Garden Bug Killer II	478-101-9688
Black Flag Flying Insect Killer I	475-214
Combat Room Fogger 1	478-126-64240
Dexol Aphid MIte and Whitefly Killer	192-153
Dexol Aphid, Mite & Whitefly Killer	192-153
Enforcer Wasp and Yellow Jacket Foam V	40849-4
Green Thumb Home Insect Fogger	5887-118-12140
Holiday Tick And Flea Killer	475-220
Hot Shot Flying Insect Killer Formula 411	8845-63
Hot Shot Fogger 3	478-126-8845
Hot Shot House & Garden Bug Killer Formula 721	721 8845-68
Ortho Ant-Stop Ant Killer Spray	239-2524
Ortho Flea-B-Gon Flea Killer Formula II	239-2523-AA
Ortho Home & Garden Insect Killer Formula II	239-2524-AA
Ortho Household Insect Killer Formula II	239-2525-AA
Quick Knock Down Wasp and Hornet Killer XI	40849-52
Raid Flea Killer	4822-73
Raid Flea Killer Plus Egg Stop Formula	4822-273
Raid House & Garden Formula 11	4822-279
Raid Indoor Fogger II	4822-180
Raid Wasp and Hornet Killer III	822-224
Raid Wasp & Hornet Killer X	4822-333
Spectracide Indoor Fogger 2	478-126-8845
Thrifty Flying Insect Killer	10900-60-8744
Thiophanate-methyl (Fungicide)	
Black Leaf Rose & Ornamental Fungicide	1001-63-5887
Thiomyl Turf & Ornamental Systemic Fungicide	1001-63-829

Over-the-Counter Pesticides
Brand Names by Pesticide Active Ingredient

Active Ingredient	EPA Reg. No.
Thiram (Repellent)	
Chacon Animal Repellent	5719-86
Chacon Repel Dog & Cat Repellent	20215-1-5719
Cooke Rootone	264-29-909
Cooke Rootone Brand Rooting Hormone	264-499-909
Lilly Miller Rootone Brand Rooting Hormone	264-499-802
Thymol (Repellent)	
Ro-Pel Garbage Protector	457-35-2
Tralomethrin (Synthetic Pyrethroid Insecticide)	
Hot Shot Indoor Flea Fogger	9688-78-5845
Hot Shot Rid-a-Bug	9688-80-8845
Hot Shot Rid-a-Bug Flea and Tick Killer	9688-81-8845
Hot Shot Roach and Ant Killer 2	9688-86-8845
Hot Shot Roach and Ant Killer 2 Unscented	9688-86-8845
Triadimefon (Fungicide)	
Green Light Fung Away	3125-370-869
Triclopyr (Herbicide)	
Ferti-lone Brush Killer Stump Killer	62719-226-7401
Ortho Brush-B-Gon Brush Killer	239-2491-AA
Ortho Brush-B-Gon Poison Ivy & Poison Oak Killer	239-2587
Ortho Poison Ivy & Poison Oak Killer Formula II	239-2515-ZA
Triethanolamine (Insecticide)	
Dexol Tender Leaf Plant Insect Spray	192-45-ZA
Trifluralin (Herbicide)	
Greenview Preen	961-280
KGro Garden Weed Preventer	2217-480-49585
Lesco Ornamental Preemergence Herbicide	9198-60-10404
Scotts Flower and Garden Weed Preventer	9198-60-538
Triforine (Fungicide)	
Orthenex Rose and Flower Spray	239-2476-ZA
Ortho Funginex Rose Disease Control	239-2435-AA
Orthonex Insect & Disease Control Formula III	239-2594-AA
Orthonex Rose and Flower Spray	239-2496-0947
Vinclozolin (Fungicide)	
Lesco Touche Flowable Fungicide	7069-62-10404

Over-the-Counter Pesticides
Brand Names by Pesticide Active Ingredient

Active Ingredient	EPA Reg. No.
Warfarin (Rodenticide)	
d-Con Pellets Kills Rats & Mice	3282-15-ZA
Hot Shot Mouse & Rat Killer	8845-39
Z-9 Tricosene (Insecticide)	
Apache Fly Bait	270-255
Apache Fly Bait	270-255
Apache TP Fly Bait Station	270-255
Zinc (Fungicide)	
Dithane M-45	829-286
Lilly Miller Moss-Kil	802-553
Lilly Miller Moss-Kil	802-508
Zinc Phosphide (Rodenticide)	
Dexol Gopher Killer Pellets	12455-30-192
Sweeneys Poison Peanuts Pellets	30-25
Ziram (Repellent)	
Chacon Animal Repellent	5719-86
Chacon Repel Dog & Cat Repellent	20215-1-5719

Appendix D

Petroleum Products in Brand Name Pesticides *

Ingredient	EPA Reg. No.
Petroleum aromatics	
Black Leaf Cygon 2E Soil Drench Systemic Insecticide	5887-128
Chacon Malathion Spray	5719-41
Ortho Fruit & Vegetable Insect Control	239-2350-AA
Ortho Lawn Insect Spray	239-2423-AA
Rid-A-Bug Flea & Tick Killer Brand TF5	845-31
Zodiac Pro Dip II	2727-169-11786
Petroleum distillates	
Ace Hardware Flying Insect Killer II	478-93-9688
Ace Hardware House & Garden Bug Killer II	478-101-9688
Black Flag Insect Spray	475-156-AA
Carpet Magic Household Flea & Tick Killer	10350-8-2596
Enforcer Flea & Tick Shampoo for Pets	40849-14
Hartz 2 In 1 Dog Flea Soap	2596-18
Hartz 2 in 1 Flea & Tick Dip	2596-86
Hartz 2 In 1 Luster Bath for Cats	2596-23
Lassie Flea & Tick Pump Spray for Dogs	11715-115-8220
Ortho Lawn Insect Spray	239-2423-AA
Ortho Tomato & Vegetable Insect Killer	239-2497-AA
Pet Gold Flea & Tick Dip	51793-3-57286
Raid Flea Killer	4822-73
Raid Max Roach & Ant Killer	121-40-4822
Tomlyn Flea Tick And Lice Shampoo	50414-4
Victory Carpet & Household Spray with Dursban	9688-47-8220
Victory Vetrinary Formula Indoor Fogger with Dursban	9688-63-8220
Zema Super Flea & Tick Spray For Dogs, Fast Acting	45087-35
Zodiac Flea & Tick Shampoo for Dogs & Cats	29909-2-11786

Petroleum Products in Brand Name Pesticides *	
Ingredient	EPA Reg. No.
Petroleum hyrdrocarbons	
Walgreens House & Garden Bug Killer	334-381-43428
Zema Super Flea & Tick Spray For Dogs, Fast Acting	45087-35
Xylene	
Adams Flea And Tick Dip	37425-9
Cooke Garden Insect Spray Containing Thiodan	802-516-909
Xylene range aromatics	
Do It Best Home Pest Insect Control	9688-42
KXL Malathion-50	33955-394-58866
Victory Carpet & Household Spray with Dursban	9688-47-8220
Victory Household Flea and Tick Killer	8220-32
Victory Vetrinary Formula Indoor Fogger with Dursban	9688-63-8220

* The products in this table state on the label that they contain petroleum aromatics, petroleum distillates, petroleum hydrocarbons, xylene, or xylene range aromatics. Other pesticides may also contain similar petroleum products, without being listed on the label.

Appendix E

Brand Name and Common Name
Cross References

A

Aatrex (atrazine)
Abamectin (Avid)
Acephate (Orthene, Orthenex)
Aciflurofen (Blazer)
Agri-Mycin (streptomycin sul fate)
Alar (daminozide)
Allethrin (Pynamin)
Altosid (methoprene)
Aluminum phosphide (Fumitoxin, Phostoxin)
Amdro (hydramethylnon)
Anilazine (Dyrene)
Answer Gopher Bait (diphacinone)
Arsenal (imazapyr)
Asulam (Asulox)
Asulox (asulam)
Atrazine (Aatrex)
Atrimmec (dikegulac sodium)
Avid (abamectin)
Azadirachtin (neem)

B

B.T. (Bactospeine, Dipel, Gnatrol)
B-Nine (daminozide)
Bactospeine (B.T.)
Banner (propiconazole)
Banol (propamocarb)
Banrot (etridiazole w/T-M)
Banvel (dicamba)
Barricade (prodiamine)
Basagran (bentazon)
Basamid (dazomet)

Baygon (propoxur)
Bayleton (triadimefon)
Baythroid (cyfluthrin)
Bendiocarb (Ficam, Turcam)
Benefin (benfluralin)
Benfluralin (benefin)
Benlate (benomyl)
Benomyl (Benlate)
Bentazon (Basagran)
Bitrex (denatonium benzoate)
Borax (sodium metaborate, sodium polyborate)
Bordeaux mixture (copper)
Boric acid (Borid, Drax Ant Kill, PT-240)
Borid (boric acid)
Botran (dicloran)
Brodifacoum (Talon)
Bromacil (Hyvar)
Bromadiolone (Maki)
Bromo-Gas (methyl bromide)

C

Cacodylic acid (Montar)
Calcium polysulfides (limesulfur)
Carbaryl (Sevimol, Sevin)
Casoron (dichlobenil)
Chlor-O-Pic (chloropicrin)
Chlorfenethol (DMC, Qikron)
Chlormequat (Cyocel)
Chlorophacinone (Rozol, Mouse Out, Liphacone)
Chloropicrin (Chlor-O-Pic)

Chlorothalonil (Bravo, Daconil)
Chlorpyrifos (Dursban, Equity,
    Empire, PT-270)
Chlorsulfuron (Telar)
Chlorthal-dimethyl (DCPA)
Copper (Bordeaux mixture)
Copper - chelated (Cutrine)
Copper hydroxide (Kocide)
Cutrine (copper - chelated)
Cybolt (flucythrinate)
Cyfluthrin (Baythroid,
    Decathalon, Optem, Tempo)
Cygon (dimethoate)
Cynoff (cypermethrin)
Cyocel (chlormequat)
Cypermethrin (Cynoff, Demon)

D

2,4-D (Weed-b-Gon)
2,4-DP (dichlorprop, Weedone)
Daconil (chlorothalonil)
Dacthal (DCPA)
Daminozide (Alar, B-Nine)
Dazomet (Basamid)
DCNA (dicloran, Botran)
DCPA (chlorthal-dimethyl,
    dacthal)
DDVP (dichlorvos)
Deadline (metaldehyde)
Decathalon (cyfluthrin)
Demon (cypermethrin)
Denatonium benzoate (Bitrex)
Devrinol (napropamide)
Di-Block (diphacinone)
Diazinon (Knox-Out 1500A,
    Knox-Out 2FM)
Dibrom (naled)
Dicamba (Banvel)
Dichlobenil (Casoron, Dyclomec)
Dichlorprop (Weedone, 2,4-DP)
Dichlorvos (DDVP)
Diclofop-methyl (Hoelon,
    Illoxan)

Dicloran (Botran, DCNA)
Dicofol (Kelthane)
Dicrotophos (Insecticide B,
    Maoget)
Dienochlor (Pentac)
Dikegulac sodium (Atrimmec)
Dimension (dithiopyr)
Dimethoate (Cygon)
Dinocap (Karathane)
Dipel (B.T.)
Diphacinone (Answer Gopher
    Bait, Di-Block)
Direx (Diuron)
Disulfuton (DiSyston)
DiSyston (disulfuton)
Dithane (mancozeb)
Dithiopyr (Dimension)
Diuron (Direx, Karmex)
DMC (chlorfenethol)
Dragnet (permethrin)
Drax Ant Kill (boric acid)
Drione (silica gel)
Dual (metolachlor)
Duosan (thiophanate-methyl and
    maneb)
Dursban (chlorpyrifos)
Dyclomec (dichlobenil)
Dyrene (anilazine)

E

Embark (mefluidide)
Empire (chlorpyrifos)
Endosulfan (thiodan)
Enstar (kinoprene)
Eptam (EPTC)
EPTC (Eptam)
Ethephon (Ethrel)
Ethrel (ethephon)
Etridiazole (Banrot)

F

Fenamiphos (Nemacur)
Fenarimol (Rubigan)

Fenbutatin oxide (hexakis, Vendex)
Fenoxycarb (Logic, Torus)
Fenvalerate (Pyrid, Tribute)
Ficam (bendiocarb)
Fluazifop-butyl (Fusilade)
Flucythrinate (Cybolt)
Fluvalinate (Mavrik)
Flytek Fly Bait (methomyl)
Fumi-cel (magnesium phosphide)
Fumitoxin (aluminum phosphide)
Funginex (triforine)
Fungo Flo (thiophanate methyl)
Fusilade (fluazifop-butyl)

G

Gallery (isoxaben)
Gamma-Mene (lindane)
Gardona (tetrachlorvinphos)
Garlon (triclopyr)
Gencor (hydroprene)
Glyphosate (Kleenup, Roundup)
Gnatrol (B.T.)
Goal (oxyfluorfen)

H

Hexakis (fenbutatin oxide, Vendex)
Hoelon (diclofop-methyl)
Hydramethylnon (Amdro)
Hydroprene (Gencor)
Hyvar (bromacil)

I

IBA (Seradix)
Illoxan (diclofop-methyl)
Imazapyr (Arsenal)
Imazaquin (Scepter)
Imidan (phosmet)
Insecticide B (dicrotophos)
Isazofos (Triumph)
Isofenphos (Oftanol)
Isotox (lindane)
Isoxaben (Gallery)

K

Karate (lambda-cyhalothrin)
Karathane (dinocap)
Karmex (diuron)
Kelthane (dicofol)
Kerb (pronamide)
Kinoprene (Enstar)
Kleenup (glyphosate)
Knox-Out 1500A (diazinon)
Knox-Out 2FM (diazinon)
Kocide (copper hydroxide)
Kung Fu (lambda-cyhalothrin, Karate, Schimitar)

L

Lambda-cyhalothrin (Karate, Kung Fu, Scimitar)
Lexone (Metribuzin)
Lime-sulfur (calcium polysulfides)
Lindane (Gamma-Mene, Isotox)
Liphacone (chlorophacinone)
Logic (fenoxycarb)

M

M-Pede (soap)
Magnesium phosphide (Fumi-cel, Magtoxin)
Magtoxin (magnesium phosphide)
Maki (bromadiolone)
Maleic hydrazide (Slow-Gro)
Mancozeb (Dithane)
Maneb (Manex)
Manex (maneb)
Maoget (dicrotophos)
Margosan-O (neem)
Mavrik (Fluvalinate)
MCPP (Mecoprop)
Mecoprop (MCPP)
Mefluidide (Embark)
Mesurol (methiocarb)
Metabrom 100 (methyl bromide)
Metalaxyl (Ridomil, Subdue)
Metaldehyde (Deadline)

Metam-sodium (Vapam)
Methiocarb (Mesurol)
Methomyl (Flytek Fly Bait,
  Musca-Cide, Muscalure,
  Stimukil)
Methoprene (Altosid)
Methyl bromide (Bromo-Gas,
  Metabrom 100)
Metolachlor (Dual)
Metribuzin (Sencor, Lexone)
Montar (cacodylic acid)
Morestan (oxythioquinox)
Mouse Out (chlorophacinone)
Musca-Cide (methomyl)
Muscalure (methomyl)

N

Naled (Dibrom)
Napropamide (Devrinol)
Neem (azadirachtin, Margosan-O)
Nemacur (fenamiphos)
Neo-Pynamin (tetramethrin)
Nicofume (nicotine)
Nicotine (Nicofume, Plant Fume
  103)

O

Oftanol (isofenphos)
Optem (cyfluthrin)
Orthene (acephate)
Orthenex (acephate)
Orthoboric acid (Tim-Bor)
Oryzalin (Surflan)
Oust (sulfometuron)
Oxadiazon (Ronstar)
Oxamyl (Vydate)
Oxycarboxin (Plantvax)
Oxyfluorfen (Goal)
Oxythioquinox (Morestan)

P

PCNB (Terrachlor)
Pentac (dienochlor)
Permethrin (Dragnet, Torpedo)

Petroleum oil (Volck Oil)
Phenothrin (Sumithrin)
Phosmet (Imidan)
Phostoxin (aluminum phosphide)
Pindone (Pival, Pivalyn)
Piperalin (Pipron)
Piperonyl butoxide (Pybuthrin)
Pipron (piperalin)
Pivalyn (pindone)
Plant Fume (sulfotep)
Plant Fume 103 (nicotine)
Plantvax (oxycarboxin)
Poast (sethoxydim)
Pramitrol (prometon)
Pro Turf VIII (thiophanate
  methyl)
Pro-Control Ant Bait
  (sulfluramid)
Prodiamine (Barricade)
Prometon (Pramitol)
Pronamide (Kerb)
Propamocarb (Banol)
Propetamphos (RF-256 Aerosol,
  Safrotin)
Propiconazole (Banner)
Propoxur (Baygon)
PT 1600A (pyrethrins)
PT 565 (pyrethrum)
PT-240 (boric acid)
PT-270 (chlorpyrifos)
Purge (pyrethrins)
Pybuthrin (piperonyl butoxide)
Pynamin (allethrin)
Pyrenone (pyrethrins)
Pyrethrins (PT 1600A, Purge,
  Pyrenone, ULD BP100)
Pyrethrum (PT 565, Pyrocide F,
  Synerol)
Pyrid (fenvalerate)
Pyrocide F (pyrethrum)

Q

Qikron (chlorfenethol)

R

Redeem (triclopyr)
Resmethrin (Scourge)
RF-256 Aerosol (propetamphos)
Ridomil (metalaxyl)
Ronilan (vinclozolin)
Ronstar (oxadiazon)
Roundup (glyphosate)
Rozol (chlorophacinone)
Rubigan (fenarimol)

S

Safrotin (propetamphos)
Scepter (imazaquin)
Scimitar (lambda-cyhalothrin)
Scourge (resmethrin)
Sencor (metribuzin)
Seradix (IBA)
Sethoxydim (Poast)
Sevimol (carbaryl)
Sevin (carbaryl)
Silica gel (Drione)
Simazine (SimTrol 90)
SimTrol 90 (simazine)
Slow-Gro (maleic hydrazide)
Soap (M-Pede)
Sodium metaborate (Borax)
Sodium polyborate (Borax,
   Terro Ant Killer II)
Stimukil (methomyl)
Stirofos (tetrachlorvinphos)
Streptomycin sulfate
   (Agri-Mycin)
Subdue (metalaxyl)
Sulfluramid (Pro-Control Ant
   Bait)
Sulfometuron (Oust)
Sulfotep (Plant Fume)
Sulfuryl fluoride (Vikane)
Sumithrin (phenothrin)
Surflan (oryzalin)
Synerol (pyrethrum)

T

Talon (brodifacoum)
Telar (chlorsulfuron)
Tempo (cyfluthrin)
Terrachlor (PCNB)
Terro Ant K. II (sodium
   polyborate)
Tetrachlorvinphos (Gardona,
   Stirofos)
Tetramethrin (Neo-Pynamin)
Thiodan (endosulfan)
Thiophanate-methyl (Fungo Flo,
   Pro Turf VIII)
Thiophanate-methyl and maneb
   (Duosan)
Tim-Bor (orthoboric acid)
Torpedo (permethrin)
Torus (fenoxycarb)
Treflan (trifluralin)
Triadimefon (Bayleton)
Tribute (fenvalerate)
Triclopyr (Garlon, Redeem)
Trifluralin (Treflan)
Triforine (Funginex)
Triumph (isazofos)
Turcam (bendiocarb)

U

ULD BP100 (pyrethrins)

V

Vapam (metam-sodium)
Vendex (hexakis, fenbutatin
   oxide)
Vikane (sulfuryl fluoride)
Vinclozolin (Ronilan)
Volck Oil (petroleum oil)
Vydate (oxamyl)

W

Weed-b-Gon (2,4-D)
Weedone (dichlorprop)

Appendix F.1
Common/Chemical Name Cross Reference
Listed Alphabetically by Common Name

Common name	Chemical name
A	
Abamectin	avermectin B1a (80%) and avermectic B1b (20%)
Acephate	O,S-dimethyl acetylphosphoramidothioate
Acifluorfen	2-[4,5-dihydro-4-methyl-4-(1-methylethyl)-5-oxo-1H-imidizole-2-yl]-3-quinoline carboxylic acid
Allethrin	(RS)-3-allyl-2-methyl-4-oxocyclopent-2-enyl (IRS)-cis/trans chyrsanthemate
Anilazine	4,6-dichloro-N-2(chlorophenyl)-1,3,5-triazin-2-amine
Atrazine	2-chloro-3-ethylamino-6-isopropylamino-s-trizaine
B	
B.T. var. aizawai	bacillus thuringiensis serotype (H-7) spores and crystals
B.T. var. israelensis	bacillus thuringiensis serotype (H-14) crystalline delta endotoxin
B.T. var. kurstaki	bacillus thuringiensis serotype (HO3a3b) spores and crystalline delta endotoxin
B.T. var. morrosoni	bacillus thuringiensis serotype (8a8b) spores and crystalline delta endotoxin
Bendiocarb	2,3-isopropylidenedioxyphenyl-methyl carbamate
Bendiocarb	2,2-dimethyl-1,3-benzodioxol-4-yl methyl carbamate
Benefin, benfluralin	N-butyl-N-ethyl-α,α,α-trifluoro-2,6-dinitro-p-toluidine
Benomyl	methyl 1-(butylcarbamoyl)-2-benzimidazole-carbamate

Common name	Chemical name
Benomyl	methyl 1-[(butylamino)carbonyl])-1H-benz-imidazol-2-ylcarbamate
Bentazone	3-isopropyl-1H-2,1,3-benzothiadiazin-4(3H)-one 2,2-dioxide
Bitrex (Denatonium benzoate)	N-[2-[(2,6-dimethylphenyl)amino]-2-oxo-ethyl]-N,N-diethylbenzenemethan-`aminium benzoate
Boric acid	sodium tetraborate decahydrate
Brodifacoum	3-[3-(4'-bromo[1-1'-biphenyl]-4-yl)-1,2,3,4-tetrahydro-1-naphthalenyl]-4-hydroxy-2H-1benzopyran-2-one
Bromacil	5-Bromo-3-sec-butyl-6-methyluracil (CA)
Bromadialone	3-[3-(4'-bromo[1,1'-biphenyl]-4-yl)-3-hydroxyl-1-phenylpropyl]-4-hydroxy-2H-1-benzopyran-2-one
Bromethalin	N-methyl-2,4-dinitro-N-(2,4,6-tribromophenyl)-6-(trifluoromethyl)benzenamine

C

Cacodylic acid	dymethylarsinic acid
Cacodylic acid	hydroxydimethylarsine oxide
Captan	cis-N-trichloromethylthio-4-cyclohexene-1,2-dicarboximide
Carbaryl	1-naphthyl N-methylcarbamate
Chlorfenethol	1,1-bis(4-chlorophenyl)ethanol
Chlormequat	2-chloroethyltrimethylammonium chloride
Chloropicrin	chloropicrin nitrotrichloromethane
Chlorothalonil	tetrachloroisophthalonitrile
Chlorphacinone	2-[(p-chlorophenyl)phenylacetyl]-1,3-indandione
Chlorpyrifos	O,O-diethyl O-(3,5,6-trichloro-2-pyridinyl)phosphorothioate
Chlorsulfuron	2-chloro-N[(4-methoxy-6-methyl-1,3,5 triazin-2-yl)aminocarbonyl]-benzenesulfonamide
Cholecalciferol	9,10-seocholesta-5,7,10(19)-trein-3 beta-ol
Cholecalciferol	activated 7-dehydrocholesterol
Cyfluthrin	cyano(4-fluoro-3-phenoxyphenyl)methyl 3-(2,2-dichloroethenyl)-2-2-dimethylcyclo-propane carboxylate

Common name	Chemical name
Cypermethrin	(+/)-α-cyano-3-phenoxybenzyl (+-)-cis,trans-3-(2,2-dichlorovinyl)-2,2-dimethylcyclopropane carboxylate

D

Common name	Chemical name
D, 2,4	2,4-dichlorophenoxyacetic acid
Dalapon	2,2-dichloropropionic acid
Daminozide	succinic acid 2,2-dimethyl hydrazide
Daminozide	Butanedioic acid mono (2,2-dimethyl hydrazide)
Dazomet	tetrahydro-3,5-dimethyl-2 H-1,3,5-thiadiazine-2-thione
DCPA	dimethyl tetrachloroterphthalate
DDT	dichlorodiphenyltrichloroethane
DDT	1,1,1-trichloro-2,2-bis(p-chlorophenyl)ethane
Deet	N,N-diethyl-3-methybenzamide
Deet	N,N-diethyl-m-toluamide
Diazinon	O,O,-diethyl -(2-isopropyl-6-methyl-4-pyrimidinyl)phosphorothioate
Dicamba	2-methoxy-3,6-dichlorobenzoic acid
Dicamba	3,6-dichloro-o-anisic acid
Dichlobenil	2,6-dichlorobenzonitrile
Dichlorprop	2-(2,4-dichlorophenoxy)proprionic acid
Dichlorvos (DDVP)	2,2-dichlorovinyl dimethyl phosphate
Diclofop-methyl	methyl (RS)-2-[4-(2,4-dichlorophenoxy)-phenoxy]propionate
Dicloran	2,6-dichloro-4-nitroaniline
Dicofol	2,2,2-trichloro-1,1-bis(4-chlorophenyl)ethanol
Dicofol	4,4-dichloro-α-trichloro-methylbenzhydrol
Dicrotophos	(E)-2-dimethylcarbamoyl-1-methylvinyl dimethyl phosphate
Dienochlor	bis(pentachloro-2,4-cyclopentadien-l-yl)
Dienochlor	decachlorobis(2,4-cyclopentadien-1-yl)
Dikegulac sodium	Sodium salt of 2,3:4,6-di-O-isopropylidene-α-L-xylo-2-hexalofuranosonic acid
Dimethoate	O,O-dimethyl-S (N-methylcarbamoylmethyl) phosphorodithioate
Dinocap	2,4-dinitro-6-octyl-phenyl-crotonate
Diphacinone	(2-diphenyl-acetyl-1,3-inanedione)
Diquat	1,1'-ethylene-2,2'-bipyridylium ion
Diquat	dihydrodipyrido(1,2-a:2',1'-c)pyrazinedium ion

Common name	Chemical name
Disulfuton	O,O-diethyl S-[2-(ethylthio)ethyl] phosphoro-dithioate
Dithiopyr	S,S'-dimethyl 2-(difluoromethyl)-4-(2-methylpropyl)-6-(trifluoromethyl)-3,5-pyridinedicarbothioate

E

Endosulfan (thiodan)	6,7,8,9,10,10-hexachloro-1,5,5a,6,9,9a-hexa-hydro-6,9-methano-2,4,3-benzodioxa-thiepin-3-oxide
Endosulfan (thiodan)	hexachlorohexahydromethano-2,4,3-benzo-dioxathiepin oxide
Eptam (EPTC)	S-ethyl dipropylthiocarbamate
Ethephon	(2-chloroethyl)phosphonic acid
Ethion	O,O,O',O'-tetraethyl S,S'-methylene bis-(phosphorodithioate)
Etridiazole	5-ethoxy-3-trichloromethyl-1,2,4-thiadiazole

F

Fenamiphos	ethyl 3-methyl-4-(methylthio)phenyl (1-methylethyl)phosphoramidate
Fenarimol	α-(2-chlorophenyl)-α-(4-chlorophenyl)-5-pyrimidinemethanol
Fenbutatin oxide	(2-methyl-2 phenylpropyl)-distannoxane
Fenoxycarb	ethyl(2-[4-phenoxyphenoxy]ethyl) carbamate
Fenvalerate	α cyano-3-phenoxybenzyl 2-(4-chlorophenyl)-3-methylbutyrate
Fenvalerate	(RS)-α-cyano-3-phenoxybenzyl (RS)-2-(4-chlorophenyl)-3-methylbutyrate
Fenvalerate	cyano(3-phenoxyphenyl)methyl-4-chloro-α-(1-methyl)benzeneacetate
Fluazifop-butyl	butyl (R)2-[-[4[[5-(trifluoromethyl)-2-pyridinyl]oxyl]phenoxy] propanoate
Flucythrinate	cyano-(3-phenoxyphenyl)methyl(+)-4-(difluororomethoxy)-α-(1-methylethyl)-benzeneacetate
Fluvalinate	(α-RS,2R)-fluvalinate [(RS)-α-cyano-3-phenoxybenzyl(R)-2-[2-chloro-4-(trifluoromethyl)anilino]-3-methyl-butanoate

Common name	Chemical name
Fosetyl-aluminum	aluminum tris (O-ethyl phosphonate)

G

Glyphosate	isopropylamine salt of N-(phosphono-methyl)-glycine

H

Hexakis	(2-methyl-2 phenylpropyl)-distannoxane
Hydramethylnon	tetrahydro-5,5-dimethyl-2(1H)-pyrimidinone [3-[4-(trifluromethyl) phenyl] ethenyl]-2-propenylidene] hydrazone
Hydroprene	ethyl (2E,4E)-3,7,11-trimethyldodeca-2,4-dienoate

I

IBA	indole-3-butyric acid
Imazapyr	2-(4-isopropyl-4-methyl-5-oxo-2-imidazolin-2-yl)nicotinic acid
Imazaquin	Ò2-[4,5-dihydro-4-methyl-4-(1-methylethyl)-5-oxo-1H-imidazol-2-yl]-3-quinoline-carboxylic acid
Iprodione	3-(3,5-dichlorophenyl)-N-(1-methylethyl)-2,4-dioxo-1-imidazolidinecarboxamide
Isazofos	O-5-chloro-1-isopropyl-1H-1,2,4-triazol-3-yl O,O-diethyl phosphorothioate
Isophenfos	1-methylethyl-2-[[ethoxy[(1-methylethyl)-amino]phosphinothioyl]oxy]benzoate
Isoxaben	N-[3-(1-ethyl-1-methylpropyl)-5-isoxazolyl]-2,6-dimethoxybenzamide

K

Kinoprene	2-propynl (E,E)-3,7,11-trimethyl-2,4-dode-cadienoate

L

Lambda-cyhalothrin	α-cyano-3-phenoxybenzyl 3-(2-chloro-3,3,3-trifluoroprop-1-enyl)-2,2-dimethylcyclo-propanecarboxylate
Lethane	b-butoxy-b'-thiocyanodiethyl ether
d-Limonene	1-methyl-4-(1-methylethenyl)cyclohexene
Linalool	3,7-dimethyl-1,6-octadien-3-ol
Lindane	γ-hexachlorocyclohexane

Common name	Chemical name
M	
Malathion	O,O-dimethyl phosphorodithioate of diethyl mercaptosuccinate
Malathion	diethyl mercaptosuccinate, S-ester
Maneb	manganese ethylenebis dithiocarbamate
MCPA	(4-chloro-2-methylphenoxy) acetic acid
MCPP	2-2(2-methyl-4-chlorophenoxy) propionic acid
Mefluidide	N-[2,4-Dimethyl-5-[(trifluoromethyl)-sulfonyl]amino]phenyl]acetamide
Metalaxyl	N-(2,6-dimethylphenyl)-N-(methoxyacetyl)-alanine methyl ester
Metaldehyde	(2,4,6,8-tetramethyl-1,3,5,7-tetraoxycyclo-octane), polymer of acetaldehyde
Metaldehyde	meta-cetaldehyde
Metam-sodium	sodium N-methyldithiocarbamate
Methiocarb	3,5-dimethyl-4-(methylthio)phenyl methylcarbamate
Methomyl	S-methyl N-[(methylcarbamoyl)oxy]thioacetimidate
Methoprene	isopropyl(2E-4E)-11-methoxy-3,7,11-trimethyl-2,4-dodecadienoate
Methoxychlor	2,2-bis (p-methoxyphenyl)-1,1,1-trichloro-ethane
Metolachlor	2-chloro-N-(2-ethyl-6-methylphenyl)-N-(2-methoxy-1-methylethyl)acetamide
Metribuzin	4-amino-6-(1,1-dimethylethyl)-3-(methylthio)-1,2,4-triazin-5(4H)-one
MITC	methylisothiocyanate
MGK 264	N-octylbicycloheptene dicarboximide
MSMA	monosodium methanearsonate
N	
NAD	naphthaleneacetamide
Naled	1,2-dibromo-2,2-dichloroethyl dimethyl phosphate
Naphthalene	naphthalene
Naphthylacetic acid	1-naphtaleneacetic acid
Napropamide	2-(1naphthoxyl)-N,N-diethylpropionamide
Napropamide	N-N-diethyl-2-(1-naphthyloxy)-propionamide

Common name	Chemical name
Neem	azadirachtin

O

Oryzalin	3,5-dinitro-N^4,N^4-dipropylsulfanilamide
Oxadiazon	2-tert-butyl-4(2,4-dichloro-5-isopropoxy-phenyl)-delta^2-1,3,4-oxadiazolin-5-one
Oxamyl	S-methyl N',N'-dimethyl-N-(methyl-carbamoyloxy)-1-thio-oxamimidate
Oxycarboxin	5,6-dihydro-2-methyl-N-phenyl-1, 4-oxathiin-3-carboxamide 4,4-dioxide
Oxyfluorfen	2-chloro-1-(3-ethoxy-4-nitrophenoxy)-4-(tri-fluoromethyl)benzene
Oxythioquinox	6-methyl-1,3-dithiolo[4,5-b]quinoxalin-2-one

P

PCNB	Pentachloronitrobenzene
Permethrin	3-(phenoxyphenyl)methyl)(+/-)cis,trans-3-(2,2-dichloroethenyl)-2,2-dimethylcyclo-propanecarboxylate
Permethrin	m-phenoxybenzyl)(+-)-cis,trans-3-(2,2-dichlorovinyl)-2,2-dimethylcyclopropane-carboxylate
Phenothrin	3-phenoxybenzyl (1R)-cis/trans chrysanthemate
Phenothrin	2,2-dimethy-3-(2-methyl-1-propanil)cyclopropanecarboxylic acid (3-phenoxyphenyl) methyl esther
Phosmet	O,O-dimethyl phosphorodithioate -S-ester with N-(mercaptomethyl)phthalimide
Pindone	2-Pivalyl-1,3-indandione
Piperalin	3-(2-methylpiperidino)propyl 3, 4-dichloro-benzoate
Piperonyl butoxide	3,4-methylenedioxy-6-propylbenzyl (heptyl) diethylene glycol ether
Piperonyl butoxide	butyl carbitol 6-propylpiperonyl ether
Piperonyl butoxide	α-[2-(2-butoxyethoxy)ethoxy]-4,5-methylene-dioxy-2-propyltoluene
Prodiamine	5-dipropylamino-α,α,α-trifluoro-4,6-dinitro-o-toluidine
Prometon	2-methoxy-4,6-bis(isopropyamino)s-triazine
Prometon	2,4-bis(isopropylamino)-6-methoxy-s-triazine

Common name	Chemical name
Pronamide	3,5-dichloro-N-(1,1-dimethyl-2-propynyl)-benzamide
Propamocarb	propyl 3-(dimethylamino)propylcarbamate-hydrochloride
Propetamphos	(E)-O-2-isopropoxycarbonyl-1-methylvinyl O-methyl ethylphosphoramidothioate
Propiconazole	1-[[2-(dichlorophenyl)-4-propyl-1,3-dioxolan-2-yl]methyl]-1H-1,2,4-triazole
Propoxur	2-(1-methyleneoxy)phenyl methylcarbamate
Propoxur	O-isopropoxyphenyl N-methylcarbamate
Pyrethroid	5-benzyl-3-furyl)methyl 2,2-dimethyl-3-(2-methylproperyl)cyclopropanedecarboxylate
Pyrethroid	3-phenoxybenzyl-(1RS,3RS;1RS,3SR)-2,2-dimethyl-3-(2 methyl prop-1-enyl)-cyclo-propanecarboxylate

R

Resmethrin	([5-(phenylmethyl)-3-furanyl] methyl 2,2-dimethyl-3(2-methyl-1-propenyl) cyclopro-pane carboxylate
Resmethrin	5-benzyl-3-furyl-methyl (1RS)-cis,trans-chyrsanthemate

S

Sethoxydim	2[1-(ethoxyimino)butyl]-5-[2-(ethylthio)-propyl]-3-hydroxy-2-cyclohexen-1 -one
Simazine	2-chloro-4,6-bis(ethylamino)-s-triazine
Soap	potassium salts of fatty acids
Sulfluramid	N-ethyl perfluorooctanesulfonamide
Sulfometuron-methyl	Methyl 2[[[[(4,6-dimethyl-2-pyrimidinyl)-amino]carbonyl]amino]sulfonyl] benzoate

T

Tetrachlorvinphos	2-chloro-1-(2,4,5-trichlorophenyl)-vinyl dimethyl phosphate (Z) isomer
Tetramethrin	3,4,5,6-tetrahydrophthalimidomethyl chrysanemate
Tetramethrin	(3,4,5,6-tetrahydrophthalimidomethyl (1RS)-cis,trans-chrysanthemate
Thiophanate-methyl	Dimethyl 4,4-0-phenylenebis-(3-thio-allophanate)
Thiram	bis(dimethylthio-carbamoyl)disulfide

Common name	Chemical name
Thiram	tetramethylthiuram disulfide
Tralomethrin	(1R,3S)3[(1' RS)(1',2',2',2',-tetrabromoethyl)]-2,2-dimethylcyclopropanecarboxylic acid (S)-α-cyano-3-phenoxybenzyl ester
Triadimefon	1-(4-chlorophenoxy)-3,3-dimethyl-1(1H-1,2,4-triazol-1-yl)-2-butaneone
Triclopyr	3,5,6-trichloro-2-pyridinyloxyacetic acid
Trifluralin	α,α,α-trifluoro-2,6-dinitro-N,N-dipropyl-p-toluidine
Triforine	(N,N'-1,4-piperazinediylbis(2,2,2-trichloro-ethylidene)-bis-[formamide])

V

Vinclozolin	3-(3,5-dichlorophenyl)-5-vinyl-5-methyl-1,3-oxazolidine-2,4-dione

Z

Zinc phosphide	zinc phosphide
Ziram	zinc dimethyldithiocarbamate

Appendix F-2

Chemical/Common Name Cross Reference
Listed Alphabetically by Chemical Name

Common name	Chemical name
A	
Cholecalciferol	activated 7-dehydrocholesterol
Allethrin	(RS)-3-allyl-2-methyl-4-oxocyclopent-2-enyl (1RS)-cis/trans chyrsanthemate
Fosetyl-aluminum	aluminum tris (O-ethyl phosphonate)
Metribuzin	4-amino-6-(1,1-dimethylethyl)-3-(methylthio)-1,2,4-triazin-5(4H)-one
Abamectin	avermectin B1a (80%) and avermectic B1b (20%)
Neem	azadirachtin
B	
Resmethrin	5-benzyl-3-furyl-methyl (1RS)-cis,trans-chyrsanthemate
Pyrethroid	5-benzyl-3-furyl)methyl 2,2-dimethyl-3-(2-methylproperyl)cyclopropanedecarboxylate
Bromadialone	3-[3-(4'-bromo[1,1'-biphenyl]-4-yl)-3-hydroxyl-1-phenylpropyl]-4-hydroxy-2H-1-benzopyran-2-one
Brodifacoum	3-[3-(4'-bromo[1-1'-biphenyl]-4-yl)-1,2,3,4-tetrahydro-1-naphthalenyl]-4-hydroxy-2H-1benzopyran-2-one
Bromacil	5-Bromo-3-sec-butyl-6-methyluracil (CA)
B.T. var. aizawai	bacillus thuringiensis serotype (H-7) spores and crystals
B.T. var. israelensis	bacillus thuringiensis serotype (H-14) crystalline delta endotoxin
B.T. var. kurstaki	bacillus thuringiensis serotype (HO3a3b) spores and crystalline delta endotoxin

Common name	Chemical name
B.T. var. morrosoni	bacillus thuringiensis serotype (8a8b) spores and crystalline delta endotoxin
Daminozide	Butanedioic acid mono (2,2-dimethyl hydrazide)
Piperonyl butoxide	α-[2-(2-butoxyethoxy)ethoxy]-4,5-methyl-enedioxy-2-propyltoluene
Lethane	b-butoxy-b'-thiocyanodiethyl ether
Piperonyl butoxide	N-butyl-N-ethyl-α,α,α-trifluoro-2,6-dinitro-p-toluidine
Fluazifop-butyl	butyl (R)2-[-[4[[5-(trifluoromethyl)-2-pyri-dinyl]oxyl]phenoxy] propanoate

C

Simazine	2-chloro-4,6-bis(ethylamino)-s-triazine
Oxyfluorfen	2-chloro-1-(3-ethoxy-4-nitrophenoxy)-4-(trifluoromethyl)benzene
Atrazine	2-chloro-3-ethylamino-6-isopropylamino-s-trizaine
Metolachlor	2-chloro-N-(2-ethyl-6-methylphenyl)-N-(2-methoxy-1-methylethyl)acetamide
Ethephon	(2-chloroethyl)phosphonic acid
Chlormequat	2-chloroethyltrimethylammonium chloride
Isazofos	O-5-chloro-1-isopropyl-1H-1,2,4-triazol-3-yl O,O-diethyl phosphorothioate
Chlorsulfuron	2-chloro-N[(4-methoxy-6-methyl-1,3,5 triazin-2-yl)aminocarbonyl]-benzenesulfonamide
Mcpa	(4-chloro-2-methylphenoxy) acetic acid
Triadimefon	1-(4-chlorophenoxy)-3,3-dimethyl-1(1H-1,2,4-triazol-1-yl)-2-butanone
Fenarimol	α-(2-chlorophenyl)-α-(4-chlorophenyl)-5-pyrimidinemethanol
Chlorfenethol	1,1-bis(4-chlorophenyl)ethanol
Chlorphacinone	2-[(p-chlorophenyl)phenylacetyl]-1,3-indandione
Chloropicrin	chloropicrin nitrotrichloromethane
Tetrachlorvinphos	2-chloro-1-(2,4,5-trichlorophenyl)-vinyl dimethyl phosphate (Z) isomer
Cyfluthrin	cyano(4-fluoro-3-phenoxyphenyl)methyl 3-(2,2-dichloroethenyl)-2-2-dimethyl-cyclopropane carboxylate

Common name	Chemical name
Fenvalerate	α-cyano-3-phenoxybenzyl 2-(4-chlorophenyl)-3-methylbutyrate
Fenvalerate	(RS)-α-cyano-3-phenoxybenzyl (RS)-2-(4-chlorophenyl)-3-methylbutyrate
Lambdacyhalothrin	α-cyano-3-phenoxybenzyl 3-(2-chloro-3,3,3-trifluoroprop-1-enyl)-2,2-dimethylcyclo-propanecarboxylate
Cypermethrin	(+/)-α-cyano-3-phenoxybenzyl (+-)-cis,trans-3-(2,2-dichlorovinyl)-2,2-dimethylcyclo-propane carboxylate
Fenvalerate	cyano(3-phenoxyphenyl)methyl-4-chloro-α-(1-methyl)benzeneacetate
Flucythrinate	cyano-(3-phenoxyphenyl)methyl(+)-4-(difluoromethoxy)-α-(1-methylethyl)-benzeneacetate

D

Common name	Chemical name
Dienochlor	decachlorobis(2,4-cyclopentadien-1-yl)
Naled	1,2-dibromo-2,2-dichloroethyl dimethyl phosphate
Dicofol	4,4-dichloro-α-trichloro-methylbenzhydrol
Dichlobenil	2,6-dichlorobenzonitrile
Anilazine	4,6-dichloro-N-2(chlorophenyl)-1,3,5-triazin-2-amine
Pronamide	3,5-dichloro-N-(1,1-dimethyl-2-propynyl)benzamide
DDT	dichlorodiphenyltrichloroethane
Dicloran	2,6-dichloro-4-nitroaniline
Dicamba	3,6-dichloro-o-anisic acid
Dichlorprop	2-(2,4-dichlorophenoxy)proprionic acid
Iprodione	3-(3,5-dichlorophenyl)-N-(1-methylethyl)-2,4-dioxo-1-imidazolidinecarboxamide
Propiconazole	1-[[2-(dichlorophenyl)-4-propyl-1,3-dioxolan-2-yl]methyl]-1H-1,2,4-triazole
Vinclozolin	3-(3,5-dichlorophenyl)-5-vinyl-5-methyl-1,3-oxazolidine-2,4-dione
Dalapon	2,2-dichloropropionic acid
Dichlorvos (DDVP)	2,2-dichlorovinyl dimethyl phosphate
D, 2,4	2,4-dichlorophenoxyacetic acid

Common name	Chemical name
Disulfuton	O,O-diethyl S-[2-(ethylthio)ethyl] phosphoro-dithioate
Diazinon	O,O,-diethyl -(2-isopropyl-6-methyl-4-pyrimidinyl)phosphorothioate
Malathion	diethyl mercapto-succinate, S-ester
Deet	N,N-diethyl-3-methybenzamide
Napropamide	N-N-diethyl-2-(1-naphthyloxy)-propionamide
Deet	N,N-diethyl-m-toluamide
Chlorpyrifos	O,O-diethyl O-(3,5,6-trichloro-2-pyridinyl)-phosphorothioate
Diquat	dihydrodipyrido(1,2-a:2',1'-c)pyrazinedium ion
Imazaquin	Ò2-[4,5-dihydro-4-methyl-4-(1-methylethyl)-5-oxo-1H-imidazol-2-yl]-3-quinoline-carboxylic acid
Acifluorfen	2-[4,5-dihydro-4-methyl-4-(1-methylethyl)-5-oxo-1H-imidizole-2-yl]-3-quinoline carboxylic acid
Oxycarboxin	5,6-dihydro-2-methyl-N-phenyl-1, 4-oxathiin-3-carboxamide 4,4-dioxide
Acephate	O,S-dimethyl acetylphosphoramidothioate
Cacodylic acid	dymethylarsinic acid
Bendiocarb	2,2-dimethyl-1,3-benzodioxol-4-yl methyl carbamate
Dicrotophos	(E)-2-dimethylcarbamoyl-1-methylvinyl dimethyl phosphate
Dithiopyr	S,S'-dimethyl 2-(difluoromethyl)-4-(2-methylpropyl)-6-(trifluoromethyl)-3,5-pyridinedicarbothioate
Dimethoate	O,O-dimethyl-S (N-methylcarbamoylmethyl) phosphorodithioate
Methiocarb	3,5-dimethyl-4-(methylthio)phenyl methyl-carbamate
Phenothrin	2,2-dimethy-3-(2-methyl-1-propanil)cyclo-propanecarboxylic acid (3-phenoxyphenyl) methyl ester
Linalool	3,7-dimethyl-1,6-octadien-3-ol
Bitrex (Denatonium	N-[2-[(2,6-dimethylphenyl)amino]-2-benzoate)oxoethyl]- N,N-diethylbenzene-methanaminium benzoate

Common name	Chemical name
Thiophanate-methyl	Dimethyl 4,4-0-phenylenebis-(3-thio-allophanate)
Metalaxyl	N-(2,6-dimethylphenyl)-N-(methoxyacetyl)-alanine methyl ester
Malathion	O,O-dimethyl phosphorodithioate of diethyl mercaptosuccinate
Phosmet	O,O-dimethyl phosphorodithioate-S-ester with N-(mercaptomethyl)phthalimide
DCPA	dimethyl tetrachloroterphthalate
Thiram	bis(dimethylthio-carbamoyl)disulfide
Mefluidide	N-[2,4-Dimethyl-5-[(trifluoromethyl)-sulfonyl]amino]phenyl]acetamide
Oryzalin	3,5-dinitro-N^4,N^4-dipropylsulfanilamide
Dinocap	2,4-dinitro-6-octyl-phenyl-crotonate
Diphacinone	(2-diphenyl-acetyl-1,3-inanedione)
Prodiamine	5-dipropylamino-α,α,α-trifluoro-4,6-dinitro-o-toluidine

E

Sethoxydim	2[1-(ethoxyimino)butyl]-5-[2-(ethylthio)-propyl]-3-hydroxy-2-cyclohexen-1 -one
Etridiazole	5-ethoxy-3-trichloromethyl-1,2,4-thiadiazole
Eptam (EPTC)	S-ethyl dipropylthiocarbamate
Diquat	1,1'-ethylene-2,2'-bipyridylium ion
Fenamiphos	ethyl 3-methyl-4-(methylthio)phenyl (1-methylethyl)phosphoramidate
Isoxaben	N-[3-(1-ethyl-1-methylpropyl)-5-isoxazolyl]-2,6-dimethoxybenzamide
Sulfluramid	N-ethyl perfluorooctanesulfonamide
Fenoxycarb	ethyl(2-[4-phenoxyphenoxy]ethyl) carbamate
Hydroprene	ethyl (2E,4E)-3,7,11-trimethyldodeca-2,4-dienoate

F

Fluvalinate	(α-RS,2R)-fluvalinate [(RS)-α-cyano-3-phenoxybenzyl(R)-2-[2-chloro-4-(trifluoro-methyl)anilino]-3-methyl-butanoate

G

Lindane	gamma-hexachlorocyclohexane

Common name	Chemical name

H

Endosulfan (thiodan)	hexachlorohexahydromethano-2,4,3-benzo-dioxathiepin oxide
Endosulfan (thiodan)	6,7,8,9,10,10-hexachloro-1,5,5a,6,9,9a-hexa-hydro-6,9-methano-2,4,3-benzo-dioxathiepin-3-oxide
Cacodylic acid	hydroxydimethylarsine oxide

I

IBA	indole-3-butyric acid
Propetamphos	(E)-O-2-isopropoxycarbonyl-1-methylvinyl O-methyl ethylphosphoramidothioate
Propoxur	O-isopropoxyphenyl N-methylcarbamate
Glyphosate	isopropylamine salt of N-(phosphono-methyl)-glycine
Prometon	2,4-bis(isopropylamino)-6-methoxy-s-triazine
Bentazone	3-isopropyl-1H-2,1,3-benzothiadiazin-4(3H)-one 2,2-dioxide
Dikegulac sodium	Sodium salt of 2,3:4,6-di-O-isopropylidene-α-L-xylo-2-hexalofuranosonic acid
Bendiocarb	2,3-isopropylidenedioxyphenyl-methyl carbamate
Methoprene	isopropyl(2E-4E)-11-methoxy-3,7,11-trimethyl-2,4-dodecadienoate
Imazapyr	2-(4-isopropyl-4-methyl-5-oxo-2-imidazolin-2-yl)nicotinic acid

M

Maneb	manganese ethylenebis dithiocarbamate
Metaldehyde	meta-cetaldehyde
Dicamba	2-methoxy-3,6-dichlorobenzoic acid
Prometon	2-methoxy-4,6-bis(isopropyamino)s-triazine
Methoxychlor	2,2-bis (p-methoxyphenyl)-1,1,1-trichloro-ethane
Benomyl	methyl 1-[(butylamino)carbonyl])-1H-benz-imidazol-2-ylcarbamate
Benomyl	methyl 1-(butylcarbamoyl)-2-benzimidazole-carbamate
Mcpp	2-2(2-methyl-4-chlorophenoxy) propionic acid
Diclofop-methyl	methyl (RS)-2-[4-(2,4-dichlorophenoxy)-phenoxy]propionate

Common name	Chemical name
Oxamyl	S-methyl N',N'-dimethyl-N-(methyl-carbamoyloxy)-1-thio-oxamimidate
Sulfometuron-methyl	Methyl 2[[[[(4,6-dimethyl-2-pyrimidinyl)-amino]carbonyl]amino]sulfonyl] benzoate
Bromethalin	N-methyl-2,4-dinitro-N-(2,4,6-tribromophenyl)-6-(trifluoromethyl)-benzenamine
Oxythioquinox	6-methyl-1,3-dithiolo[4,5-b]quinoxalin-2-one
Piperonyl butoxide	3,4-methylenedioxy-6-propylbenzyl (heptyl) diethylene glycol ether
Propoxur	2-(1-methyleneoxy)phenyl methylcarbamate
Isophenfos	1-methylethyl-2-[[ethoxy[(1-methylethyl)amino]phosphinothioyl]oxy]benzoate
Methomyl	S-methyl N-[((methylcarbamoyl)oxy]thio-acetimidate
Limonene -d	1-methyl-4-(1-methylethenyl)cyclohexene
Hexakis	(2-methyl-2 phenylpropyl)-distannoxane
Fenbutatin oxide	(2-methyl-2 phenylpropyl)-distannoxane
Piperalin	3-(2-methylpiperidino)propyl 3, 4-dichloro-benzoate
Msma	monosodium methanearsonate

N

Naphthalene	naphthalene
NAD	naphthaleneacetamide
Naphthylacetic acid	1-naphtaleneacetic acid
Napropamide	2-(1naphthoxyl)-N,N-diethylpropionamide
Carbaryl	1-naphthyl N-methylcarbamate

O

MGK 264	N-octylbicycloheptene dicarboximide

P

Dienochlor	bis(pentachloro-2,4-cyclopentadien-l-yl)
PCNB	Pentachloronitrobenzene
Phenothrin	3-phenoxybenzyl (1R)-cis/trans chrysanthemate
Pyrethroid	3-phenoxybenzyl-(1RS,3RS;1RS,3SR)-2,2-dimethyl-3-(2 methyl prop-1-enyl)-cyclo-propanecarboxylate

Common name	Chemical name
Permethrin	m-phenoxybenzyl)(+-)-cis,trans-3-(2,2-dichlorovinyl)-2,2-dimethylcyclopropane-carboxylate
Permethrin	3-(phenoxyphenyl)methyl)(+/-)cis,trans-3-(2,2-dichloroethenyl)-2,2-dimethylcyclo-propanecarboyxlate
Resmethrin	([5-(phenylmethyl)-3-furanyl] methyl 2,2-dimethyl-3(2-methyl-1-propenyl) cyclo-propane carboyxylate
Triforine	(N,N'-1,4-piperazinediylbis(2,2,2-trichloro-ethylidene)-bis-[formamide])
Pindone	2-Pivalyl-1,3-indandione
Soap	potassium salts of fatty acids
Propamocarb	propyl 3-(dimethylamino)propylcarbamate-hydrochloride
Kinoprene	2-propynl (E,E)-3,7,11-trimethyl-2,4-dode-cadienoate

S

Cholecalciferol	9,10-seocholesta-5,7,10(19)-trein-3 beta-ol
Metam-sodium	sodium N-methyldithiocarbamate
Boric acid	sodium tetraborate decahydrate
Daminozide	succinic acid 2,2-dimethyl hydrazide

T

Oxadiazon	2-tert-butyl-4(2,4-dichloro-5-isopropoxy-phenyl)-delta^2-1,3,4-oxadiazolin-5-one
Tralomethrin	(1R,3S)3[(1' RS)(1',2',2',2',-tetrabromoethyl)]-2,2-dimethylcyclopropanecarboxylic acid (S)-α-cyano-3-phenoxybenzyl ester
Chlorothalonil	tetrachloroisophthalonitrile
Ethion	O,O,O',O'-tetraethyl S,S'-methylene bis(phosphorodithioate)
Hydramethylnon	tetrahydro-5,5-dimethyl-2(1H)-pyrimidinone [3-[4-(trifluromethyl) phenyl] ethenyl]-2-propenylidene] hydrazone
Dazomet	tetrahydro-3,5-dimethyl-2 H-1,3,5-thiadiazine-2-thione
Tetramethrin	3,4,5,6-tetrahydrophthalimidomethy chrysanemate

Common name	Chemical name
Tetramethrin	(3,4,5,6-tetrahydrophthalimidomethyl (1RS)-cis,trans-chrysanthemate
Metaldehyde	(2,4,6,8-tetramethyl-1,3,5,7-tetraoxycyclo-octane), polymer of acetaldehyde
Thiram	tetramethylthiuram disulfide
DDT	1,1,1-trichloro-2,2-bis(p-chlorophenyl)ethane
Dicofol	2,2,2-trichloro-1,1-bis(4-chlorophenyl)ethanol
Captan	cis-N-trichloromethylthio-4-cyclohexene-1,2-dicarboximide
Triclopyr	3,5,6-trichloro-2-pyridinyloxyacetic acid
Trifluralin	α,α,α-trifluoro-2,6-dinitro-N,N-dipropyl-p-toluidine

Z

Ziram	zinc dimethyldithiocarbamate
Zinc phosphide	zinc phosphide

Appendix G

Chronic Toxicity of Active Ingredient Pesticides in Over-the-Counter Products
(animal data)

The table which follows list the crhonic toxicity potential for the listed active ingredients to cause cancer (Can.), reproductive damage (Repro.), and genetic damage (Gen.) The active ingredients are classified by the following groups.

Carbamates (nerve-gas type)   Organophosphates (nerve-gas type)
Chlorinated hydrocarbons   Plant Growth Regulators
Fumigants   Pyrethrins, Pyrethrum
Fungicides   Repellents
Herbicides   Rodenticides
Insect Growth Regulators   Synergists
Insecticides.(not classified elsewhere) Synthetic pyrethroids

You will notice that we do not list the brand names for these active ingredient pesticides. This is because chronic toxicity studies are performed using the technical pesticide chemical. The active ingredient pesticide can end up in hundreds of different final products in many different types of formulations.

Because the toxicity rating are based on active ingredient pesticides and not on brand name products, we list them in the table by their common name. If you want to know the brand name of a pesticide in the table below, see Appendix E on page ..., which cross references brand names, with common names.

Key to the Table

(X) = Possible adverse effect.

(-) = Either no data or information available is not
 sufficient to make a determination.

(0) = Adequate data and no adverse effect noted.

Common Name	Cancer	Repro.	Gen.
Carbamates (nerve-gas type)			
Bendiocarb	o	x	x
Methomyl	o	o	o
Carbaryl	x	o	x
Propoxur	x	o	o
Chlorinated hydrocarbons			
Dicofol	x	x	o
Dienochlor	-	-	-
Endosulfan (thiodan)	o	o	o
Lethane	-	-	-
Lindane	x	x	x
Methoxychlor	o	x	-
Fumigants			
Dichlorvos (DDVP)	x	o	x
Metam-sodium	x	x	x
Paradichlorobenzene (mothballs)	x	x	o
Zinc phosphide	-	-	-
Fungicides			
Anilazine	o	o	x
Benomyl	x	x	x
Calcium polysulfides	-	-	-
Captan	x	o	x
Chlorothalonil	x	o	x
Copper	-	-	-
Copper pentahydrate	-	-	-
Copper sulfate	-	-	-
PCNB (pentachloronitrobenzene)	x	o	x
Sulfur	o	o	o
Thiram	-	x	o
Triadimefon	x	x	o
Triforine	x	o	o
Ziram	x	x	-
Herbicides			
Acifluorfen	x	o	x
Ammonium thiosulfate	-	-	-
Benefin, benfluralin, balan	-	-	-

Common Name	Cancer	Repro.	Gen.
Herbicides (continued)			
2,4-D	x	x	x
Dalapon	-	x	o
DCPA (chlorthal dimethyl, dacthal)	x	o	o
Dicamba (Banvel)	o	o	x
Dichlorprop	-	-	-
Diquat	x	x	x
EPTC (Eptam)	o	x	x
Ferric sulfate (Iron salts)	-	-	x
Fluazifop-butyl	-	-	-
Glyphosate	x	o	o
MCPA	o	x	x
MCPP (Mecoprop)	-	x	-
MSMA	-	o	-
Napropamide	x	o	x
Octyl ammonium methanearsonate	-	-	-
Oryzalin	x	o	o
Potassium nitrate	x	-	-
Prometon	o	o	o
Sodium chlorate	-	-	-
Sodium nitrate	x	-	-
Triclopyr	o	o	x
Zinc salts	-	x	x
Insect Growth Regulators			
Fenoxycarb	-	-	o
Hydroprene	-	-	-
Kinoprene	-	-	-
Methoprene	o	o	o
Insecticides (not classified elsewhere)			
Anhydrous soap	-	-	-
Arsenic trioxide	x	x	o
B.T.	o	o	o
Boric acid	x	x	x
Calcium carbonate	-	-	-
Diatomaceous earth (amorphous silica)	o	o	o
Garlic (allium sativum)	o	o	o
Hydramethylnon	o	x	o

Common Name	Cancer	Repro.	Gen.

Insecticides (continued)

Common Name	Cancer	Repro.	Gen.
Linalool	o	o	o
Naphthalene	-	-	o
Neem (azadirachtin)	-	-	-
Nicotine	-	-	-
Pennyroyal	-	x	-
Petroleum oil	x	-	-
Potassium salts of fatty acids (soap)	o	o	o
Rotenone	x	-	x
Silica gel (silicon dioxide)	o	o	o
Sulfluramid	-	-	-

Organophosphates (nerve-gas type)

Common Name	Cancer	Repro.	Gen.
Acephate	x	o	x
Chlorpyrifos	o	o	x
Diazinon	o	x	x
Dichlorvos (DDVP)	x	o	x
Dimethoate	o	x	x
Disulfuton	-	-	x
Malathion	o	o	o
Naled	x	x	o
Phosmet	x	x	x
Tetrachlorvinphos	x	o	x

Plant Growth Regulators

Common Name	Cancer	Repro.	Gen.
IBA (indole-3-butyric acid)	o	o	o
Naphthaleneacetamide (NAD)	-	-	-

Pyrethrins/Pyrethrum

Common Name	Cancer	Repro.	Gen.
Pyrethrins	x	x	x
Pyrethrum	-	-	-

Repellents

Common Name	Cancer	Repro.	Gen.
Alkyl pyridines	-	-	-
Bitrex (denatonium benzoate)	-	-	-
Citric acid (citronella,citrus aromatics)	o	o	o
Deet (N,N-diethyl-m-toluamide)	-	x	o
Flower & vegetable oils	o	o	o
d-Limonene	o	o	o

Common Name	Cancer	Repro.	Gen.
Repellents (continued)			
Methyl nonyl ketone	-	-	-
Thymol	o	o	o
Rodenticides			
Brodifacoun	-	-	-
Bromadialone	-	-	-
Chlorophacinone	-	-	-
Diphacinone	-	-	o
Strychnine	-	-	-
Warfarin	o	x	o
Zinc phosphide	-	-	-
Synergists			
MGK 264	-	x	o
Piperonyl butoxide	o	o	o
Synthetic Pyrethroids			
Pyrethrum	-	-	-
Allethrin	o	o	o
Cyfluthrin	o	x	o
Fenvalerate	x	o	o
Permethrin	x	x	o
Phenothrin	x	o	o
Pyrethroid (unspecified)	-	-	-
Resmethrin	x	x	o
Tetramethrin	x	x	o

Appendix H

References

This is not a complete set of references for all of the topics discussed, which would take a book in itself. The references for the childhood cancer and breast cancer studies that were described in chapter five on chronic health effects, and the dog cancer study metioned in chapter eight are included. There are selected references for acute health effects and poisoning, particulary for lindane and deet which are discussed in chapter nine on human use pesticides. Some general references are also included.

Exposure

Fenske, R.A., Lu, C. 1994. Determination of handwash removal efficiency: incomplete removal of the pesticide chlorpyrifos from skin by standard handwash techniques. American Industrial Association Journal 55(5):425-432.

Lewis, R.G., Fortmann, R.C., Camann, D.E. 1994. Evaluation of methods for monitoring the potential exposure of small children to pesticides in the residential environment. Archives Environmental Contamination Toxicology 26(1): 37-46.

Schiller-Scotland, C.F., Hlawa, R., Gebhart, J. 1994. Experimental data for total deposition in the respiratory tract of children. Toxicology Letters 72(1-3):137-144.

Acute Effects

Borowitz, S.M. 1988. Prolonged organophosphate toxicity in a twenty-six month old child. Journal Pediatrics 81:121-126.

Centers for Disease Control. 1987. Fatalities resulting from sulfuryl fluoride exposure after home fumigation--Virginia. Journal American Medical Association 258:2041/2044.

Crowley, R.J., Geyer, R., Muir, C.G. 1986. Analysis of N,N-diethyl-m-toluamide (DEET) in human postmortem specimens. Journal Forensic Science 31:280-282.

Davies, M.H., Soto, R.J., Stewart, R.D., et al. 1988. Toxicity of diethyltoluamide - containing insect repellents (letter). Journal American Medical Association 259:2239-2240.

Deschamps, D., Questel, F., Baud, F.J., et al. 1994. Persistent asthma after acute inhalationof organophosphate insecticide. Lancet 344:1712.

Mortensen, M.L. 1986. Management of acute childhood poisonings caused by selected insecticides and herbicides. Pediatric Clinics North America 33:421-445.

Pramanik, A.K., Hansen, R.C. 1979. Transcutaneous gamma benzene hexachloride absorption and toxicity in infants and children. Archives Dermatology 115:1224-1225.

Roland, E.H., Jan, J.E., Rigg, J.M. 1985. Toxic encephalopathy in a child after brief exposure to insect repellents. Canadian Medical Association Journal 132:155-156.

Snyder, J.W., Poe, R.O., Stubbins, J.F., et al. 1986. Acute manic psychosis following the dermal application of N,N-diethyl-m-toluamide (DEET) in an adult. Journal Toxicology Clinical Pathology 24:429-439.

Tenenbein, M. 1987. Severe toxic reactions and death following the ingestion of diethyltoluamide - containing insect repellents. Journal American Medical Association 258:1509-1511.

Breast Cancer

Davis, D.L., Bradlow, H.L., Wolff, M., et al. 1993. Medical hypothesis: xenoestrogens as preventable causes of breast cancer. Environmental Health Perspectives 101(5):372-377.

Falck, F., Jr., Andrew, R., Jr., Wolff, M.S., et al. 1992. Pesticides and polychlorinated biphenyl residues in human breast lipids and their relation to breast cancer. Archives of Environmental Health 47:143-146.

Kreiger, N., Wolff, M.S., Hiatt, R.A., et al. 1994. Breast cancer and serum organochlorines: a prospective study among white, black, and Asian women. Journal of the National Cancer Institute 86(8):589-599.

Mussalo-Rayganaam H., Hasanen, E., Pyysalo, H., et al. 1990. Occurrence of beta-hexachlorocy-clohexane in breast cancer patients. Cancer 66:2124-2148.

Westin, J.B., Richter, E. 1990. The Israeli breast-cancer anomaly. Annals of the New York Academy of Science 609:269-279.

Wolff, M.S., Toniolo, P.G., Lee, E.W., et al. Blood levels of organochlorine residues and risk of breast cancer. 1993. Journal of the National Cancer Institute 85(8):648-652.

Childhood Cancer and Aplastic Anemia

Buckley, J.D., Robinson, L.L., Swotinsky, R., et al. 1989. Occupational exposures of parents of children with acute nonlympho-cytic leukemia: a report from the Children's Cancer Study Group. Cancer Research 49:4030-4037.

Davis, J.R., Brownson, R.C., Garcia, R., et al. 1993. Family pesticide use and childhood brain cancer. Archives of Environmental Contamination and Toxicology 24:87-92.

Gold, E., Gordis, L., Tonascia, J., et al. 1979. Risk factors for brain tumors in children. American Journal of Epidemiology 109(3):309-319.

Hemminki, K., Saloniemi, I., Salonen, T., et al. 1981. Childhood cancer and parental occupation in Finland. Journal of Epidemiology and Community Health 35:11-15.

Holly, E.A., Aston, D.P., Ahn, P.K.A., Kristiansen, J.J. 1992. Ewing's bone sarcoma, parental occupational exposures and other factors. American Journal of Epidemiology 135(2):122-129.

Infante, P.F., Epstein, S.S., Newton, W.A.Jr. 1978. Blood dyscrasias and childhood tumors and exposure to chlordane and heptachlor. Scandinavian Journal of Work Environment and Health 4:137-150.

Kishi, R., Katakura, Y., Yuasa, J., et al. 1993. [Association of parents' occupational exposure to cancer in children: a case-control study of acute lymphoblastic leukemia]. Sangyo Igaku, Japan Journal of Industrial Health 35(6):515-529. [Japanese with English Abstract].

Leiss J.K., Savitz, D.A. 1995. Home pesticide use and childhood cancer: a case-control study. American Journal Public Health 85(2):249-52.

Lowengart, R.A., Peters, J.M., Cicioni, C., et al. 1987. Childhood leukemia and parents' occupational and home exposures. Journal of the National Cancer Institute 79(1):39-46.

Rauch, A.E., Kowalsky, S.F., Lesar, T.S., et al. 1990. Lindane (Kwell)-induced aplastic anemia. Archives of Internal Medicine 150:2393-2395.

Reeves, J.D. 1982. Household insecticide-associated blood dyscrasias in children (letter). American Journal of Pediatric Hematology/Oncology 4:438-39.

Schwartzbaum, J.A., George, S.L., Pratt, C.B., et al. 1991. An exploratory study of environmental and medical factors potentially related to childhood cancer. Medical Pediatric Oncology 19(2):115-121.

Shu, X.O., Gao, Y.T., Brinton, L.A., et al. 1988. A population-based case-control study of childhood leukemia in Shanghai. Cancer 62:635-644.

Wilkins, J.R. III, Sinks, T. 1990. Parental occupation and intracranial neoplasms of childhood: results of a case-control interview study. American Journal of Epidemiology 132:275-292.

Parkinson Disease

Barbeau, A., Roy, M., Bernier, G., et al. 1987. Ecogenetics of Parkinson's Disease: Prevalence and environmental aspects in rural areas. Canadian Journal Neurological Science 14:36-41.

Bocchetta, A., Corsini, G.U. 1986. Parkinson's disease and pesticides (letter). Lancet 2:1163.

Butterfield, P.G., Valanis, B.G., Spencer, P.S., et al. 1993. Environmental antecedents of young-onset Parkinson's disease. Neurology 43(6):1150-1158. NEW

Golbe, L.I. 1993. Risk factors in young-onset Parkinson's disease. (Editorial). Neurology 43(9):1641-1643. NEW

Hertzman, C., Wiens, M., Snow, B., et al. 1994. A case-control study of Parkinson's disease in a horticultural region of British Columbia. Movement Disorders 9(1):69-75.

Koller, W., Vetere-Overfield, B., Gray, C., et al. 1990. Environmental risk factors in Parkinson's disease. Neurology 40(8):1218-1221.

Rajput, A.H., Uitti, R.J., Stern, W., et al. 1986. Early onset Parkinson's disease in Saskatchewan - environmental considerations for etiology. Canadian Journal Neurological Science 13:312-316.

Rajput, A.H., Uitti, R.J., Stern, W., et al. 1987. Geography, drinking water chemistry, pesticides and herbicides and the etiology of Parkinson's disease. Canadian Journal Neurological Science 14:414-418.

Sechi, G.P., Agnetti, V., Piredda, M., et al. 1992. Acute and persistent Parkinsonism after use of diquat. Neurology 42:261-263.

Semchuk, K.M., Love, E.J., Lee, R.G. 1992. Parkinson's disease and exposure to agricultural work and pesticide chemicals. Neurology 42:1328-1335.

Cancer in Dogs

Sternberg, S.S. 1992. Canine malignant lymphoma and 2,4-dichlorophenoxyacetic acid herbicides (letter). Journal National Cancer Institute 84(4):271.

General References

S. Budavari (Editor). *The Merck Index, An Encyclopedia of Chemicals, Drugs, and Biologicals.* 11th Edition. Merck & Co., Inc. Rahway, N.Y. 1989.

Rachel Carson. *Silent Spring.* Houghton Mifflin. Boston. 1962

The Farm Chemicals Handbook '95. Meister Publishing Company. Willoughby, OH. 1995.

D.P. Morgan. *Recognition and Management of Pesticide Poisonings.* Fourth Edition. U.S. Environmental Protection Agency, Washington, D.C., U.S. Government Printing Office. 1992.

Robert van den Bosch, *The Pesticide Conspiracy.* University of California Press. Berkeley and Los Angeles, CA. 1978

Appendix I

Units of Measurement

To give you a idea of the magnitude of the differences in numbers, consider how long it would take someone to count one-dollar bills at the rate of one per second.

- ◆ One million dollars — 12 days
- ◆ One billion dollars — 32 years
- ◆ One trillion dollars — 31,688 years

The amount of pesticides (and other chemicals) present in human and environmental samples are often reported as parts per million (ppm), parts per billion (ppb), or parts per trillion (ppt). These numbers are based on grams, a unit of the metric system.

- ◆ 1 gram is equal to 1,000 milligrams
- ◆ 1,000 grams is equal to 1 kilogram
- ◆ 1 kilogram is equal to 2.2 pounds

These units are too large for chemicals present in thousandths of a gram or less. These amounts are expressed as:

- ◆ Milligrams (mg) - thousandths of a gram or 10^{-3} grams
- ◆ Micrograms (μg) - millionths of a gram or 10^{-6} grams
- ◆ Nanograms (ng) - billionths of a gram or 10^{-9} grams
- ◆ Picograms (pg) - trillionths of a gram or 10^{-12} grams

Different ways of reporting the same units are in the table below.

Units of Measurement Different Ways of Reporting the Same Amount				
Parts per million (ppm)	mg/kg	μg/g	mg/l	μg/ml
Parts per billion (ppb)	μg/kg	ng/g	μg/l	ng/ml
Parts per trillion (ppt)	ng/kg	pg/g	ng/l	pg/ml

Appendix J

Further Information and Resources

Books

Common-Sense Pest Control: Least-toxic solutions for your home, garden, pets and community. by William Olkowski, Sheila Daar, and Helga Olkowski. Taunton Press Newton, CT. 1991. 715 pages.

Rodale's Chemical-free Yard & Garden: The Ultimate Authroity on Successful Organic Gardening. by Anna Carr, Miranda Smith, Linda A. Gilkeson, Joseph Smillie, Bill Wolf. Rodale Press. Emmaus, PA. 1991. 456 pages.

The Organic Gardener's Handbook of Natural Insect and Disease Control: A Complete Problem-solving Guide to Keeping your Garden & Yard Healthy without Chemicals. by Barbara W. Ellis and Fern Marshall Bradley. Rodale Press. Emmaus, PA. 1992. 534 pages.

Services

Heat Treatment for Termites
Thermal Pest Eradication (TPE)
Isothermics
P.O. Box 6951
Orange, CA 92613
714/970-1789, 1/800/873-2912

Bio-Blast for Termites
EcoScience Corp.
377 Plantation St.
Worcester, MA 01605
508/754-0300

Sand Barriers - Termites
Live Oak Structural
801 Camelia St.
Berkeley, CA 94710
Telephone: 510/524-7101
Fax: 510/524-7240

Sand Barriers - Termites
Term-Trol Exterminating Co.
Box 4915
Austin, TX 78765
512/451-9638

Products

Boric Acid Paste
Statpleton's Magnetic Roach Food
Blue Diamond Manufacturing
Box 10001 Old Highway 11W
Mooresburg, TN 37811
1/800/237-5705

Groups and Organizations

See the order form on the last page for how to reach Dr. Moses or the Pesticide Education Center.

Bio-integral Resource Center (BIRC)
P.O. Box 7414
Berkeley, CA 94707
Telephone: 510/524-2567
Fax: 510/524-1758

Breast Cancer Action
1280 Columbus
San Francisco, CA 94133
Telephone: 415-922-8279
Fax: 415/922-3253

Citizens Clearinghouse for Hazardous Wastes
P.O. Box 6806
Falls Church, VA 22040
Telephone: 703/237-CCHW
Fax: 703/237-7449

Mothers and Others for a Livable Planet
40 W. 20th Street, 9th floor
New York, NY 10011
Telephone: 212-242-0010, ext. 305
Fax: 212/242-0545

National Coalition Against the Misuse of Pesticides
701 E. Street, NW. Suite 200
Washington, DC 20003
Telephone: 202-543-5450
Fax: 202/543-4791

National Pediculosis Associaton (NPA)
P.O. Box 149
Newton, MA 02161
617/449-NITS
1/800/446-4NPA

Northwest Coalition for Alternatives to Pesticides
P.O. Box 1393
Eugene, OR 97440
Telephone: 503/344-5044
Fax: 503/344-6923

Pesticide Action Network North America Regional Office
116 New Montgomery St., Suite 810
San Francisco, CA 94105
Telephone: 415/541-9140
Fax: 541-1253

Pesticide Watch
116 New Montgomery, Suite 530
San Francisco, CA 94105
Telephone: 415/543-2627
Fax: 415/543-1480
e-mail: pestiwatch@igc.apc.org

Washington Toxics Coalition
4516 University Way, NE
Seattle, WA 98105
Telephone: 206/652-1545
Fax: 632-8661

Index

G

H

I

J

K

How to Order this Book

By fax: 415/391-9159

By telephone: Call Toll Free: 800/PEC-FREE (732-3733).
Have your VISA or MasterCard ready.

By *e-mail:* pec@igc.apc.org

By mail: Pesticide Education Center,
P.O. Box 420870, San Francisco, CA 94142-0870.
Telephone: 415/391-8511.

Name: _____

Address: _____

City: _____ State: _____ Zip: _____

Telephone: (_____)_____

Please send _____ copies @ $19.95 each $_____

California sales tax (see below)   _____

Shipping and handling (see below)   _____

                                    Total $_____

Sales tax: Only for books shipped in California - add 7.25%;
    San Francisco and Los Angeles counties - add 8.5%;
    Alameda and Contra Costa counties - add 8.25%.
Shipping: First-class: $5 per book   Book rate: $4 per book

Contact us for bulk order discounts, or for international
shipping charges.

Payment: ☐ Check

☐ VISA/MasterCard number:_____

Name on card: _____

Expiration date: _____

Call toll free and order now

How to Order this Book

By fax: 415/391-9159

By telephone: Call Toll Free: 800/PEC-FREE (732-3733).
Have your VISA or MasterCard ready.

By *e-mail:* pec@igc.apc.org

By mail: Pesticide Education Center,
P.O. Box 420870, San Francisco, CA 94142-0870.
Telephone: 415/391-8511.

Name: _____

Address: _____

City: _____ State: _____ Zip: _____

Telephone: (_____)_____

Please send _____ copies @ $19.95 each $_____

California sales tax (see below)   _____

Shipping and handling (see below)   _____

                                    Total $_____

Sales tax: Only for books shipped in California - add 7.25%;
     San Francisco and Los Angeles counties - add 8.5%;
     Alameda and Contra Costa counties - add 8.25%.
Shipping: First-class: $5 per book   Book rate: $4 per book

Contact us for bulk order discounts, or for international
shipping charges.

Payment: ☐ Check

☐ VISA/MasterCard number:_____

Name on card: _____

Expiration date: _____

Call toll free and order now